by the same authors

The Functional Nutrition Cookbook
Addressing Biochemical Imbalances through Diet
Lorraine Nicolle and Christine Bailey
Foreword by the Institute of Functional Medicine
ISBN 978 1 84819 179 2
eISBN 978 0 85701 125 1

Biochemical Imbalances in Disease
A Practitioner's Handbook
Edited by Lorraine Nicolle and Ann Woodriff Beirne
Foreword by David S. Jones M.D.
ISBN 978 1 84819 033 7
eISBN 978 0 85701 028 5

of related interest

Vital Face
Facial Exercises and Massage for Health and Beauty
Leena Kiviluoma
ISBN 978 1 84819 166 2
eISBN 978 0 85701 130 5

Make Yourself Better
A Practical Guide to Restoring Your Body's Wellbeing through Ancient Medicine
Philip Weeks
ISBN 978 1 84819 012 2
eISBN 978 0 85701 077 3

Regrowing Hair Naturally
Effective Remedies and Natural Treatments for Men and Women with Alopecia
Areata, Alopecia Androgenetica, Telogen Effluvium and Other Hair Loss Problems
Vera Peiffer
ISBN 978 1 84819 139 6
eISBN 978 0 85701 118 3

Sleep Better with Natural Therapies
A Comprehensive Guide to Overcoming Insomnia,
Moving Sleep Cycles and Preventing Jet Lag
Peter Smith
ISBN 978 1 84819 182 2
eISBN 978 0 85701 140 4

EAT TO GET YOUNGER

EAT TO GET YOUNGER

Tackling inflammation and other ageing processes for a longer, healthier life

LORRAINE NICOLLE AND CHRISTINE BAILEY

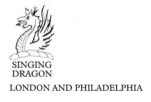

SINGING
DRAGON

LONDON AND PHILADELPHIA

First published in 2014
by Singing Dragon
an imprint of Jessica Kingsley Publishers
73 Collier Street
London N1 9BE, UK
and
400 Market Street, Suite 400
Philadelphia, PA 19106, USA

www.singingdragon.com

Library of Congress Cataloging in Publication Data
Nicolle, Lorraine.
  Eat to get younger : tackling inflammation and other ageing processes for a longer, healthier life /
Lorraine Nicolle and Christine Bailey.
    pages cm
  Includes index.
  ISBN 978-1-84819-179-2 (alk. paper)
  1. Longevity--Nutritional aspects. 2. Aging--Prevention. 3. Nutritionally induced diseases--Prevention.
  I. Bailey, Christine, 1970- II. Title.
  RA776.75.N535 2014
  613.2--dc23
                    2013049415

British Library Cataloguing in Publication Data
A CIP catalogue record for this book is available from the British Library

ISBN 978 1 84819 179 2
eISBN 978 0 85701 125 1

Printed and bound in Great Britain

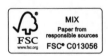

CONTENTS

DISCLAIMER

Every effort has been made to ensure that the information in this book is correct, but it should not in any way be used as an alternative to seeing your doctor, nor should it be viewed as a diagnostic tool for any condition. You should visit your doctor if you suspect that you may have a medical condition or if you have undiagnosed symptoms. Moreover, you should not discontinue, nor alter the dosage of, any medication without the knowledge of your doctor.

Neither the author nor the publisher takes any responsibility for the consequences of any decision made as a result of the information contained in this book.

CHAPTER 1

YOUR LIFE IN YOUR HANDS

Picture yourself in ten years' time. How long will you have lived by then – 40, 60, 80, or even 90 years? Imagine how you'll look and feel, the condition of your skin and hair, your body shape, whether or not you are likely to be in any pain, how your mood will be, your memory and your sharpness of mind.

Getting older is inevitable. But whatever your current chronological age, you can still take action to slow the rate of degeneration that accompanies the passing years.

This is a somewhat provocative claim. You're probably wondering whether it can possibly be true, whether certain nutrition and lifestyle strategies may truly be endowed with the power to help you hold back the advancing years. Well, here's what the cutting edge scientists are saying…

YOU CAN CHANGE THE WAY YOU AGE

It is common to worry about developing the age-related diseases of your parents, and their parents before them, but the fate of your forebears is not necessarily your destiny. Although certain diseases may be in your genes, 'waiting to happen', most of your genes lie dormant, not doing anything much, unless something in your environment switches them on. Hence, your genetic inheritance isn't the most powerful determinant of the way that you age.

Of more importance are the *epi*genetic changes that your genes accumulate as you progress through life. Epigenetic changes modify the way that genes function. The *structure* of your DNA doesn't necessarily alter; what does alter is the extent to which your genes are switched on and off ('expressed').

Epigenetic changes have far-reaching effects on both the rate and the type of ageing that you experience. Those that switch off cancer-controlling genes, for example, tend to have catastrophic results. If a tumour suppressor gene is epigenetically silenced, cancer cells are able to multiply unchecked.[1] Epigenetic changes can also speed cell death: the ends of the chromosomes on your cells' DNA are capped with tiny structures called telomeres. As you age, the telomeres gradually erode, getting shorter and shorter. If they get too short, the cell either shuts down or self-destructs. Scientists tell us that telomere shortening causes our organs to gradually lose their function, leading eventually to chronic diseases such as cardiovascular disease, cancer, Alzheimer's disease and diabetes. Scientists also tell us that epigenetic changes can speed up the telomere erosion process.

So, epigenetic changes can cause genes that accelerate ageing to be turned *on*. And they can also turn *off* genes that prevent cancer and other degenerative diseases from taking hold.

What's the point of knowing all this? The point is that these epigenetic changes are caused by environmental triggers – by aspects of your diet and lifestyle. The type of food you commonly eat and how much of it, the amount of alcohol you drink, whether you smoke, what nutritional supplements you take, how physically active you are, your stress levels, your exposure to traffic pollution and other toxins, how frequently you feel joyful or loving, or, alternatively, sad, angry or frustrated – it's these types of factors that determine which of your genes are active and which are silent. This, in turn, drives the rate at which you age, and the extent to which you will suffer the pain and disability of chronic disease along the way.

And this means that epigenetic changes are probably reversible. With the right diet and lifestyle modifications, there is the potential to switch back the damaging changes to the way your genes function.[2]

EPIGENETIC ANTI-AGEING STRATEGIES

Not surprisingly, 'nutri-epigenetics' is now a major focus of scientific research. Restricting calorie intake, for example, is thought to reverse certain epigenetic changes that cause premature ageing. (The proposed mechanism is that calorie restriction activates anti-ageing genes called 'sirtuins'.[3]) In fact, the practice of calorie restriction has attracted so much interest for its potential to promote healthy ageing that the US government is currently funding a research programme on the effects of a two-year 25 per cent reduction in calories.[4] You can read more about calorie restriction in Chapters 2 and 3.

Other studies are looking at so-called 'epigenetic nutrients'. These are vitamins, minerals and plant chemicals whose powerful potential for reducing the risk of cancer and other age-related diseases may turn out to lie in their ability to reverse epigenetic changes.[5] Nutrients with the most evidence to date include the plant chemicals curcumin (from the turmeric spice),[6] epigallocatechin gallate (EGCG, found in green tea),[7] sulforaphane (from cruciferous vegetables such as broccoli, cabbage and cauliflower)[8] and resveratrol (from the skins of grapes and particularly from red wine), as well as the B vitamin folate and the mineral selenium.[9] As you read through this book, you'll see that these special nutrients feature time and time again as potentially helpful interventions in all sorts of age-related health issues.

OTHER PROCESSES INVOLVED IN AGEING

Epigenetic changes can also cause inflammation and other damaging processes that speed ageing.[10] Age-accelerating processes include poor digestive function, inadequate detoxification, excessive oxidation and glycation, hormone imbalances, problems with fat metabolism, failing energy production, slow methylation and disruptions to brain chemicals. You may not yet recognize all of these terms but they'll be explained as you go through the book and you'll start to see exactly how they drive premature ageing and disease.

Such drivers of ageing are in fact normal, healthy body processes that are no longer working properly. If you're like most people, you probably tend to ignore minor symptoms of ill-health, such as disrupted sleep, frequent headaches, colds that seem to go on for ages, creaky joints, a stuffy nose, poor memory, or gastrointestinal wind and bloating. These types of symptoms indicate imbalances in body processes which may be relatively easy to correct. If they are ignored, however, such imbalances can become entrenched and the symptoms become so severe that they progress into degenerative diseases.

Healthy ageing means looking at these seemingly minor symptoms in order to identify the body processes that need support. The earlier you do this, the better – before things break down to such an extent that they are hard to rescue.

This type of approach to health is one of *proactive* prevention and is often more effective than *reactive* treatment. If you can keep all your body processes functioning well, identifying and supporting any that are struggling, you'll age far better and will be less likely to succumb to degenerative diseases.

ALL ROADS LEAD TO INFLAMMATION

Another reason to address dysfunctional body processes is that they eventually cause inflammation – the type of low-grade, systemic, chronic inflammation that can't be seen on the outside, but which all the while is insidiously damaging your body and your brain. It's now thought that this type of inflammation is the basis of most age-related diseases,[11] such as cardiovascular disease, Alzheimer's disease, Parkinson's disease, some cancers, osteoporosis, diabetes and even depression. What's more, inflammation speeds the rate of telomere erosion.[12] And this, as we've seen, goes hand in hand with premature ageing.

This is why you'll see a great many references to inflammation throughout this book. We'll be explaining how chronic inflammation makes you age prematurely, and we'll reveal the many potential causes of such 'inflamm-ageing'. This way, you can better identify and address them, for a longer, healthier life.

HEALTHY AGEING REQUIRES OPTIMAL NUTRIENT LEVELS

Reversing epigenetic changes and chronic inflammation involves getting your body processes back into tip-top condition. To do this, you need to remove the diet and lifestyle practices that are hampering their function; and feed them the nutrients they need.

Now, if you eat a standard 'healthy' diet, you may be assuming that you're unlikely to be low in any vital nutrients. But did you know that you don't have to be officially 'deficient' in a nutrient in order to be at levels that are too low to keep your body systems fully functioning?

Most governments set recommended intake levels for vitamins and minerals – in the UK we have recommended daily allowances

(RDAs). But some scientists claim these are probably too low for healthy ageing. If you get your RDAs of nutrients every day, you may prevent short-term diseases such as scurvy (from lack of vitamin C) but, as you'll see throughout this book, these levels may not be quite sufficient to keep each and every one of your biological pathways in tip-top working order.[13]

You may go on for years, or even decades, without realizing you have minor shortfalls in certain crucial nutrients. Nevertheless, behind the scenes, these seemingly insignificant insufficiencies may be aggravating one or more of your body systems. As we've seen, once these body processes start to struggle, they promote inflammation and other problems that accelerate the ageing process and increase your risk of degenerative disease.

IT'S NEVER TOO LATE TO MAKE CHANGES

So, we've said that your rate of ageing is determined not so much by the genes you have inherited as by the changes to their function brought about by aspects of your diet and lifestyle. We've also said that, when it comes to ageing well, prevention is better than cure. But it's also important to know that it's never too late to make a difference to your rate of ageing.

A small pilot study of men with low-risk prostate cancer found that those who made lifestyle changes for five years had lengthened telomeres in their immune system cells, whereas the telomeres in the men who did not make the changes became shorter over the same time period.[14] (The lifestyle changes comprised a healthy diet, good levels of physical activity, stress management and social support.) Larger trials are needed to confirm this result but the findings are promising.

We have clients in their 40s, 50s, 60s and beyond who feel a great deal more healthy and energized than they did 10 or 20 years previously. Their cells may not have become physiologically younger but their body systems are working far better. And these individuals are reaping the benefits, in terms of more energy, better mood and sleep, fewer headaches, colds, flu and other infections, maintaining a healthier weight and requiring fewer medical drugs.

WHY HASN'T MY DOCTOR TOLD ME THIS?

Many doctors do give diet and lifestyle advice but the most common medical approach to age-related problems is to prescribe pharmaceutical drugs. These drugs become available after having been 'proved' safe and effective in large studies called randomized controlled trials (RCTs). There are many arguments about whether or not RCTs do indeed provide such proof, but the point we want to make here is that RCTs are, in the main, the only type of scientific evidence that medics will recognize.

Nutrition and lifestyle changes don't carry the safety risks of pharmaceutical drugs. Hence, there is not such a burning need for RCTs, nor is there the financial incentive. (Most diet and lifestyle interventions cannot be marketed to make the financial profit of drugs, since they cannot be patented.)

WHERE'S THE PROOF?

As diet, lifestyle and nutritional supplements lack the RCT evidence that justifies the prescribing of drugs, your doctor may not always be aware of the most cutting-edge thinking on such interventions. However, there is plenty of scientific support for making the sorts of changes we recommend throughout this book, as you'll see by the number of reference points we've included. Most of these references are to peer-reviewed studies that have been published in scientific journals. They may include observations of different populations, small preliminary human trials (like the one on telomeres in men with early prostate cancer mentioned above), studies on animals, laboratory experiments of nutrient effects on human cells, or even opinions by widely recognized scientific experts.

If you want to, you can read the summaries ('abstracts') of these papers yourself. Simply log on to the US National Institutes of Health database Pubmed (www.ncbi.nlm.nih.gov/pubmed). If you are attached to a university, you can usually get access to the full papers. Otherwise, you may need to pay a fee, although an increasing number are now 'open access', which means they can be downloaded in full, at no charge.

More examples of the immense power of diet and lifestyle on ageing are found in studies of the world's communities that have the highest proportions of long-lived inhabitants and the lowest incidences of age-related diseases.[15] Despite their geographic disparity (such communities are found in Europe, the US, Japan and Central America), there are certain practices that are common to all of them. These include eating a wholefood, lower-calorie diet that is predominantly plant-based, being physically active and getting plenty of daylight, engaging in stress-management behaviours, having a sense of community, spiritual belonging and strong family values, and living with a sense of purpose.

Given the commonality of such practices in these long-lived peoples, it is likely that they are powerful factors in slowing down the ageing process.

SO, WHAT'S THE KEY TO HEALTHY AGEING?

Putting all this information together, we hope that you can see that your family history is not necessarily your destiny. You do have some control over how the rest of your life is going to play out.

One of the routes to a long and healthy life is to put a stop to any chronic, low-level inflammation. Your best chance of achieving this is to take a good look at your current state of health in order to gauge which body systems may need some extra support. Getting these systems back into better working order is an end in itself because it will promote healthier ageing, but it will also help to remove the fuel that is feeding the age-accelerating inflammation.

As we said earlier, getting your body processes back into tip-top condition means removing the nutrition and lifestyle practices that are hampering their function, and feeding them the nutrients they need – at optimal, not merely adequate, doses. According to current scientific thinking, such strategies may have the power to reverse the damaging epigenetic changes that you've accumulated throughout your life – the sorts of unwanted changes that turn *on* the genes that accelerate ageing, and turn *off* those that prevent cancer and other degenerative diseases from taking hold.

The information in each of the following chapters is designed to help you make the right decisions to achieve these goals. It includes explanations of the processes involved in the most common signs and symptoms associated with ageing. It provides clear programmes of action for improving the functioning of the key body systems, and these programmes include meal plans, lifestyle advice and suggestions for nutritional supplements. What's more, we've provided the recipes for more than 100 of the healthy ageing dishes in the meal plans. Each of these recipes has been carefully constructed to support the healthy ageing processes featured in its particular chapter.

Now, read on to find out how you can change your life forever...

A NOTE BEFORE WE BEGIN

Please note that the action plans, including the meals plans and recipes, are not designed to be exhaustive or prescriptive, but to be bases to be adapted to your individual needs.

Although this book recommends nutritional supplements for you to consider, you're likely to benefit most if you agree your programme with a qualified nutrition practitioner who uses a personalized approach to optimizing health. You can find a practitioner near you by logging on to the website of the British Association for Applied Nutrition and Nutritional Therapy (www.bant.org.uk). Once you have found a practitioner, you can check his/her credentials at the register held by the Complementary and Natural Healthcare Council (www.cnhc.org.uk).

CHAPTER 2

EATING FOR A GOOD LIFE

Once you've read to the end of this chapter, you'll have mastered the fundamentals of what (and how) to eat in order to change the way you look and feel, for good. By following the guidelines below, you'll be adopting a core eating plan that gives you more energy and improves your digestion, your mood and your sleep, as well as your weight and shape.

You will develop a robust set of dietary habits that you can gradually customize to meet your own individual needs, as you select further recommendations from the later chapters that are of most interest to you. As you do this, you'll be building a personalized diet to tackle the particular aspects of ageing you are most concerned about. Your priority may be to improve any ongoing pain, for example, or you may be more interested in reducing your blood fats or cholesterol levels, looking after your skin, or smoothing the transition through the menopause, to name but a few typical issues of ageing.

Following the eating principles laid down in this chapter will not only provide you with more nourishment than the typical modern diet but will also remove some of your most burdensome sources of stress and inflammation. For many years, these have likely been preventing you from reaching your full health potential.

In this way, your new way of eating can improve the functioning of many different biological pathways, dramatically slowing the degenerative processes of ageing. You'll look and feel rejuvenated, revitalized and, ultimately, more youthful.

HOW TO GET STARTED

We recommend that you start by reading through all the dietary principles, learning about the *Eat to Get Younger* low-glycaemic load (low-GL) diet and the ideas for incorporating special foods that are antioxidant, anti-inflammatory and alkalizing.

Once you have an idea of the scale of the changes you'll need to implement, decide on the speed at which you want to do so. An eating plan for healthy ageing is one that you'll need to adopt for the rest of your life. You may adapt it as the years go by, but you'll be saying goodbye to your bad habits forever.

If this sounds daunting, remember that the transition period from old habits to new is the hardest. If you are used to relying on ready-prepared meals, commercial salad dressings, cereal bars, muffins, tinned soups, fruit yogurts, take-out sandwiches and so on, don't fall into the trap of making so many changes at once that you suddenly find yourself deprived of your favourite foods. You'll simply fall off the wagon. Take as many days or weeks as you need to gradually replace the foods doing you harm with the healthier, healing alternatives that we suggest. And if you need help with addictions to sugar, starches, caffeine or alcohol, see the tips in Chapter 10 and, in particular, consider the recommendations in that chapter (and in Chapter 4) for supplementing 5-hydroxytryptophan (5-HTP) or L-glutamine.

After you have been incorporating the *Eat to Get Younger* dietary principles for long enough to feel comfortable with them, move on to Chapters 3–10, so that you can consider the additional advice for tackling the specific areas of your health that are priorities for you as you age. The chapters do not need to be read in the order in which they appear in this book. You can read them in the order of most importance to you. For example, if your key aim is to lose weight and control your carbohydrate or sugar cravings, read Chapter 4 first, whereas if you are mostly concerned that you are feeling too tired and are overwhelmed with the stresses of day-to-day life, start with Chapter 6.

Each of the chapters carries its own example meal plan, which not only incorporates the *Eat to Get Younger* way of eating but also takes into account other special dietary measures for that particular issue. And the end of the book is packed with recipes that feature in the meal plans, making it simple to implement our recommendations.

Before you leave Chapter 2, you also have the option of learning about two increasingly popular eating regimes – calorie restriction and fasting – to see whether they could be helpful for you. If you want to try them, we've suggested some meal plans for these too.

And once you've moved on from this chapter, it's a good idea to refer back to it from time to time as you are progressing through the book. Doing so will help to keep you on track, by reminding you about the basics of what to eat and what not to eat if you want to age well. And do remember that you don't have to adhere to your new dietary principles all the time – 80 per cent of the time will do. In most cases, over-indulging in unhelpful foods and drinks once in a while is not going to do you any harm. It's the overall pattern of what you do day in and day out that matters.

We believe that our dietary recommendations for healthy ageing are tasty, filling, practical and sociable, and that following the *Eat to Get Younger* plan should not therefore become a chore. But if you do ever feel your motivation dipping, hold on to the knowledge that by working your way through this book and implementing the recommendations herein you cannot fail to significantly alter the course of your health, whatever your current chronological age.

THE EAT TO GET YOUNGER DIET
CONTROL YOUR CARB INTAKE

In Chapter 4, you'll learn about a particularly powerful driver of premature ageing called insulin resistance. Insulin resistance causes levels of sugar and insulin in the bloodstream to remain dangerously high. Too much sugar in the blood damages cells, tissues and vital organs, in a process called glycation. Chapters 4 and 5 explain more about glycation and how to find out if it is affecting you.

The potentially devastating condition of insulin resistance develops from many years of unstable blood sugar levels and also from the gradual accumulation of excess weight. Chapter 4 explains in detail the process of how blood sugar problems and insulin resistance develop. One key point to take on board now, however, is that blood sugar problems and weight gain are both promoted by eating the wrong type of carbohydrates, and both can be effectively addressed by switching to healthier carb foods.

By this we mean that you should get your carbs from foods that release their sugar (glucose) *slowly* into the bloodstream ('slow carbs') rather than from foods that cause blood sugar levels to surge ('fast carbs'). Foods that release their sugars slowly keep blood sugar levels stable and are referred to as having a low 'glycaemic load' (GL), or as being 'low-GL' foods. Conversely, foods that cause spikes in blood sugar levels are referred to as 'high-GL' foods.

Foods that contain more carbs have a higher GL than foods containing more protein, fat, fibre or water. As you might expect, the highest-GL foods are those that contain more sugars and refined/white starches. Whole grains have a lower GL than their white equivalents because they contain fibre.

One type of fibre, namely soluble fibre, is helpful not only for controlling blood sugar levels but also for reducing fat and cholesterol levels in the bloodstream.[1] The best sources of soluble fibre are beans, pulses, turnip, swede (rutabaga), okra, brown rice, oats, flaxseeds, chia seeds, xanthum gum and guar gum. These gums are often used in small amounts in gluten-free baking, pastry fillings and ice creams to combine ingredients, improve texture and add lightness. (Note that a minority of individuals, including those with coeliac disease or inflammatory bowel disease, appear to be sensitive to xanthum gum.)

Meat, poultry, fish, eggs, beans, pulses, nuts, seeds, dairy products, vegetables, fruits, fats and oils have a lower GL than grains and root vegetables, as the latter two food groups are higher in carbs.

GLs are expressed numerically: if a food has a GL of 20 or more, it is considered high; a GL of 11–19 is considered moderate; a GL of 10 or less is considered low. For healthy ageing, better energy levels and long-term weight control, the lower your GL intake, the better. Experts vary in their recommendations of what should be the daily limit for health, but around 50–60 GLs may be appropriate. Box 2.1 below shows a table of some common foods and their GLs, to give you an idea of how they vary between different categories of food.

BOX 2.1 SOME COMMON FOODS AND THEIR GL VALUES

A low-GL diet helps you to lose weight, control your blood sugar levels and improve your long-term health. To eat a low-GL diet, select foods that have a GL of 10 or less. Below are examples of some common foods so that you can get an idea of the best foods to choose on a low-GL diet. You can use this link (http://ajcn.nutrition.org/content/76/1/5. full.pdf+html) to see a list of hundreds of different foods and their GLs.[2] Values are given per typical serving size of the food.

The GLs of the foods below will vary, of course, depending on the brands and how they were prepared, especially in terms of the amount of sugar added. But these figures are designed to give you a general idea of high- and low-GL foods. Remember that foods with the highest GLs are those made from white starch – see Chapter 4 for more about the problems associated with eating these 'white' foods, as well as some ideas for healthier alternatives.

▶ Energy drink: 40

▶ Chocolate cake with icing: 20

▶ Chickpeas: 8

▶ Coke: 15

▶ Baked potato: 18

▶ Baked beans: 7

▶ Sports drinks: 12–21

▶ Croissant: 17

▶ Apple: 4–6

▶ Lemon squash: 17

▶ Pastry/French baguette: 15

▶ Orange: 3–6

▶ White/puffed rice: 14–40

▶ Apple/orange juice: 12

▶ Lentils: 3–6

▶ White bagel: 25

▶ Banana: 12–16

- Milk: 3–4

- Breakfast cereals: 12–22

- Muesli: 7–10

- Peas/carrots: 3

- Muffins: 15–30

- Rye bread/pumpernickel: 5–8

- Eggs/fish/meat: all extremely low

However, rather than laboriously keeping track of GLs consumed throughout the day, a simpler way of following the plan is to avoid all added sugar, replace white starchy foods with wholefood varieties and try to stick to no more than two portions a day. Refer to Box 2.2 below for more detailed guidelines on eating carbs for healthy ageing.

BOX 2.2 HOW TO EAT CARBS FOR HEALTHY AGEING

- Limit starchy foods to one portion, once or twice a day. Eat it either at breakfast and lunch, for example, or at lunch and dinner, or at breakfast and dinner.

  ▷ Refer to Box 2.3 to see what we mean by 'one portion'.

- The lowest-GL starchy foods are beans and pulses, including lentils and chickpeas (if you can tolerate them without digestive discomfort), and non-potato root vegetables such as celeriac, carrots, turnips, swede (rutabaga), beetroot and squash, including butternut and pumpkin.

- However, if you are happy with your current weight, and if you believe you are controlling your blood sugar levels pretty well, you can include sweet potatoes, new potatoes in their skins and whole grains such as brown, black or red rice, quinoa, oats and buckwheat (again, just one portion, once or twice a day). How do you know how well you are controlling your blood sugar levels? Answering the questions in Chapter 4 will help you assess this.

▶ Avoid refined carbs, commonly known as white starch. See Chapter 4 for in-depth information on white starch and how to make it easier to forego the foods that contain it. Below, you'll find some ideas for swapping some commonly eaten high-GL starches for lower-GL alternatives:

High GL starch	Lower GL alternative
Spaghetti, tagliatelle	Spaghetti squash, kelp noodles, Konjac noodles, spiralized courgette (zucchini) or carrot. See recipe for *Asparagus and Courgette Spaghetti with Red Pepper Marinara Sauce*
White rice	Red rice, black rice, brown basmati (a small amount only) and cauliflower or parsnip 'rice'. See recipes for *Nori Avocado Maki Rolls* and *Asian Cauliflower 'Rice' Stir Fry*
Mashed potatoes	Cauliflower or root vegetable mash
Wraps made from flour	Lettuce leaf wraps. See recipe for *Lemon Harissa Turkey Leaf Wraps*
Crisps, tortilla chips, other baked snacks	Unsalted nuts or seeds. See recipes for *Cauliflower Munchies*, *Tomato Seed Crackers* and *Onion Kale Chips*
Baked potatoes	Baked sweet potatoes, squash, carrots and/ or beetroot
Couscous, quinoa	*Asian Cauliflower 'Rice' Stir Fry* (as above)
Lasagne	Moussaka, or lasagne made with strips of courgette (zucchini) in place of pasta
Muffins, cakes, scones, breads	Same made from coconut and almond flours. See recipes for *Coconut Cinnamon Bread*, *Cacao Courgette Bread* and *Berry Muffins*
Granola	Nut and seed-based granola. See recipe for *Buckwheat Granola* and *Grain-Free Breakfast Bowl*

Box 2.3 gives you information on portion sizes. Chapter 4 has more information on white starch and how to identify it and replace it with healthier alternatives.

BOX 2.3 HOW TO CHECK YOUR PORTION SIZES

One serving is:

▸ Fruit: 1 medium piece (e.g. apple), ½ cup fresh fruit or ¼ cup (small handful) dried fruit (30g/1oz)

▸ Grains: 1 slice wholemeal bread, 2 oat cakes, or 1–2 tbsp cooked brown rice

▸ Starchy vegetables: ½ sweet potato, 2 small new potatoes, or 1 cup (250ml/8fl oz) butternut squash or pumpkin

▸ Non-starchy vegetables: 1 cup (250ml/8fl oz) raw vegetables, large bowl of green salad leaves, or ½ cup (125ml/4fl oz) cooked vegetables

▸ Meat, fish, chicken: 115g/4oz (the size of a pack of cards)

▸ Whole grains: ⅓ cup (85ml/3fl oz) cooked (a small fist size)

▸ Beans, lentils: ⅓ cup (approx. 85ml/3fl oz) cooked

▸ Nuts, seeds: a small handful

EAT PLENTY OF HEALTHY FATS

As you'll see in Chapter 4, it's crucial to include some fat in every meal if you are keen to age well. It used to be thought that the way to long-term health was to eat as little fat as possible. But we now know this way of eating can have a catastrophic effect, *promoting* degenerative conditions rather than improving them, and also causing hunger pangs that lead to weight gain. The most up-to-date evidence suggests that it is healthier to *change* the types of fat you eat rather than to severely *restrict* the overall level of fat in your diet.[3]

The main problem with low-fat diets is that they lack the special types of fat that are crucial for good health because of their anti-inflammatory and cardio- and cancer-protective effects. These are the omega 3 and omega 6 polyunsaturated fats (PUFAs), and also the omega 9 monounsaturated fats (MUFAs). The best sources of MUFAs are avocados, nuts and olive oil; indeed, we recommend that olive oil be your main source of fat. You can use it in cold dressings and also in cooking at low temperatures, such as when cooking with liquids (e.g. soups, casseroles and sauces).

The best sources of PUFAs are oily fish, nuts and seeds (and their cold-pressed oils). In particular, the omega 3 fats eicosapentaenoic acid (EPA) and docosahexaenoic acid (DHA), from oily fish, have powerful anti-inflammatory effects and are therefore a crucial part of any healthy ageing programme.

The fats that most strongly promote premature ageing are the trans-fats.[4] These are vegetable oils that have been chemically altered to make them firmer and to increase their shelf life. They are found in most processed foods, and for optimal health it is best to avoid them. (Trans-fats are already banned in Denmark, Austria, Switzerland, New York and California.)

Another age-accelerating fat is oxidised fat. Oxidised fats are created when you heat PUFAs like vegetable oils (oils typically made from corn or seeds).

It's also best to avoid *excessive* amounts of saturated fats. These are found in lard, fatty cuts of meat, farmed fatty fish, intensively farmed eggs and full-fat dairy products. Coconut fat is also a saturated fat but it has some health-promoting properties (see Chapters 4 and 8). Contrary to popular (but misguided) belief, there is a place for a small amount of saturated fat in the diet: saturated fat is the only natural fat that doesn't become toxic when it is used in baking and frying.

How much fat? The government says that 30–35 per cent of our daily calories should come from fat, and we agree. Indeed, this is likely to be the case if you are on a low-GL diet and are therefore reducing carbs. Saturated fats should be kept within 10 per cent of your overall calories for the day.

You can learn more about all these fats and their specific health effects, both positive and negative, in Chapter 8.

OTHER HELPFUL ADDITIONS TO A HEALTHY AGEING DIET
Eat natural whole foods
Base your diet on fresh vegetables, herbs, sea vegetables, spices, nuts and seeds, fermented foods, beans and pulses (if your digestive system can tolerate them). Unless you are vegan, include organic free-range eggs and fish, game, meat and poultry that is either wild-caught or naturally reared. Keep processed foods to a minimum. Avoid ready meals, take-aways, microwave meals, foods containing artificial preservatives and chemicals, trans-fats and foods containing high fructose corn syrups.

Eat organic
Organic fruit and vegetables often contain more nutrients (especially antioxidant phytochemicals) than conventionally grown produce. They are also grown without chemical fertilizers and pesticides, and they are GM-free (that is, not genetically modified). If you eat animal products, choose organic dairy, free-range eggs and naturally reared meats. This helps ensure they are free from antibiotics, genetically modified (GM) feed and added growth hormones. Organic, grass-fed meat is often richer in healthy omega 3 fats and another type of useful fat called CLA (conjugated linoleic acid), and is lower in saturated fats.

Allow alkalizing foods to dominate
When you're in optimum health, your blood is slightly alkaline. But many foods in today's processed diet make our body fluids acidic: when these foods are digested and metabolized, they leave acid residues.

For example, when animal proteins (e.g. meat, fish and eggs) are metabolized, they release acidic components such as uric acid and phosphate. Conversely, most fruits and vegetables leave alkaline residues because they release bicarbonate and alkalizing minerals such as calcium, potassium and magnesium. And while it is true that fruits do contain some acids (citric acid in oranges and lemons, for instance), fruit acids are too weak to have an acidic effect within the human body.

A predominantly acid-forming diet is one that is high in grains and flour products, fats and oils, beans and pulses, sugar, alcohol, coffee, and, as mentioned above, meat, fish and eggs. Eating a lot of these foods increases our requirement for alkalizing minerals (such as calcium, magnesium and potassium) and can place an unnecessary strain on our vital organs, including the liver and kidneys.[5]

To keep the body in a healthy acid/alkaline balance, make sure you complement such acid-forming foods with plenty of alkaline-forming fruits, vegetables and almonds. If you want to age well, alkaline-forming foods should dominate your diet. Box 2.4 lists some foods to include.

BOX 2.4 EXAMPLES OF ALKALINE-FORMING FOODS

Alkalizing foods should dominate the diet. So, eat a variety of these every day:

▸ Many fruits, such as avocado, lemon, lime, grapefruit, oranges, coconut, tomato, figs, pineapple, grapes, cherries, berries, kiwi, passionfruit, papaya.

▸ Natural flavourings such as sea salt, fresh herbs, sea vegetables, spices, chlorella, spirulina, apple cider vinegar, lecithin.

▸ Some plant protein foods, including almonds, chia seeds, chestnuts, millet, fermented tofu and tempeh, sprouted seeds.

▸ Drinks: coconut water, almond milk, herbal teas, green juices.

▸ Most vegetables, including sprouted seeds and beans (e.g. alfalfa), artichokes, asparagus, cabbage, cauliflower, broccoli, kale, chard, celery, courgette (zucchini), chicory (endive), leek, lettuce, radish, squash, garlic, beetroot, rocket (arugula), watercress, wheatgrass, sweet potato.

Eat antioxidant-rich foods

In Chapter 5 we explain the science behind a process called oxidation. Oxidation is one of the main drivers of inflammation and premature ageing. One of the ways to reduce your body's burden of oxidation is to eat lots of antioxidant-rich foods – vegetables, fruits, spices, herbs, nuts and seeds.

You may have noticed on the labels of certain health foods or dietary supplements that the product is said to contain 'ORACs' (oxygen radial absorbancy capacity) – perhaps '500 ORACs per serving', or 1000 or even 2000 ORACs. An ORAC score is a measure of a food or supplement's antioxidant power. It was developed in the 1990s by Tufts University in the US. In their studies on animals, the Tufts researchers found that foods with higher ORAC scores helped protect against long-term memory loss and age-related damage to small blood vessels.[6] Originally, Tufts assigned specific ORAC scores to antioxidant-rich foods. Prunes (100g/4oz), for example, scored 5770 ORACs, while the same weight of corn achieved a score of 400. This quantified list has, however, now been withdrawn, due to concerns that the ORAC scores on the labels of commercial food products can be prone to inaccuracies and in some cases may be inflated.

However, it is pretty easy to tell whether a food is high in ORACs: the fresher and the more deeply and brightly coloured it is, the higher its ORAC score and the greater its antioxidant power. So, fill your plate with a rainbow of fruits and vegetables – dark greens, purples, reds, oranges and yellows. Aim to eat eight or more portions of vegetables daily and 2–3 portions of fruit. We don't recommend more fruit than this because it is so high in (natural) sugar, including fructose. Too much fructose can contribute to irritable bowel syndrome (IBS), weight gain and the build-up of fat in the liver.

Check your portion sizes

Keep your portion sizes down and you will benefit not only your waistline but your overall health too. Refer back to Box 2.3 for portion sizes and see Box 2.5 for how to avoid piling too many calories on your plate. There is some evidence that restricting calories promotes longevity – see below for information about this. Reducing your portion size is a sure-fire way to restrict calories. Some people also find it helpful to eat from a smaller-sized plate.

BOX 2.5 HOW TO CONSTRUCT A HEALTHY PLATEFUL

Rather than laboriously weighing every food, it's easier to focus on your portion sizes (see Box 2.3) and also on how you fill your plate.

Half of your plate should be low-starch vegetables, such as dark green leaves, broccoli, cauliflower, Brussels sprouts, courgettes (zucchini), fennel, cucumber, tomato, cabbage, runner beans, olives, lettuce, radicchio, radishes, okra, peas, onions, garlic, leeks, aubergine (eggplant), bell peppers and mushrooms.

A quarter of your plate should include protein-rich foods, such as fish, seafood, lean meat, eggs, nuts, and, if you can tolerate them, dairy products, tofu and tempeh (and other beans and lentils if you are vegan).

On the remaining quarter, you have the option of adding one portion of cooked starchy vegetables or whole grains. These include new potatoes, sweet potato or butternut squash, or gluten-free whole grains, such as wholemeal rice, black or red rice, quinoa and buckwheat.

If you have more than 2–3 stone (15–20kg) to lose, or if you suffer from issues to do with blood sugar control (such as episodes of low blood sugar, or a diagnosis of metabolic syndrome or diabetes – see Chapter 4), replace grains and potatoes with beans and pulses (as long as they don't cause digestive discomfort) or non-potato root vegetables such as celeriac, carrots, beetroot and squash. (Note that it's harder to avoid grains if you're vegan because they complement beans, pulses, nuts and seeds to make a 'complete' protein containing all the essential amino acids.)

Eat consciously

Take your time over meals. Rather than eating on the run, sit at a table and eat slowly and mindfully. Doing so will promote healthy digestion, will slow down the release of sugar (glucose) into the bloodstream (helping to keep blood sugar levels stable) and will make you less likely to overeat.

Include fermented foods

Foods containing healthy bacteria (known as probiotic foods) are essential for our digestive wellbeing and general health. One of the best ways to increase the levels of healthy microbes in your gut is to eat fermented or cultured foods daily. These include home-made yogurt, kefir, sauerkraut, kimchi, miso, kombucha and pickled vegetables. If you've never tried making them, take a look at our recipes at the end of the book.

Add in superfoods

Fundamental to eating for a younger you is focusing on the quality and nutrient density of the foods you eat. The modern diet is often high in calories but low in nutrients. Superfoods are nutritionally dense, packed with protein, amino acids, vitamins, minerals, phytochemicals, enzymes, fibre and/or healthy fats. And they don't have to cost a fortune: many are everyday foods or foods easily available from health stores. Top of the list are the green superfoods, such as wheatgrass, spirulina and chlorella, together with green leafy vegetables like watercress, kale, spinach and rocket (arugula). Other superfoods include antioxidant-rich berries, algae and sea vegetables, maca, cacao, coconut, herbs, spices, seeds and sprouted seeds.

The recipes in this book include a range of superfoods to supercharge your health and slow down many of the biological processes of ageing.

Keep hydrated

Don't overlook the importance of fluids in your diet. This is one of the simplest and most effective ways to help turn back the clock. Water is essential for digesting and absorbing foods, transporting nutrients around the body, keeping cells functioning properly, and removing toxins via the liver and kidneys.

Keeping hydrated will promote energy levels and clear thinking. Not drinking sufficiently can make you feel tired and lead to toxic build-up. It can also cause constipation and it dries out the skin and joints. Ideally, choose filtered water and either drink it plain or in broths and herbal teas. Aim for eight glasses of such liquid a day. Eating fresh fruits and vegetables, soups and smoothies will also contribute to your fluid intake.

Include vegetable juices and/or smoothies

Another way to hydrate is by drinking vegetable juices. This is an easy way to alkalize your diet. And because juices are so readily absorbed, you swiftly assimilate the vitamins, minerals and enzymes, even if your digestive function is less than perfect. If you suffer from episodes of low blood sugar levels, however, smoothies may be more suitable than juices, in view of their higher fibre content.

Our recipes include a range of vegetable-based juices and energizing smoothies. Commercial varieties lack the most beneficial nutrients, as they are usually pasteurized or heat-processed.

Include anti-inflammatory foods and drinks

Box 2.6 lists many commonly available anti-inflammatory foods, including those that contain the omega 3 fats we introduced earlier in this chapter. We've included many of these foods in the recipes and we encourage you to eat plenty of them daily. Aim to drink 3–4 cups of green tea a day. This wonder-drink, especially matcha green tea powder, is rich in anti-inflammatory 'catechins' that have the added benefit of helping to control blood sugar levels and reduce the ageing process of oxidation in the body. If you are caffeine-sensitive, look for decaff varieties. Chapter 8 goes into more detail on constructing an eating plan high in anti-inflammatory foods.

BOX 2.6 SOME ANTI-INFLAMMATORY FOODS

▶ Oily fish: salmon, trout, mackerel, sardines, herring, anchovies. Best wild-caught. (Avoid larger fish such as tuna and swordfish, as these are higher in toxins.)

▶ Omega 3-rich seeds: flax, chia, hemp, sesame and pumpkin seeds. Include their oils and butters. Do not heat them. (Note that many of these also contain omega 6 fats.)

▶ Fatty foods containing other healthy oils and antioxidants: olives, avocados, pecans, Brazils, almonds, walnuts, hazelnuts.

- Spices: turmeric, garlic, ginger, chilli, cinnamon, nutmeg.

- Herbs: ideally fresh – for example, rosemary, oregano, thyme, mint, coriander (cilantro), basil, parsley.

- Antioxidant-rich fruits and vegetables: especially berries, cherries, citrus fruits (including the zest), dark leafy greens such as kale, rocket (arugula) and watercress, broccoli, Brussels sprouts, beetroot, peppers, onions and olives. In general, the more deeply pigmented the fruit or vegetable, the greater its antioxidant power.

- Enzyme-rich foods: pineapple core (e.g. macerated into a smoothie), papaya.

- Drinks: filtered water, tea (white, green, black and redbush/rooibos), herbal infusions, bone broths.

- Fermented foods: sauerkraut, kefir, yogurt, kombucha, miso, tempeh, natto.

- Green superfoods: chlorella, spirulina, wheatgrass, barley grass.

- Sea vegetables: kelp, kombu, wakame, arame.

- Mushrooms: shittake, maitake, enoki, oyster mushrooms.

OTHER THINGS TO REDUCE OR AVOID FOR HEALTHY AGEING

Foods that cause unpleasant reactions

If you feel worse after eating certain foods, consider eliminating them for four weeks to see if you notice any improvement. Many people may feel better avoiding dairy products, beans and pulses, or gluten, for example. Gluten is a protein found in wheat, barley and rye. There is evidence that gluten can promote inflammation in the body even if you are not a sufferer of coeliac disease.[7] As a consequence, *all* of the recipes in this book are gluten-free. See Chapter 3 for more information on how gluten and other problematic foods can cause reactions in the gut that can lead to body-wide inflammation and degenerative illnesses.

Burnt or blackened foods

Barbecuing meat or fish, or grilling, frying or griddling it at high temperatures, or for lengthy periods of time, produces polycyclic aromatic hydrocarbons (PAHs). PAHs increase oxidative stress in the body (see Chapter 5), leading to inflammation and a myriad of health problems. Poaching, stewing or slow-cooking are better ways to cook animal proteins. Blasting starchy foods at high temperatures produces carcinogenic compounds called acrylamides. These are at especially high levels in French fries and potato crisps (chips).

Excessive stimulants

Caffeine, found in tea, coffee, chocolate, 'energy drinks' and colas, is a potent stimulant. It causes your stress hormones to surge, which disrupts your blood sugar levels. Caffeine also depletes many nutrients, especially B vitamins and minerals such as iron, zinc, calcium and magnesium. Yet, as you'll see in Chapter 4, various healthy ageing benefits have, in recent years, been associated with consuming tea and coffee (both green and black varieties) and dark chocolate.

Our advice, then, is simply to minimize your caffeine intake to a level at which you are not experiencing any negative side-effects (these can include headache, hyperactivity, jitteriness, poor sleep, racing heartbeat, gastric reflux, abdominal pain and high blood pressure). You can use decaff varieties of both tea and coffee, without missing out on their beneficial plant chemicals. You could also consider alternatives such as roasted dandelion root and/or chicory root, and rooibos tea.

Toxins

Toxic metals and chemicals in foods are widespread and can place additional burden on your liver and kidneys, as well as influence your mood and behaviour. By keeping your diet as natural and unprocessed as possible, you can reduce your intake. Avoid 'E' numbers and monosodium glutamate (MSG), a flavour enhancer that can influence mood. MSG is commonly found in packet soups, sauces, crisps and take-aways. Other foods may contain hormones, pesticides and heavy metals: larger fish, such as shark, marlin and tuna, can be contaminated with mercury and dioxins. For this reason, we suggest you consume only wild-caught, smaller fish such as salmon, mackerel, sardines and anchovies.

Alcohol

While some people may gain some benefits from drinking regular, small amounts of alcohol, there is no getting away from the fact that it confers many negative effects on health. Drinking too much will lead to weight gain, blood sugar and insulin problems, fatty liver, elevated levels of blood fats and homocysteine, and increased oxidative stress. See Chapter 7 for the problems associated with raised homocysteine, and see Chapter 5 for the damage that is caused by oxidative stress. Alcohol also burdens the digestive and detoxification systems.

Although it's true that red wine includes antioxidants, we are sceptical about the supposed health benefits of drinking alcohol regularly. A little red wine does indeed feature in the lives of many of the populations known for their high percentage of long-lived, healthy inhabitants,[8] but these communities adopt a wide range of health-promoting activities and therefore may suffer less from the negative effects of alcohol. Such health-promoting activities include a good diet, exercise, stress management and a strong sense of purpose, family, friendship and community. See Chapter 10 for more on these beneficial lifestyle habits.

If you want to drink alcohol, do it for pleasure, rather than thinking of it as an aid to good health, and drink it in small quantities only. Alcohol can be addictive; if you feel you have to drink daily or if you have a history of addiction, you may want to re-evaluate the role it plays in your life and seek professional help if necessary. And, according to the World Cancer Research Fund,[9] if you are concerned about your risk of developing cancer, or if you have had cancer in the past, you may wish to avoid alcohol altogether.

If these risks do not affect you and you would like to include alcohol for pleasure, we recommend abstaining for at least three days a week and, on the days that you do drink, sticking to two units a day for women and three for men.

TWO ALTERNATIVE PLANS TO CONSIDER

CALORIE RESTRICTION: THE SECRET TO HEALTHY AGEING?

Restricting calorie intake has been used as a weight-loss strategy for decades. Our clinical experience has shown us, however, that it is easier to stick to a healthy weight loss plan long-term by following a low-GL diet than by focusing on restricting calories.

Today, the practice of calorie restriction (CR) is gaining a new-found popularity amongst a different sector of the population, namely lean people who are looking for ways to slow down the ageing process. Indeed, CR has more evidence behind it for increasing longevity than any other nutritional or lifestyle practice.

The bulk of the findings so far are from studies of yeasts, insects, fish and rodents – there is less evidence for the effects of CR in humans because there are difficulties with encouraging enough people to participate in a study that so heavily restricts their diet over the long term. Having said this, there are ongoing observations of lean individuals who have chosen to practise CR and have been doing so for some years. So far, it appears that their blood levels of glucose, insulin, cholesterol and some other markers of cardiovascular ageing are lower than they are in people on a more typical diet, as are their levels of thyroid and sex hormones.[10] (This type of blood profile is associated with improved longevity.) What's more, none of these individuals (some as old as 82 years) reportedly takes any medication nor has yet developed any chronic disease. Improved blood pressure and markers of inflammation and glycation (damage to cells caused by sugars) have also been reported.[11]

The key to this type of diet is to eat less, without suffering malnutrition. Thus, the people who practise it usually supplement their diet with micronutrients. If you want to try CR, we recommend, at the very least, a good multivitamin and mineral supplement, plus fish oil and gamma linolenic acid (GLA) and some extra vitamin C, vitamin D and magnesium.

How low should you go?

CR can typically involve reductions of about 30–40 per cent from the general government guideline levels of 2500 calories a day for men and 2000 for women. However, recent evidence suggests that benefits may be obtained with a less restrictive calorie intake. The US government-funded CALERIE studies, for example, have been looking at the effects of a 25 per cent calorie restriction on normal-weight and moderately overweight people, over a period of two years. (For more information on these studies see the CALERIE website at http://calerie.dcri.duke.edu/index.html.) Results reported so far do indeed indicate improvement in some signs of healthier ageing.[12] The diet of the world's longest-lived people, in a community on the Japanese island of Okinawa, is naturally restricted to about 1800 calories a day.[13]

CR is a very restrictive way of eating, requiring a great deal of discipline and willpower. In our experience, most people find it easier and more satisfying to adopt the low-GL approach to healthy ageing, which is explained in the section above. But we have introduced the idea of CR because of the promising results on longevity published in the scientific literature, for those of you who feel robust enough to give it a try and for whom there are no contraindications (see below). We'd recommend you enlist the help of a nutrition practitioner or other healthcare provider to ensure that you don't miss out on any vital nutrients. And, just to reiterate, the results for improved signs of ageing in CR participants have been found in lean to moderately overweight people, rather than in those with significant weight to lose. Hence, you won't find a recommendation for CR for weight loss in Chapter 4.

CR is *not* recommended if you are a child or teenager, pregnant or breastfeeding, or if you have an eating disorder or are currently underweight. In addition, you should seek medical advice if you have a long-term medical condition and/or you are on medication, particularly for blood sugar or blood pressure control. If you are in any of these categories, or if you suffer from regular low mood, intense cravings or binge-eating episodes, you'll probably do better on the low-GL diet.

What's the science behind CR and healthier ageing?

Nobody really knows why CR improves signs and symptoms of healthy ageing. But it is thought that it may help in a number of different ways:

▶ CR helps to keep glucose and insulin low – high levels of both are common in middle-aged people eating a typical Western diet and they both contribute to ageing (see Chapter 4).[14]

▶ CR reduces the everyday damage to cells that is caused by the process of 'oxidation'. This is because most oxidation arises from the metabolic process of burning food for energy. With less food available, your metabolic rate slows down (and this is evident from the lower levels of thyroid hormones in the blood of people on calorie-restricted diets) and fewer 'free radicals' are produced.[15] For an explanation of oxidative stress and how it contributes to the ageing process, see Chapter 5.

▶ CR is a low-level 'stressor', which helps to build up tolerance to potential higher-intensity stressors[16] and also enhance repair and renewal processes during the ageing process.[17]

▶ CR helps to slow down, or even reverse, harmful changes to our gene function that we accumulate as we go through life. These changes are called 'epigenetic' changes and they are now considered to have great influence over the rate at which we age.[18] For an explanation of how these epigenetic changes are involved in the ageing process, see Chapter 1.

The ideal calorie intake varies between individuals, according to your unique biochemistry and also your levels of physical activity. Even if you decide *not* to significantly restrict your calories, aim to take in less than the government's recommended 'average' allowance of 2000 calories a day for women and 2500 calories a day for men. Adopt a low-GL routine. Don't deprive yourself if you are genuinely hungry, but don't 'overeat' at any one sitting as doing so can push blood sugar levels up too high.

FASTING FOR WEIGHT LOSS AND HEALTHY AGEING

Done properly, fasting is not only extremely effective in shifting those extra pounds, but it may also reduce signs of inflammation and various risk factors for cardiovascular disease,[19] including improving blood glucose control, particularly in women.[20] The results from studies on animals indicate fasting may be as effective as CR at reducing the risk of age-related chronic diseases.[21] Another benefit of fasting is that it can be effective in changing your relationship with food, allowing you to understand the difference between *real hunger* and eating out of habit or for emotional reasons.

If you are interested in this way of eating, you could complement your low-GL diet with regular, short periods of fasting. As it can be quite restrictive, however, we recommend you enlist the help of a nutrition practitioner or other healthcare provider to ensure that you don't miss out on any vital nutrients.

There are two types of fasting that you could consider:

▶ Lifestyle fasting: This is a way to incorporate fasting into your daily routine. It is sometimes referred to as the 16/8 fast because you fast for 16 hours and eat within a window of eight hours only. Essentially, you follow the same pattern every day: instead of eating a morning breakfast, you break the fast around noon with lunch and then finish your eating for the day by 8pm. You don't need to restrict your calories from the standard recommended intake of 2000 a day for women and 2500 a day for men – the health benefits are thought to be due to the restricted period of eating having a stabilizing effect on blood glucose and insulin levels – but also don't overeat.

▶ Intermittent fasting: This is also known as 5/2 fasting. You select two days each week that will be your fast days. On these days your food intake will be restricted to 500–600 calories a day. Fast days should be separated by at least one day. For best effects, we suggest eating lunch and then an early dinner to allow sufficient fasting hours (ideally 20 hours). On non-fast days you can eat normally – we suggest following the low-GL diet on these days. Ultimately, there is no one 'correct' way to practise intermittent fasting. If you prefer, you could try it just once a week. You may decide to do it long term, or for a few weeks or months only, perhaps to help you move on from a plateau you have reached in your weight-loss programme.

If you enjoy high-intensity or endurance exercise, take a break on fasting days. High levels of physical activity put a greater demand on your recovery processes. Exercising too intensively on fasting days can put a strain on the adrenal glands and eventually lead to 'burnout'.

Initially, you may feel irritable, light-headed or tired on fasting days. In most cases, these symptoms soon diminish or disappear. Ensure you keep hydrated (using the advice above).

As with the practice of calorie restriction, there are some people for whom fasting is not recommended. Do not fast if you are a child or teenager, pregnant or breastfeeding, or if you have an eating disorder or are currently underweight. In addition, you should seek medical advice before fasting if you have a long-term medical condition and/or you are on medication, particularly for blood sugar or blood pressure control. If you are in any of these categories, or if you suffer from regular low mood, intense cravings or binge-eating episodes, you'll probably do better on the low-GL diet, without trying to incorporate fasting.

MEAL PLANS

We have included three different six-day meal plans in this chapter to get you started. In general we recommend the *Eat to Get Younger* meal plan, which focuses on a low-GL, antioxidant-rich diet. It includes an optional snack, but only eat it if you are genuinely hungry. We have also included a meal plan for each of the two options for fasting outlined above. We have not included a meal plan for CR; we recommend that if you want to try this, you should ideally do so with supervision from a nutrition or medical practitioner, and, as we've said above, you will most certainly also need to take dietary supplements.

LIFESTYLE FASTING

This meal plan is referred to as the 16/8 fast. With this plan you follow the same pattern every day. Instead of eating a morning breakfast, you break the fast around noon with lunch and then finish your eating for the day by 8pm.

Breakfast	N/A
Lunch	*Broccoli Pear Soup*
	Almond bread
	Kale Salad with Sweet Tahini Dressing with slices of roast chicken
	Seeded Fattoush Salad with 50g/2oz low-fat goat's cheese
	Mexican Lettuce Wrap
	Seared Beef Salad with Coriander Pesto
	Prawn and Sea Vegetable Salad with Umeboshi Dressing
Dinner	*Macadamia Dukkah-Crusted Sea Bass with Green Beans and Rocket*
	Asian Cauliflower 'Rice' Stir Fry
	Saffron Chicken Skewers with Chimmichuri Sauce with mixed salad
	Grilled Mackerel with Sweet and Sour Mushrooms with steamed leafy greens
	Tempeh Coconut Curry with wholegrain rice
	Slow-Cooked Za'atar Lamb Shoulder with Green Beans and Rocket
Snack	*Supergreen Gut Healer Smoothie*
	Spiced Glazed Nuts
	Beet Mint Dip with carrot sticks
	Handful of berries
	Salted Vinegar and Onion Kale Chips
	Tropical Goji Sorbet
	Courgette Hummus with vegetable sticks
	Tropical Protein Smoothie
	Superfood Fudge
	Wedge of melon
	Fruit Parfait

INTERMITTENT FASTING

Breakfast	Fast day
	Soaked Chia Muesli with blueberries
	Fast day
	Persimmon Carrot Ginger-Aid
	Grain-Free Breakfast Bowl
	Anti-Inflammatory Turmeric Shake
	Super Greens Frittata
	Longevity Cashew Latte
	Cacao Courgette Bread
Lunch	*Asian Chicken Noodle Soup*
	Roasted Baby Beets with Tempeh and Walnut Dressing
	Broccoli Pear Soup
	One *Tomato Seeded Cracker*
	Quinoa Tabbouleh with Pomegranate
	Vietnamese Chicken Salad with Chilli Lime Dressing
	Watercress, Apple and Walnut Salad with Creamy Mustard Dressing
Dinner	*Baked Halibut with Spiced Tomato Relish* with salad
	Moroccan Beef Tagine with steamed vegetables
	Chilli and Lime Spiced Sardines with salad
	Miso Ginger Baked Chicken with roasted vegetables and sweet potato
	Thai Salmon Fishcakes with mixed salad
	Parchment-Baked Fish with Tamarind and Lime with mixed salad
Snack	Fast day
	Handful of *Spiced Glazed Nuts*
	Lime Mint Cleanser
	Fast day
	Lime Guacamole with vegetable sticks
	Handful of berries
	Chocolate Lime Mousse
	Roasted Banana, Caramel Kefir Ice Cream

THE EAT TO GET YOUNGER BASIC PLAN

Breakfast	*Antioxidant Green Burst*
	Handful of nuts
	Lime Mint Cleanser
	Cacao Courgette Bread with nut butter
	Soaked Chia Muesli
	Matcha Green Tea Chia Pudding
	Berry Muffin
	Quick Mexican Baked Eggs
Lunch	*Greek Chicken Salad with Roasted Olives*
	Rich Greens Soup
	One *Tomato Seeded Cracker*
	Seared Beef Salad with Coriander Pesto
	Super Greens Frittata with mixed salad
	Bitter Greens with Grapefruit and Avocado with slices of roast chicken
	Pineapple Gazpacho
	Flaxseed crackers
Dinner	*Thai Salmon Fishcakes* with mixed salad
	Asian Cauliflower 'Rice' Stir Fry
	Asparagus and Courgette Spaghetti with Red Pepper Marinara Sauce with slices of poached or roast chicken
	Korean Spiced Venison with wilted greens
	Grilled Mackerel with Sweet and Sour Mushrooms with steamed leafy greens
	Grain-Free Pizza with mixed salad
Snack	*Omega Vanilla Shake*
	Lime Guacamole with vegetable sticks
	Handful of berries
	Salted Vinegar and Onion Kale Chips
	Roasted Herb and Lemon-Scented Olives
	Grapefruit

Tomato Nut Cheese with flaxseed crackers
Handful of berries

Handful of Brazil nuts and goji berries
Coriander Detox Juice

Longevity Cashew Latte
Spiced Glazed Nuts

If you do nothing else, do this...

▶ Adopt a low-GL diet, swapping sugars and white starches for beans, pulses, non-potato root vegetables and occasionally whole grains, sweet potatoes and boiled new potatoes in their skins. Limit these carbs to one portion, once or twice a day.

▶ Include plenty of the special anti-inflammatory, antioxidant, fermented and alkalizing foods that have been mentioned above.

▶ Eat organic where possible.

▶ Keep hydrated with at least 1.5 litres (3 pints) of caffeine-free natural fluids a day, including vegetable juices or smoothies.

▶ Avoid foods that cause unpleasant reactions, burnt or blackened foods, excessive stimulants, toxic additives and alcohol.

▶ If you need help with addictions to sugar or starches, see the tips in Chapter 10 and consider supplementing 5-HTP or L-glutamine.

▶ Optional: consider implementing either calorie restriction or fasting, if you have no contraindications.

▶ Introduce the new eating plan gradually, making changes at your own pace.

▶ After you've become comfortable with it, move on to Chapters 3–9, so that you can consider the additional advice for tackling the particular areas of health risk that are relevant to you.

CHAPTER 3

HOW TO HAVE A HAPPY GUT

The most obvious life-sustaining roles of your digestive system include the absorption of vital nutrients and the expulsion of toxins. When it comes to healthy ageing, however, the gastrointestinal (GI) tract has another vital role to play: it helps to regulate immune function throughout the entire body, including your propensity towards chronic, long-term inflammation. As we saw in Chapter 1, unresolved inflammation leads to premature ageing and degenerative diseases. Good gut health is crucial in keeping this 'inflamm-ageing' in check, as you'll see as you progress through this chapter.

The GI tract starts in the mouth and runs through the oesophagus (the tube that connects the stomach to the throat), the stomach, the small intestine and the large intestine, before finally reaching the rectum. It is often perceived as being part of our 'insides' but, in fact, it is technically outside the body. Indeed, one of its main roles is to act as a barrier, preventing food-borne toxins from entering the bloodstream.

You may be reading this in full knowledge that your digestion needs some help. We have seen clients who can no longer fit into their clothes, so bloated are their abdomens; people who dread eating socially because they seem to be intolerant to most everyday foods; people who can't travel far because they never know when they will need to rush to the loo; or people whose sleep is interrupted night after night, with acid reflux and painful heartburn. We've had clients who have had to put their sex lives on hold, as well as their social lives and even their careers, because their digestive problems are so distressing and confining.

Even if your symptoms have not yet reached such an extreme level, perhaps you are tired of feeling bloated, or maybe you have never felt quite right since that bout of gastroenteritis you suffered months ago. These are some of the sorts of complaints to look out for:

- frequent belching or flatulence

- heartburn or acid reflux

- bloating shortly after eating, or a sense of excessive fullness after meals

- finding it difficult to move the bowels/needing to strain, loose bowels, or alternating between the two

- undigested food in the loo bowl

- 'churning' feeling in the gut

- lower abdominal pain from trapped wind

- regular nausea

- stools that are pale in colour, greasy or shiny.

If you suffer from even just one of these on a regular basis, your GI tract is likely to need some support. This chapter will help you to work out a plan of action.

If, on the other hand, you have been lucky enough to stay relatively free from digestive complaints, you may think this chapter is not for you. But before you skip over it entirely, take a moment to consider whether you are affected by any of the following issues.

Tick the box for each statement that applies to you.

☐ Have taken antibiotics, antacids or pain medications (e.g. ibuprofen or aspirin) within the last five years

☐ Prone to asthma, sinusitis or stuffy nose

☐ A gut infection within the last five years

☐ Diagnosed with an autoimmune illness (e.g. rheumatoid arthritis, multiple sclerosis, autoimmune hypothyroidism, type 1 diabetes)

☐ Feeling extraordinarily tired all the time, even after a good night's sleep

☐ Unexplained muscle aches

☐ Unexplained stiff joints or pains in joints

☐ Feel spacey or unreal: 'brain fog'

☐ Regularly crave bread or other starchy or sugary foods

☐ Fungal skin or nail infection

☐ Eczema, hives or psoriasis

☐ Long periods of feeling as if you are, 'coming down with something'

Total score _____

If you scored 5 or above, you are almost certainly in need of digestive support. Poor gut health can cause these types of whole-body symptoms, even in the absence of digestive problems. Some people with the serious GI condition of coeliac disease, for example, have no or only minimal symptoms in the gut.[1]

Gastrointestinal problems become more common as we get older. Although some of this is because we are ageing, many other factors can play a part. Certain frequently used medications (such as antibiotics, aspirin, ibuprofen and steroids), for example, can injure the gut, interfere with digestion and absorption, and paradoxically promote inflammation in the body. (We say 'paradoxically' because most of these medications are used as anti-inflammatories.)

The good news, though, is that by taking active steps, you can improve your digestive health without resorting to drugs. And getting your gut health back into balance will not only improve your digestion but will put your entire body into more of an anti-inflammatory state.

WHAT'S CAUSING THESE SYMPTOMS?

The most common underlying causes of all the symptoms mentioned above (both in the gut and elsewhere in the body) are two troublesome culprits known as 'dysbiosis' and 'leaky gut'. Food allergies also cause significant inflammation (in the gut and elsewhere) but true allergies are not as common as you might think – see Box 3.1.

BOX 3.1 DO YOU HAVE A FOOD ALLERGY/INTOLERANCE?

Do you experience symptoms of food allergy or intolerance? Maybe you get gas, diarrhoea or pain in the stomach or abdomen after eating certain foods, or perhaps you feel exhausted, headachy or stuffy-nosed later that day or the following morning? Do you try to avoid eating in social situations, for fear of producing rather unsociable reactions such as belching or flatulence?

When this happens, it is natural to want to identify the offending food and avoid it. But this can be difficult if the problem food is one that you eat regularly, such as bread, milk, onions, garlic or even apples – all these foods commonly cause unpleasant reactions.

Well, now for some good news. Did you know that relatively few people are genuinely allergic or intolerant to specific foods? Far more common are other problems occurring in the gut, which cause symptoms that look and feel very much like allergies and intolerances. The most common of these problems are dysbiosis (or microbial imbalances), insufficient production of stomach acid or digestive enzymes, and leaky gut (sometimes referred to as intestinal hyperpermeability). Many people find that once these underlying problems are sorted out, they can go back to enjoying the foods to which they had assumed they were 'allergic'.

You can tackle the problems of dysbiosis, leaky gut and low digestive secretions by following the advice in this chapter. If, after so doing, you still have symptoms, it may be that you are one of the minority of people who have either a genuine food allergy or an intolerance. True allergies tend to cause immediate, acute, inflammatory reactions and can be diagnosed through a test for the presence of inflammatory chemicals called IgE antibodies. Once identified, you will most likely need to avoid that food for the rest of your life.

Food intolerances differ from allergies in that they do not involve an immune response driven by the IgE antibody. You may have coeliac disease, for example, which is an autoimmune intolerance to a protein called gluten, found in wheat, spelt, rye and barley. (Coeliac disease is estimated to affect 1 in 100 people.[2]) Or you may have a gluten 'sensitivity'. This is different to coeliac disease, although it still means you have to avoid the same grains. Other types of intolerances may be due to insufficient production of digestive enzymes. If you are not producing enough of the lactase enzyme, for example, you'll be intolerant to milk and other dairy products that contain the sugar lactose.

Food intolerances can be harder to diagnose than food allergies because the symptoms can be less specific and they may be delayed for hours or even days. Intolerances can be identified by using any of these tests:

▶ A coeliac disease blood test. (Remember, coeliac differs from other intolerances in that it is a serious autoimmune disease.)

▶ A gluten sensitivity blood test.

▶ A lactose breath test (for suspected intolerance of lactose, found in dairy products).

▶ A fructose breath test (for suspected intolerance of fructose, found in fruit, some vegetables and some processed foods).

▶ Blood tests for immune reactions to many types of foods or food additives. These tend to measure antibodies such as IgG and other chemicals produced by immune system cells that are typically involved in sensitivities.

You may find that a more reliable (and cheaper) way of identifying the culprit foods is to avoid them for 3–4 weeks and then reintroduce them, one at a time, and see if you experience any symptoms. (Coeliac disease is an exception – if you suspect this, you should be appropriately tested.) Trying to identify the offending foods can, however, be a tricky business and you may find it easier to do it with the help of a nutritionist or nutritional therapist. You can find appropriately qualified and regulated nutrition practitioners near you by using these websites:

▶ British Association for Applied Nutrition and Nutritional Therapy: www.bant.org.uk.

▶ Complementary and Natural Healthcare Council: www.cnhc.org.uk.

Your GI tract is home to more than 100 trillion microbial cells, encoding 100 times more genes than your own genome.[3] Your overall health is just as much determined by these microbes as by your own body cells. They're tremendously important for controlling your digestion, for example, as well as for producing certain vitamins, other beneficial nutrients and also chemical messengers that affect your emotional health. And recently it's been found that your gut microflora may even help to determine your body weight and the extent to which you are predisposed to unintentionally pile on excess pounds.[4]

GUT DYSBIOSIS

If the delicate ecobalance between the many different types of gut microbes becomes disrupted, you are said to have the condition gut dysbiosis. Essentially, your microbial balance depends on what you eat: feed these microbes too much junk food, for example, and you will find that harmful bugs flourish (bacteria, yeasts or both), crowding out the helpful microbes in the large bowel. Another type of dysbiosis is where microbes from the colon have somehow managed to migrate higher up the gut, to the small intestine. Here, they ferment the sugars and carbohydrates in your food, in much the same way as yeasts ferment sugars to produce beer in a brewery. This type of dysbiosis (called a small intestinal bacterial overgrowth, or SIBO) causes uncomfortable gas and bloating within an hour or two of eating. It's also thought to be a factor in many cases of irritable bowel syndrome (IBS).

Dysbiosis is a common cause of inflammatory conditions, and several diseases have been associated with the condition, including Crohn's disease, colon cancer, asthma, diabetes and obesity.[5]

LEAKY GUT

Leaky gut (also known as intestinal hyperpermeability) is where the cells of the gut lining (sometimes referred to as the epithelial cells) lose their ability to stick together tightly. This means they no longer form an effective barrier – they can't prevent harmful molecules from moving through the gut lining to the inside of the body. Once such toxins get through the gut lining and into the bloodstream, they activate an attack by your immune system. This causes inflammatory and allergic-like symptoms that can manifest anywhere in the body. Over the long term, a leaky gut can even lead to inflammatory autoimmune conditions such as rheumatoid arthritis.[6] Box 3.2 describes in more detail the ways in which problems in the GI tract can promote chronic inflammation and premature ageing.

BOX 3.2 HOW CAN INFLAMM-AGEING START IN THE GUT?

In Chapter 8 you'll learn about the importance of having a good level of 'immune tolerance'. A tolerant immune system is a healthy immune system. It's on constant surveillance and can easily differentiate between harmful invaders and molecules that are foreign but 'friendly' (pollen, for example). A tolerant immune system will launch an attack when necessary but has the intelligence to suppress reactions to foreign molecules that are not in themselves harmful to the body. In this way, the job of a healthy immune system is, for most of the time, to *not* respond to things.

The older we get, the more likely it is that our immune system starts to lose this 'tolerance'. It starts to overreact to things, mounting unnecessary inflammatory responses and not being able to shut them off again. When this happens, you gradually become pushed towards a state of ongoing inflammation, or 'inflamm-ageing' – the type of chronic, low-grade, whole-body inflammation that can't be seen on the outside but which is causing long-term damage and increasing your risk of premature ageing and chronic disease.

If you want to maintain your immune tolerance as you age, you need a strong and intact gut lining. This is because in the gut lining there are special cells and antibodies that prevent foreign molecules from getting through the mucus barrier into the underlying tissues. If these invaders manage to get through, they trigger the immune cells in the underlying tissue to launch an inflammatory attack.

So, if you have a leaky gut, you lose your immune tolerance. (In fact, poor gut health is considered the most common reason for losing your immune tolerance.[7]) And if you lose your immune tolerance, you end up overreacting to perfectly benign substances – pollen, perfumes, cat and dog dander, various foods and many others. The sorts of inflammatory reactions you might experience can range from a stuffy nose to hayfever, sinusitis, painful joints or headaches; or it may be that you are simply fatigued, or your mood is low and you have a general feeling of malaise. In the long term, unresolved inflammation increases your risk of age-related chronic illnesses.[8] Maintaining optimal immune tolerance also relies on a healthy microbial balance in the GI tract. This is because friendly microbes help the gut's immune system to work properly. They also help to prevent your gut lining from becoming leaky.

So dysbiosis and leaky gut can lead to inflamm-ageing: the chronic, low-grade, body-wide inflammation that causes premature ageing and degenerative diseases.

The links between gut problems and body-wide inflammation are now so well documented in the scientific journals that some doctors are beginning to view their patients as human–microbe hybrids. They believe that everyone with a chronic condition of ill-health should be investigated for undiagnosed problems in the GI tract.[9] For example, there is some evidence that an infection in the gut of a bacterium called *Klebsiella* may be a trigger for the autoimmune disease ankylosing spondylitis.[10] What's more, a stomach infection of *Helicobacter pylori* (*H. pylori*, a leading cause of gastritis and stomach ulcers) may increase your risk of cardiovascular disease.[11] And inflammatory bowel diseases such as ulcerative colitis can lead to all sorts of other problems, including various types of arthritis and inflammatory conditions in the eyes and skin.[12]

TOP TIPS FOR A HAPPY GUT

A few years ago, a group of forward-thinking doctors and scientists in the US devised a five-pronged approach for getting a dysfunctional digestive tract back into full working order. They were working within a new type of healthcare paradigm for tackling premature ageing, which they called Functional Medicine (FM), and they strived to find alternative strategies to what they saw as an over-reliance on medical drugs. You can read more about FM at www.functionalmedicine.org. Their five-pronged approach is shown below.

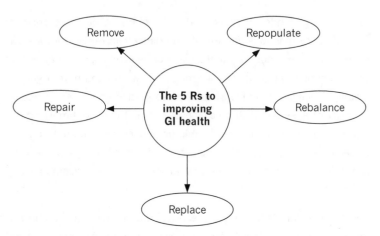

We use this '5 R' framework in our clinics. In this chapter, we have outlined the most effective of our specially devised recommendations for implementing each of the 5 Rs. These are powerful interventions and the ones that we have had the most success with. And you can put them into practice right now.

REMOVE IRRITANTS AND TOXINS

The first thing to do is *remove* the factors that are *causing* your problems. Put the following recommendations into action for a month before you start to incorporate changes from the other Rs.

Are your drugs to blame?

Discuss with your doctor whether you can safely reduce or remove drugs that are notorious for hampering gut health. The most common culprits are aspirin, ibuprofen and other non-steroidal anti-inflammatory drugs (NSAIDs), antacids, proton pump inhibitors (PPIs), antibiotics, codeine and the contraceptive pill.

Dysbiosis is common after periods of antibiotic use, as these drugs destroy all types of bacteria in the gut – the good and the bad. That's why we recommend to all our clients that if they have to take antibiotics, they should also take steps to replenish the good bacteria. The simplest way to do this is by taking a supplement of some beneficial types of bacteria. These supplements are known as probiotics and are discussed in more detail later in this chapter.

Another class of drug to be aware of is acid blockers, as they can also promote dysbiosis. Antacids and PPIs work either by neutralizing your stomach acid or by inhibiting its production. In the short term, this stops the irritation to the gastric lining, providing some relief from the acid-induced pain. But the downside is that, with the lack of stomach acid, food is left undigested in the gut. This is a veritable feast for the colonies of unwanted bacteria waiting on the sidelines. And the more they get to eat, the more they proliferate.

Then there are the NSAIDs. These are notorious for damaging the gut lining, causing not only leaky gut but also more immediately apparent problems such as gastritis and gastric ulcers. Chapter 8 includes more information on NSAIDs.

If you are taking any of these medications, it's worth talking with your doctor about their risks and benefits as they affect your individual situation.

Might bacterial or yeast overgrowths (dysbiosis) be the main problem?

If you have excess wind, bloating or cramping, try avoiding the sugars and starches that readily ferment in the gut, producing gases. These are found in processed and refined foods such as pastries, biscuits and white bread, and also in alcohol (dysbiosis is far more common in heavy drinkers[13]). However, you might be surprised to learn that some healthy foods are high in fermentative sugars and starches. Box 3.3 lists the most troublesome of these, along with more gut-friendly alternatives.

BOX 3.3 YOUR GUIDE TO FOODS THAT DO AND DON'T CAUSE WIND AND BLOATING IN THE GUT

Many people with IBS symptoms such as wind and bloating see dramatic improvements when they follow an eating plan that controls the type of sugars and starches (carbohydrates) consumed. This way of eating tends to help because:

▶ Certain types of sugars and starches are devoured (fermented) by 'unfriendly' microbes in the gut, producing gas. Excess gas in the gut leads to belching, flatulence, pain, constipation and/or diarrhoea (depending on the type of gas produced).

▶ Eating too much sugar causes inflammation. Inflammation damages the gut lining, making it become too leaky. This can lead to whole-body symptoms such as joint pain, fatigue, 'brain fog' and even depression.[14]

There are many different types of carbohydrate-controlled diets. They have names like the GAPs Diet, the Atkins Diet, the Specific Carbohydrate Diet, the Low FODMAPs diet, the Caveman/Paleolithic Diet, the Anti-Candida Diet and the gluten-free and lactose-free diet. They are notoriously difficult to follow because they require you to give up some of your favourite foods.

Having worked with all these diets, our recommendation is to temporarily avoid the foods listed below. These contain the sugars and starches that commonly ferment in the gut, triggering uncomfortable and unsociable symptoms:

▶ Wheat, rye and barley. Swap to oats, buckwheat, quinoa, polenta and rice.

▶ Onions, garlic, leeks, cauliflower, broccoli, Brussels sprouts, Jerusalem artichokes, asparagus and mushrooms. Swap to rocket (arugula), salad leaves, courgette (zucchini), olives, tomatoes, peppers, peas, beansprouts, aubergine (eggplant), pattypan squash, seaweed, spinach, water chestnut, fresh herbs, celery, okra, radishes and cucumber.

▶ Beans and pulses, including chickpeas (and hummus) and soy products (e.g. tofu and soy milk). Swap to nuts and seeds and butters made from these.

▶ Animal dairy products: milk, cream, commercial yogurt, crème fraîche and cheese. Swap to coconut milk, cream and yogurt, oat milk and cream, and milks made from hemp, rice or almonds. (Some dairy-intolerant people find they are fine on lactose-free versions.)

▶ Apples, pears, plums, cherries and apricots. Swap to oranges, tangerines, strawberries, melon, papaya and blueberries.

▶ Certain added sugars, especially honey, fructose, xylitol and sorbitol. Swap to stevia or a small amount of maple syrup.

Note that meat, fish, eggs and seafood are fine to eat.

Reduce or avoid these foods until you feel significantly better and for at least two weeks (but could be up to three months). Then challenge yourself by reintroducing one food at a time and monitoring how you feel over the next three days. Make sure you eat large and regular portions over the day of the food you are testing. If you get no reaction, you can go back to eating it after you have completed the entire challenge. If you do get a reaction, keep avoiding it for now. You may want to test it again at some point in the future. Leave at least three days between challenges of different foods.

The above exclusion plan is based on the principles of a 'low-FODMAP' diet, for which there is scientific evidence on its use in IBS.[15]

You can also tackle microbial overgrowths head-on by using antimicrobial agents: good foods to eat are cloves, oregano, licorice, turmeric, olive oil and coconut oil. For a truly therapeutic effect, take two tablets of concentrated oregano oil immediately after each meal. At the right dose, oregano oil is a powerful anti-bacterial and anti-fungal and may also help to eradicate certain troublesome parasites.[16]

If you have heartburn or gastritis, ask your doctor for a test for the *H. pylori* bacterium that can damage the lining of the stomach. Your doctor may prescribe antibiotics if the test result is positive. (If you decide to take these, remember to take probiotics as well.)

Avoid man-made fats and reduce saturated fats. Lower-fat meals tend to digest more quickly, minimizing the chance of dysbiosis and also of reflux. Man-made fats are known as *trans-*, hydrogenated and partially hydrogenated fats. These are found in processed foods, baked goods such as croissants and pastries, and commercial salad dressings. Saturated fats are found naturally in cheese, cream and fatty cuts of meat. Government guidelines are that saturated fats should be kept within 10 per cent of total calorie intake. This means that if you are eating 2000 calories a day, you need to eat no more than 20g saturated fat. When reading food labels, any containing 5g or more of saturated fat per 100g of the food is too high. We have a range of lower-fat recipes such as *Lime Guacamole, Cauliflower Munchies, Vietnamese Chicken Salad with Chilli Lime Dressing, Turmeric Glazed Fish with Cucumber Pickle,* and *Tropical Goji Sorbet.*

Could food allergens or intolerances be damaging the gut? Although food allergies and intolerances are less common than bacterial or yeast overgrowths, they do affect some people. See Box 3.1 for information on how to identify allergies and intolerances.

If you suffer from gastric reflux, experiment with avoiding alcohol, chocolate, coffee, tea and mint. These foods and drinks tend to relax the muscle at the bottom of the oesophagus (known as the cardiac sphincter), making reflux from the stomach more likely.[17] Reflux is not usually caused by having too much stomach acid (see Box 3.4).

Any change to your caffeine intake is best done gradually – for example, by replacing half of your coffee with alternatives, such as dandelion and/or chicory root coffee, or with (organic) decaffeinated coffee. Drinking decaff coffee means you can continue benefitting from the healthful phytochemicals in coffee. (Chapter 4 has more information on the potential healthy ageing benefits of coffee.)

Remove foods that can make the gut lining become too leaky. The main culprits are gluten grains (wheat, rye and barley) and foods that are high in lectins, such as beans (especially soy), pulses and peanuts.[18] Many of these foods also contain the types of carbs that cause excess fermentation in the gut, leading to wind and bloating (see Box 3.3).

BOX 3.4 ACID ATTACK?

Many people mistakenly believe that their heartburn and reflux is caused by producing too much acid. In fact, this is rarely the case. This common misconception is an understandable one, given that you are likely to have been prescribed acid-blocking medication by your doctor.

The most typical reason for reflux and its associated pain (technically known as gastro-oesophageal reflux disease, or GORD – GERD in the US) is that the cardiac sphincter has become too flabby, opening too readily and allowing the stomach's contents to regurgitate back up to the oesophagus.

This can happen if there is too much food in the stomach, perhaps because you have over-indulged – it's best to stop eating before you are completely full. Or it could be because the food in the stomach is not being efficiently processed and passed on to the small intestine. This may be due to *insufficient* production of gastric acid rather than too much! Other common causes of reflux are stress, food sensitivities, obesity or a hiatus hernia. Damaged mucosa can also worsen reflux and heartburn.[19] (Gastric infections like *H. pylori* – see page 53 – can easily damage the mucosa.)

REPLACE DIGESTIVE HELPERS

After you have been following the 'remove' recommendations for about a month, you can start to introduce actions from this section. Stick with it for about 3–4 weeks, after which you can move on to the third 'R' – repopulate.

This stage is about *replacing* anything you might be missing for optimum digestion.

Fibre

Make sure you are eating plenty of soluble fibre. Good sources are brown rice, oats, flaxseeds, chia seeds, turnip, swede (rutabaga), okra and, to a lesser extent, other vegetables. Soluble fibre is also present in beans, pulses and xanthum and guar gums, but these foods can cause wind and bloating in some people with compromised digestion.

Soluble fibre helps the friendly bacteria to set up home in the gut, rather than just passing straight through. It can provide long-lasting relief from constipation and diarrhoea and it also produces special molecules that reduce inflammation in the colon and keep it healthy.[20] If you have a tendency towards constipation, follow the advice in Box 3.5 on how best to use linseeds, chia seeds and psyllium. Steer clear of soluble fibre supplements called fructo-oligosaccharides and inulin because they can increase gas production.

BOX 3.5 SOME TIPS FOR CONSTIPATION

▶ Soak 1–2 teaspoons of cracked linseeds (flaxseeds) in 125ml/half a cup of room-temperature water overnight. Drink the mixture in the morning, followed by another half-cup of warm water. Wait at least 30 minutes before breakfast.

▶ Alternatively, soak 1 tbsp ground linseed in 125ml/half a cup of 100 per cent prune juice overnight. Eat it in the morning with a spoon, followed by a glass of warm water. (Don't use this tip if you have dysbiosis, as the natural sugars may increase uncomfortable wind and bloating.)

▶ You can also soak 2 tbsp of chia seeds in 125ml/half a cup of water and leave to soak for 15–30 minutes, stirring with a whisk to prevent clumping. This can then be added to smoothies.

▶ Instead of linseeds or chia seeds, you could try psyllium husk powder. Mix 2 tsp into 125ml/half a cup of warm water first thing in the morning. Follow with another glass of warm water.

▶ Include plenty of whole grains, fruit and vegetables in your diet.

▶ Wake up your bowel with some exercise – aim for at least 30 minutes a day of brisk walking, cycling, swimming, dancing or aerobics.

▶ Soluble fibre can only work its magic if fluid intake is also increased. Many people make the well-intentioned change to increased fibre intake, only to find that their symptoms become worse, due to lack of water. So make sure you are drinking 1.5 litres (approximately 3 pints) of non-caffeinated fluids a day, more in hot weather or if you are very physically active. If you're not keen on cold water, try warm water (which is better for constipation) or herbal teas, decaff tea and coffee, very diluted fruit juices, coconut water or unsweetened milks made from hemp, almond, oat, rice or coconut.

▶ Try taking some magnesium and vitamin C supplements – up to 500mg a day magnesium oxide and 3g a day vitamin C, in six divided doses (of 500mg), spaced by approximately 30 minutes. (This level of vitamin C is not advised for more than a few days.)

▶ Ask your family doctor for a thyroid function test.

▶ Trial a course of probiotics: buy one that includes a combination of *Lactobacillus* and *Bifidobacterium* species, with at least 10 billion live organisms in each daily dose.

▶ Stimulate sluggish bile flow by taking a supplement of artichoke extract shortly before each meal. We recommend taking one that is standardized to provide 32mg of the active phytochemical cynarin per meal.

Digestive secretions

As we age, and especially during times of stress or if we are rushing meals, our production of digestive secretions can suffer. If levels of stomach acid or digestive enzymes become too low, the digestive tract can become burdened with undigested food molecules. These tend to attract troublesome yeasts and bacteria that devour the food, producing a lot of gas along the way. This leads to the pain and bloating of 'trapped wind' or the embarrassment of excessive flatulence.

Some foods naturally contain enzymes that may help to break down food in the gut. These include fresh pineapple core and green papaya. See our recipes for *Supergreen Gut Healer, Anti-Inflammatory Turmeric Shake, Nori Avocado Maki Rolls* and *Kale Salad with Sweet Tahini Dressing.*

Alternatively, you can take enzymes in supplement form. Unless you have gastritis or ulceration, digestive enzymes can safely be supplemented with each meal. You can buy animal-derived pancreatic enzymes or, alternatively, plant-derived enzymes such as bromelain (from pineapple), papain (from papaya) and many others. You could experiment by purchasing one pot and monitoring any improvement in your gut symptoms.

Some people find it more effective to take tablets containing hydrochloric acid (HCl). HCl is the type of acid produced by the stomach to digest food and kill harmful microbes – see Box 3.6.

BOX 3.6 MIGHT HYDROCHLORIC ACID SUPPLEMENTS HELP YOUR DIGESTION?

As you age, the parietal cells in your stomach lining gradually produce less stomach acid (also known as hydrochloric acid, or HCl). If you are not producing enough HCl, your absorption of vitamin B12 and minerals from food will be compromised – this includes iron, calcium, magnesium, zinc and copper. What's more, you'll be left with undigested food molecules in the gut. These attract unwanted bacteria and yeasts, promoting the growth of these bugs. Hence, low HCl leads to dysbiosis and gut infections.

It's not only advancing age that causes a decline in HCl production. Other causes include pernicious anaemia, chronic *H. pylori* infection (the main bacterium that causes gastritis and ulceration), periods of stress, taking antacids or PPI medications (proton pump inhibitors such as lansoprazole and omeprazole) and having low zinc levels.

Some people find that taking supplements of HCl (sold as betaine hydrochloride) dramatically reduces IBS symptoms because the increased acidity in the gut leads to more efficient protein digestion. It also exterminates any bugs and toxins that may have hitched a ride with the food. You can gauge your need for such supplementation by doing the following simple test. (Do not attempt this test if you have any heartburn, gastritis, ulceration or black, tarry blood in the stool, as the tablets could make these conditions worse. See your family doctor in the first instance if you have any of these complaints.)

Start by taking one tablet of betaine hydrochloride (350–750mg) with a protein-containing meal. These tablets are widely available from pharmacies and health food shops. (Swallow the tablets whole, with a glass of water. Do not chew them or empty them on to food, as they can be corrosive to teeth.) If you are producing enough stomach acid, you should experience some discomfort or heartburn – if this is the case, you should *not* take HCl tablets, as you are already producing enough yourself. (You can neutralize the acid by taking a teaspoon of bicarbonate of soda in a little water.)

If, however, there is no burning sensation, start taking two tablets with each protein-containing meal. If you experience no burning sensation, increase this by one tablet every two days, up to a maximum of eight tablets with each protein-containing meal. This may seem like a large dose to take but it is not nearly as much acid as a healthy stomach normally produces. Once you reach the dosage level where you feel warmth, tingling or any type of stomach discomfort, including burning, reduce the dose by one capsule per meal. Stick with this dose until you begin to feel the discomfort at this dose and then reduce it again. (With smaller meals, you may require less HCl, so take fewer capsules.)

If you are consistent with your supplementation, and if you address the underlying causes of your low HCl levels (e.g. stress, pernicious anaemia, *H. pylori* infection, acid-suppressing drugs or inadequate zinc intake), you should find that you can gradually reduce the dose, as you become more intolerant to the acid supplements. This could indicate a return to more normal levels of acid secretion by your stomach.

This test for low stomach acid was devised by the Institute for Functional Medicine. While it has not been scientifically validated, it is widely used by FM doctors and other healthcare practitioners using FM. If you're able to improve your HCl levels, you will absorb your nutrients much better and you will reduce your risk of gut infections.

One final point: if you are going to do this test, do be aware that the symptoms of burning or discomfort should be short-lived, as they are simply an indication that you do not need the level of acid that you are supplementing. If these symptoms continue, it is likely that there is another reason. In this case, you should stop taking the supplements and discuss your symptoms with your doctor.

If you suspect you are not digesting protein foods such as meat, poultry, fish and eggs very well – maybe they are lying heavy on your stomach after eating – try adding lemon or lime juice, vinegars or wine to your cooking. (See the recipe for *Grilled Mackerel with Sweet and Sour Mushrooms*.) The extra acidity starts to break down the proteins, giving your digestive system a helping hand. Alternatively, you could take a teaspoon of apple cider vinegar in a little water just before meals.

Another trick is to use a slow-cooker. Nowadays, these are modestly priced. They are also extremely energy-efficient, using only the same amount of electricity as a standard light bulb. But their real benefit lies in the way that the long, slow cooking process breaks down the tough collagen fibres in meat and fish, producing a delicious 'melt-in-the-mouth' consistency, which is amazingly easy on the digestive tract. See our recipe for *Slow-Cooked Za'atar Lamb Shoulder*.

Zinc

Find out about your zinc levels. Anybody looking for optimum digestion needs good levels of this mineral, the most important nutrient for stomach acid production. If you don't have enough of it, your gastric acid levels could suffer. Low zinc status can also cause leaky gut.[21]

You can easily check your zinc status by challenging your taste buds with a zinc solution. For this, you'll need to purchase a small bottle of zinc sulphate, available from some pharmacies, health food shops and online. Follow the instructions on the bottle for the 'taste test'. Essentially, if you can't taste the metal in the solution, your zinc levels are likely to be insufficient for optimal health.

Don't be persuaded into doing similar tests for the status of other minerals, such as calcium or magnesium. This test only works with zinc, due to zinc's crucial role in enabling the taste buds to work properly.

Good food sources of zinc are oysters, beef, crab, pork and chicken. Vegan sources include seeds, seaweeds and whole grains. See the recipes for *Prawn and Sea Vegetable Salad with Umeboshi Dressing, Seared Beef Salad with Coriander Pesto* and *Soaked Chia Muesli*. Adequate levels of zinc are found in most multivitamin and mineral supplements.

Digestive bitters

Once you have worked on your zinc levels, you can help to stimulate your digestive juices by adding in foods that have a bitter taste.[22] The easiest way to do this is to start every lunch and dinner with a salad of bitter leaves, such as chicory (endive), watercress, dandelion and rocket (arugula). Such bitters used to be widely eaten until relatively recently – now they seem to appear only on the most fashionable menus of the most expensive restaurants. If you can't always find bitter leaves, you could carry a small bottle of Swedish herbal bitters in your bag. These concoctions typically contain dandelion, gentian, licorice and other digestive herbs. A few drops can be drunk or sprinkled on to the tongue shortly before food. Pickled Japanese fruits called umeboshi plums (found in healthfood stores) can have a similar effect. See the recipe for *Prawn and Sea Vegetable Salad with Umeboshi Dressing*.

REPOPULATE WITH THE HEALTHY BACTERIA

If you have got to this stage in the quest for a healthy gut, you will already have made fantastic progress – well done! You've undertaken a great deal to get rid of the rampaging undesirables – the bugs that cause the problems. And you are likely to be digesting your meals a lot better because you are focusing on the foods that you tolerate well and are supporting your digestion with better eating practices and, if necessary, supplements of digestive herbs, enzymes or betaine hydrochloride.

Now is the time to entice back the microbes that are helpful in the gut – the good guys such as *Lactobacillus* and *Bifidobacteria*. These do an amazing job in keeping us healthy, improving not only our digestion but also the health of the entire body. As we saw earlier in this chapter, dysbiosis can cause inflammation anywhere in the body. A healthy microbial balance, then, promotes an anti-inflammatory effect.

At this stage of the programme, you can stop taking any antimicrobials you may have started, such as oregano supplements, as long as you have been taking them daily for at least four weeks. Continue with the other interventions you have been so diligently undertaking, if you are feeling the benefit. Here's what you should also be doing to *repopulate*.

Fermented foods

Eat foods that have been cultured to contain healthy bacteria. These include home-made live yogurt, coconut milk kefir, kimchi and sauerkraut. By making these yourself, using the recipes in Chapter 11, you can ensure they contain the helpful bacteria, whereas some commercial varieties are lacking.

Probiotics

Take a supplement containing friendly microbes. These supplements are known as probiotics. Look for those that contain *Lactobacillus acidophilus* or *casei* and *Bifidobacteria*, at combined levels of at least 10 billion live organisms. Probiotics help to wipe out dysbiosis, so it is hardly surprising that they have been so successful in certain types of diarrhoea and constipation, and in reducing IBS symptoms.[23]

Take three capsules a day of a yeast probiotic called *Sacchromyces boulardii*. This fights overgrowths of problematic yeasts, such as *Candida albicans*. It also increases levels of an important antibody in the gut called secretory IgA (sIgA). SIgA is a crucial component of the gut's immune system, preventing harmful molecules from getting past the mucous barrier and into the bloodstream. It is often depleted in situations of leaky gut.

REPAIR YOUR GUT LINING

Congratulations – you have reached stage four of your Happy Gut Programme! Here, we focus on *repairing* the delicate mucous membrane of the gut lining. This enables it to resume its important tasks of protecting the body from harmful toxins and orchestrating the immune system to help keep you free of unwanted inflammation and allergic-like reactions. And according to expert opinion, one of the most powerful ways to improve the course of inflammatory autoimmune diseases (rheumatoid arthritis, for instance) is to heal a leaky gut.[24] Once the gut's barrier function is restored, potential invaders cannot get from the gut into the underlying immune system and no inflammation will occur.

You can implement this 'repair' stage at the same time as the 'repopulate' stage if you want to, or you can leave it until you've been taking the probiotics for a couple of months, stopping the probiotics before you start this fourth stage. Whenever you choose to implement it, keep going with the 'repair' stage for at least three months to get the full benefit.

Meat stocks

The most magical repair food for the gut lining is fresh stock made from the bones of chicken, turkey or red meat. Fresh, organic stocks can now be found at many supermarkets and are excellent sources of collagen and glucosamine, which are restorative nutrients for the gut lining. Stocks make tasty bases for soups, casseroles, sauces and gravies. See our recipes for a basic stock and for *Asian Chicken Noodle Soup*.

L-glutamine

We also recommend taking a teaspoon of L-glutamine powder twice a day before meals, as this has been shown to help heal a leaky gut.[25] Don't take it in the evening, as some people find it keeps the brain alert.

Vitamins and minerals

Other important nutrients for the gut lining are vitamin D (from sunlight), vitamin A (from eggs and liver), vitamin C (fruits and vegetables) and zinc (as we've seen above). You can find all these nutrients in a good multivitamin and mineral supplement, but we also recommend asking your doctor for a vitamin D test, as deficiency is so common in the UK.[26] It's a mistake to think that you can get all your vitamin A from carrots and other orange and dark green fruits and vegetables. These foods contain beta-carotene, which many people can convert into vitamin A, but almost half of us may not be able to convert enough of it for good gut health.[27]

Omega 3 fats

Eat oily fish such as sardines, mackerel, trout, salmon and kippers at least three times a week. If you can't quite manage this, you should take a fish oil supplement, ideally containing a total of 1g of the combined omega 3 fatty acids EPA and DHA. These fatty acids help to reduce inflammation. Inflammation contributes to leaky gut.[28]

Soothing phytonutrients

If you have an irritated gut lining – for example, you may have heartburn or gastritis – drink a warm herbal tea (such as chamomile) and add to it a teaspoon of a soothing concoction containing slippery elm powder, gamma oryzanol, cabbage extract (vitamin 'U') and deglycerized licorice (DGL).

REBALANCE THE MIND AND BODY

You won't be surprised to learn that there is indeed a very strong link between high stress levels and poor gut health. Stress hormones such as cortisol are well-established causes of leaky gut. Stress also depletes beneficial bacteria in the gut and worsens reflux, constipation and diarrhoea. So, learn about the cause of your stress and take action to *rebalance*. See Chapter 6 for some advice on this.

Although the 'rebalance' stage is presented as the fifth 'R' in the programme, the best results are achieved from implementing it as early on as possible and keeping going with it for life. It's all about reducing the activity of stress hormones while you are eating and increasing the production of digestive hormones.

The most effective change you can make is one that is simple and free, even if it might seem a bit daunting at first: you need to chew each mouthful of food at least 40 times. (Yes, we did say 40.) You'll get used to it and after a while you will do it without even thinking about it. Some people also find that chewing fennel seeds after meals helps to dampen down excess gas production.[29]

Here are some other changes that will help a great deal:

▸ Do not eat at your computer, or while standing up, or if you are in a rush.

▸ Before you dive into your food, spend a few moments anticipating it, allowing the delicious fragrances of the meal to trigger the release of digestive hormones.

▸ Try not to drink more than a few sips of anything while eating, not even water. Many people with digestive problems inadvertently wash food down into the stomach before there has been time to chew it fully. (Remember, each mouthful needs to be chewed 40 times.)

▸ If you have reflux, don't eat within two hours of going to bed. If you still have problems, put a thick book underneath the feet of the bed at the headboard end, to elevate the oesophagus while sleeping.

- Consider whether you need to lose weight: there is a strong link between reflux problems and obesity because obesity increases abdominal pressure, inhibiting the passage of food through the digestive system.

- And, finally, did we say you need to chew each mouthful 40 times?

These are relatively small changes but you will be amazed at the difference they make to your digestion. And good gut health makes you feel years younger...

MEAL PLAN

Breakfast	*Cocoa Coconut Waffles* with berries and lactose-free yogurt (or *Soaked Chia Muesli* if you are in the 'remove' stage of the 5 R framework and eliminating dairy)
Lunch	*Carrot Ribbon Noodles with Almond Satay Sauce* (if you have dysbiosis, omit the garlic and use the green part of the spring onion/scallion only) with slices of roast chicken
Dinner	*Slow-Cooked Za'atar Lamb Shoulder* with steamed vegetables (courgette/zucchini, red pepper, peas and pak choi)
Snack	Milk *Kefir* (made with lactose-free milk)/*Water Kefir* *Tropical Protein Smoothie*

If you do nothing else, do this...

- Discuss with your doctor the need for each of the drugs you are taking, with a view to cutting down or avoiding those that that are not absolutely necessary.

- Avoid trans-fats, found in processed foods, and reduce saturated fats, found in butter, lard, fatty meat and dairy products.

- Reduce or avoid the specific starches and sugars that tend to ferment bacteria and yeasts in the gut, causing wind and bloating.

- Reduce or avoid foods that can cause a leaky gut, especially gluten grains and soy foods.

- Take two tablets of concentrated oregano oil immediately after each meal.

- If you have heartburn, ask your doctor for an *H. pylori* test.

- Check out any suspected food allergies or intolerances.

- Eat soluble fibre and drink at least 1.5 litres (approximately 3 pints) of non-caffeinated fluid a day.

- Experiment with a digestive enzyme supplement or a betaine hydrochloride supplement with meals and see if they help your symptoms.

- Make your proteins more easily digestible by cooking them in lemon juice, vinegar or wine, or by using a slow cooker.

- Stimulate your digestive juices with bitter green leaves or with a supplement of herbal bitters.

- Eat foods that have been cultured to contain healthy bacteria and/ or take a probiotic supplement containing *Lactobacillus acidophilus* or *casei*, *Bifidobacteria* and *Sacchromyces boulardii*.

- Eat fresh stock made from the bones of chicken, turkey or red meat.

- Take a teaspoon of L-glutamine powder twice a day before meals.

- Take a good vitamin and mineral supplement containing vitamins A and C and the mineral zinc. (You can test your zinc levels with the taste challenge.)

- Get tested for your vitamin D levels and take a supplement if necessary.

- Eat oily fish three times a week and/or take a fish oil supplement.

- Review your stress levels and take action to manage them.

- Chew each mouthful of food at least 40 times.

- Eat in a relaxed state, take time to anticipate your food and don't drink while eating.

CHAPTER 4

BECOMING LEAN AND PREVENTING DIABETES

We're forever being told that obesity is a major health epidemic. Hardly a day goes by without the publication of a new shock statistic. Yet still we are getting fatter. Worldwide, the prevalence of obesity almost doubled between the years 1980 and 2008.[1] And, according to NHS figures released in 2013, only a third of men and 39 per cent of women in the UK are now considered to be a healthy weight.[2]

Up until a few decades ago, however, unwanted weight gain was not the seemingly inevitable part of ageing that it is today. For most people, life involved some sort of physical activity, whether it was pulling wet washing through a mangle, relying less on the car and more on cycling and walking, or playing ball with the children (who were not diverted by TV and computer games). There's no doubt that if you want to look after your body shape as you age, you need to engage in regular exercise. We look at this issue in Chapter 10 and give you some tips for exercising in the most beneficial ways.

Another weight-promoting factor to arise in recent decades is the ubiquitous temptation of white starch (see Box 4.3). Nowadays, if you want to stay lean into your middle and later years, you need to make a conscious effort to eat in a way that rejects many of the staple foods on offer in supermarkets, cafés and other outlets. Instead, you need to eat foods that have become less popular in recent times, as we have become less inclined to cook or prepare food ourselves. This can take courage, not least because it involves 'going against the norm' – eating in a way that may seem different to the standard Western diet and therefore different to how many of your friends and family are eating.

And as if the regular exercise and dietary changes weren't enough to be getting on with, you may also find that you are one of the many millions of people who have developed certain metabolic dysfunctions, such as insulin resistance or thyroid or sex hormone problems, which hamper even the best efforts to lose weight. Box 4.2 gives an overview of these types of underlying issues and what you can do about them.

By the time you've finished reading this chapter, you'll have gathered the most useful information about weight gain and its associated problems, about the most effective ways of eating to lose weight, and about specific supplements you may want to try, given their role in sugar metabolism, cravings and weight control.

ARE YOU CARRYING EXCESS WEIGHT?

How do you gauge whether or not you are overweight? The measurement considered most accurate involves calculating the ratio of your waist circumference to that of your hips. A healthy reading is 0.8 or less for women, and 1 or less for men. If your result is higher than this, it indicates that the amount of fat around your middle may be affecting the health of your vital organs.

This calculation is known as the waist-to-hip ratio and it is simple to work out yourself at home:

▸ Take a tape measure and put it around your waist, at the narrowest part of your torso just under the ribcage. Write down this measurement – for example, 27 inches.

▸ Then move the tape measure to your hips. Wrap it around the widest part of the hip area, also taking in your bottom. Write down this measurement – for example, 37 inches.

▸ Now divide your waist measurement by your hip measurement – 27 divided by 37 = 0.73 (a healthy ratio).

Another measurement you may have heard of is the body mass index (BMI). This is not considered as accurate a measure as the waist-to-hip ratio, as sometimes people can find they have an 'overweight' reading when really they are just very muscular or big-boned. Even so, it's worth knowing about it because some health providers still use it – see Box 4.1.

BOX 4.1 THE BODY MASS INDEX (BMI)

The BMI is your body mass divided by the square of your height. To calculate your own BMI, use this equation:

Weight (kg) $\div$ Height (m)^2

Then check your result against the following list of readings:

Underweight: less than 18.5

Healthy weight: 18.5–25

Overweight: 25–30

Moderately obese: 30–35

Severely obese: 35–40

Very severely obese: over 40

Some people can tell that they are overweight simply by looking in the mirror or by the tightness of their clothes. For them, there is little value in calculating their waist-to-hip ratio. But you may be one of the many people who do not necessarily look particularly overweight. This is where the waist-to-hip ratio becomes particularly useful because it can alert you to the fact that, although you may not be carrying as much extra fat as some, it is enough to be affecting your health. This is because it's not just about how overweight you are but *where* you are carrying the extra pounds. Excess fat around the tummy area is considered far more dangerous than excess fat around the hips and bottom. This is because your heart, kidneys, liver and other vital organs are situated in the middle of your torso, making them vulnerable to the damaging effects of fat deposited in this area. We'll find out about these damaging effects in the next section.

WHAT'S WRONG WITH BEING OVERWEIGHT?

Obesity shortens life span by between three and ten years, depending on its severity,[3] and it causes many debilitating health problems along the way. Figures indicate that the number of UK hospital admissions caused by weight-related issues tripled within the five years to 2012.[4]

INSULIN RESISTANCE AND DIABETES: ARE YOU HEADING IN THIS DIRECTION?

One of the main problems with being overweight is that it massively increases your risk of developing insulin resistance (sometimes referred to as 'pre-diabetes') and diabetes. Both of these conditions cause premature ageing and shorten lifespan. It has been suggested that insulin resistance may be the single most important dysfunction underlying the development of chronic disease.[5]

These life-threatening conditions are preceded by years, sometimes decades, of a gradual decline in your ability to control the level of sugar (glucose) in your bloodstream. You can take the following short questionnaire to gauge how well you are currently controlling your blood sugar levels.

How often do you experience the following? Tick the box for each statement that applies to you.

☐ Awaken a few hours after falling asleep, finding it hard to get back to sleep

☐ Crave sweets, starches or stimulants

☐ Eat desserts or sugary snacks daily or almost daily

☐ Bingeing or uncontrolled eating

☐ Excessive appetite

☐ Sleepy in afternoon

☐ Regular headaches

☐ Fatigue that is relieved by eating

☐ Headache, irritability, loss of concentration or shakiness if meals are skipped or delayed

- [ ] Premenstrual syndrome

- [ ] Waist-to-hip ratio (see above) greater than 0.8 if female and 1 if male

- [ ] Blood results that show elevated levels of fasting triglycerides (see page 73)

- [ ] Blood results that show elevated LDL-cholesterol and/or low levels of HDL-cholesterol (see page 73)

- [ ] Blood results that show elevated haemoglobin A1c (Hb A1c) (see page 72)

- [ ] Family members with diabetes (tick once for each family member affected)

- [ ] Frequent thirst

- [ ] Frequent urination

- [ ] Unintended weight loss or weight gain

This set of questions is designed to give you an initial indication of how well your body is able to process dietary carbohydrates and sugar, by using the hormones insulin and glucagon.

Low blood sugar levels: hypoglycaemia

If you scored between 8 and 20, you may have what is known as 'dysglycaemia'. Typically, the first you're likely know of this is when you start suffering from episodes of plummeting blood sugar levels (known as 'hypoglycaemia'), giving you the sorts of symptoms mentioned above.

What causes hypoglycaemia? A common sequence of events goes like this. You eat something that has a high glycaemic load (GL) – see Chapter 2 for an explanation of high- and low-GL foods – typically a sugary or starchy food, such as white bread, a muffin, croissant or biscuit. This floods the blood with the sugar glucose. Such a lot of glucose in the bloodstream triggers a massive release of insulin from the pancreas – so much insulin, in fact, that it rushes glucose into the cells at turbo-charged speed. This leaves the blood with an inadequate back-up supply of glucose to allow you to function properly.

High blood sugar levels: hyperglycaemia

If this blood sugar 'rollercoaster' situation continues for years, your cells gradually become less able to accept the insulin being pushed at them. The insulin receptors become tired and weak, and they fail to open and allow insulin and sugar into the cells. This situation is called insulin resistance. There is nowhere for the sugar to go and so it stays in the blood, where it starts to cause damage to body tissues, leading to premature ageing. You may be heading for this if you scored 12 or more in the questionnaire above.

Sugar's devastating damage

This type of damage occurs when glucose in the blood attaches itself to proteins – for example, to collagen. This process is called glycation and it damages the proteins, making them dysfunctional. Glycated collagen in the skin causes wrinkles. In the walls of the arteries, collagen glycation leads to the build-up of plaque and the subsequent narrowing of the arteries, increasing your risk of heart attack and stroke.

People with excess sugar in the blood (hyperglycaemia), due to insulin resistance, are particularly vulnerable to glycation and thus to premature ageing. You can find out whether glycation is damaging your tissues by asking your doctor for a haemoglobin A1c (Hb A1c) blood test. This measures the extent to which the haemoglobin protein within your red blood cells has been glycated (damaged) by elevated blood sugar levels.

The process of glycation produces molecules called advanced glycation end products (AGE products). AGE products are also caused by smoking cigarettes and are found in some foods, including browned foods: caramelized toppings, roasted coffee, toasted bread and especially grilled or fried high-fat meat and fish.[6]

If we accumulate AGE products, either because of hyperglycaemia or by eating AGEs in foods, we become more prone to premature ageing. Refer to Chapter 5 for more on AGE products and how they cause tissue degeneration.

Other blood test results that can indicate problems with blood sugar control are:

▶ Elevated low density lipoprotein-cholesterol (LDL-c): This is often referred to as the 'bad' type of cholesterol. In fact, it isn't bad at all – it is vital for health – but it can be unhealthy to have too much of it, so ideally you want it to be less than 3mmol/L.

▶ Low levels of high density lipoprotein-cholesterol (HDL-c): This is a marker of how well the body is transporting excess cholesterol from the arteries to the liver, where it can be detoxified and excreted. You want to have good levels of this – 1.2mmol/L or above.

▶ A total cholesterol-to-HDL-c ratio of 4.5 or above: This is a more useful indicator of health than simply looking at total cholesterol, HDL-c or LDL-c in isolation.

▶ Elevated triglycerides: This is a measure of the amount of fat in the bloodstream and is a good indicator of excess sugar and white starch intake because these foods are converted to saturated fat in the body (see Box 4.3). You want your reading to be less than 1.7mmol/L.

It is also worth being aware that uncontrolled diabetes is a gateway into a whole raft of severe health issues, such as failing sight and even blindness (retinopathy), nerve problems that can include severe unremitting pain (neuropathy) and failing kidneys (renal disease).

INSULIN RESISTANCE LEADS *NOT ONLY* TO DIABETES

As we've seen, your sugar-control system is more likely to fail and cause insulin resistance if you are overweight. Insulin resistance makes you more vulnerable not only to diabetes but also to other age-related diseases, such as:

▶ Non-alcoholic fatty liver disease.[7]

▶ Cardiovascular disease: The term 'metabolic syndrome' (MetS) refers to a cluster of symptoms that increase your risk of a heart attack or a stroke, and which are caused by insulin resistance. The diagnostic criteria for MetS vary slightly between health organizations but they tend to include some or all of the following signs: central obesity, high blood pressure, raised triglycerides, low HDL-cholesterol and elevated fasting glucose levels. MetS is estimated to affect 25 per cent of all adults in Europe, while in the US as many as 40 per cent of the adult population are thought to be affected by the age of 60.[8]

▶ Increased cancer risk.[9]

▶ Loss of memory and cognition, including dementia[10] and possibly depression.[11] (See Chapter 7 for more about improving your memory, mind and mood.)

OTHER SIGNS OF PREMATURE AGEING CAUSED BY EXCESS WEIGHT

▶ Inflammation: Far from being simply a passive source of stored energy, excess fat around the middle is now known to cause chronic, low-level inflammation, the type of inflammation that drives the progression of so many age-related, degenerative diseases. The most dangerous type of fat is that known as 'visceral adipose tissue' (VAT), especially that around the tummy area. This is because VAT surrounds our vital organs, whereas subcutaneous fat is confined to the area just underneath the skin.

How can something as seemingly benign as fat have such a devastating effect on health? It all comes down to the fact that excessive fatty tissue produces and releases high levels of inflammatory molecules[12] such as tumour necrosis factor alpha (TNF-a) and interleukin-6 (IL-6). In scientific papers these are sometimes referred to as adipokines. Not only do they cause inflammation, but they also stop insulin working properly, contributing to insulin resistance,[13] and they get the liver to release chemicals (such as C-reactive protein, or CRP, and fibrinogen) that promote cardiovascular disease.

In 2010 Diabetes UK released figures claiming that 97 per cent of Britons are unaware that their 'beer bellies' and 'muffin tops' are promoting their risk of age-related diseases such as cancer, diabetes and cardiovascular disease.[14]

▸ Arthritis: Excess weight puts additional stress on joints. Being overweight or obese has been associated with osteoarthritis risk.[15]

▸ Gastro-oesophageal reflux disease (GORD; see Chapter 3 for more on this).[16]

▸ Sleep disorders: Obesity is commonly connected with sleep apnoea, a breathing disorder that causes restless, interrupted sleep, partly due to low oxygen levels in the blood. Obesity-associated GORD can also disrupt sleep. And while obesity can lead to sleep deprivation, this can then increase your appetite the following day,[17] making it difficult to control your calorie intake. Thus poor sleep and obesity can become a vicious cycle. Improving sleep can often help in weight-loss programmes. Chapter 10 suggests some ideas for you to try.

▸ Out-of-control appetite: Even if you are sleeping well, excess fatty tissue adversely affects the metabolism of a very useful hormone called leptin.[18] Leptin's role is to signal the brain to reduce your appetite. Leptin is produced by fat cells, so the more fat you are carrying, the more leptin you will produce. On the face of it, you would think this sounds like a good thing. And in the days of old, before constant food abundance, this system worked well. If you were fat enough to be healthy, leptin would signal the brain to reduce your appetite. Then, once you had been eating less for a while, your fat cells would diminish and leptin's curb on appetite would be lifted, making you want to fatten up again.

But the problem is that if you keep continuously overproducing leptin (because you are overweight and possibly addicted to fattening foods such as sugar, white starch and alcohol), the brain cells become resistant to this important hormone. This renders the brain unable to hear the signal to reduce appetite.[19] Leptin resistance may be one of the reasons that it is so much harder for obese people to stick to weight-loss diets than it is for people who are carrying less fat.

- Oestrogen-related problems: If you are overweight, you have more of a tendency to produce too much of the female hormone oestrogen. This situation has been termed 'oestrogen dominance' and it can lead to many health problems in women, such as endometriosis and fibroids. One of the typical signs of this occurring in men is the appearance of 'man boobs'.

  Fatty tissue produces a potent enzyme called aromatase. In both men and women, aromatase targets male sex hormones (androgens), produced by the adrenal glands, and converts them into oestrogen.[20] This fat-derived oestrogen production tends to increase both with weight gain and also with age.[21] This is one of the reasons obesity is considered a risk factor for some hormonally driven types of cancer, such as cancer of the breast, bowel and ovaries.

- Increased heart attack and stroke risk: We saw on page 73 how insulin resistance leads to cardiovascular disease because of MetS. But even if you're not yet insulin resistant, the increased inflammation that arises from being overweight is a key driver of hardening and narrowing of the arteries. What's more, increased fatty tissue also causes the hormone adiponectin to plummet.

  If you don't have enough adiponectin, you tend to more easily develop insulin resistance and also the build-up of dangerous arterial plaque.[22] Plaque build-up, otherwise known as atherosclerosis, causes the arteries to narrow, restricting blood flow to the heart and brain. If some of the plaque becomes dislodged, this can cause a blockage within the artery, leading to a heart attack or a stroke, depending on the site of the blockage.

- Hypertension: Fat-derived hormones are also implicated in the epidemic of high blood pressure (known as hypertension). Hypertension has been described as the most common obesity-related health problem.[23]

BOX 4.2 WHY CAN'T I LOSE WEIGHT?

One way to lose weight is to eat fewer energy units (calories) than you are burning. The rate at which you burn calories depends on the speed of your metabolism. People who do regular physical exercise have faster metabolisms. So, if you are looking to lose weight, you need to work on both sides of the equation – eat less food (fewer calories in) and take more exercise (more calories burned).

But that's only part of the story. If it really was that simple, we'd all be satisfyingly svelte. In reality, there are a great many underlying biological factors that can hamper your best efforts to shift the pounds. Here are some of the most common issues that we come across in our clinics – consider whether any of them might be affecting you:

▶ Eating too much starch and sugar is a sure-fire way to pile on the pounds. Did you know, for example, that you manufacture as much as 15–20g of fat every day, simply by eating more carbohydrates than you need?[24]

▶ Too high an intake of sugars and starches also causes sharp peaks and troughs in blood sugar levels, eventually leading to insulin resistance (see page 72 for more on this condition). Insulin resistance intensifies the swings in blood sugar levels, leaving you plagued with cravings for more starchy and sugary foods. It's almost impossible to control your calorie intake under these circumstances. The best solution is to adopt the low-GL diet described in Chapter 2. Also see Boxes 4.3 and 4.4 in this chapter for more information on the most problematic foods and how to switch to healthier alternatives.

▶ Could your weight gain be stress-related? Stress causes your levels of cortisol and other stress hormones to surge, and this leads to blood sugar disruption and the associated cravings. Cortisol surges also alter brain chemistry so that fatty and sugary foods seem more rewarding – meaning that, for many people, reaching for the biscuit barrel is a natural reaction to feeling stressed. What's more, cortisol acts as a trigger for fat cells to grow and for more dietary fat to be stored. See Chapter 6 for an action plan to improve your stress levels.

- A significant cause of stress is lack of sleep. Poor sleep also disrupts leptin and other hormones that help us to control appetite (see page 75).[25] Chapter 10 has more information on sleep and how to improve it.

- Stress can also make you more likely to become addicted to foods that raise your levels of endorphins, the body's natural pleasure providers. Again, these foods are usually sugary, starchy foods,[26] and once you're addicted, it becomes far harder to shift unwanted weight gain. The low-GL diet (see Chapter 2) is a powerful tool for regaining control over your eating habits. Chapter 10 has further information on how to beat addictions.

- If you have been trying unsuccessfully to lose weight, it may be that your levels of the 'happy' brain chemical serotonin are on the low side. This is often the case in people with a history of attempted weight loss because the raw material needed to make serotonin (called tryptophan) is one of the first nutrients to be depleted by dieting.[27] Just like blood sugar problems, addictions, poor sleep and stress, low serotonin can lead to cravings for starchy and sugary foods.[28] If this is the case with you, one option may be to supplement serotonin's precursor 5-hydroxytryptophan (5-HTP), as this can help to curb appetite, naturally reducing the amount you are eating.[29]

- The thyroid regulates calorie burning, and a well-established effect of an under-functioning thyroid is unwanted weight gain. A blood test can establish your levels of thyroid hormones. Nutrition and lifestyle can do a lot to support thyroid function – see Chapter 6 for guidelines.

- As we age, our levels of growth-promoting (anabolic) hormones begin to fall. Low levels of DHEA (dehydroepiandrosterone) and testosterone can lead to increases in fat mass, at the expense of muscle tissue, in both men and women. Other imbalances in the sex hormones can also make it difficult to lose weight. Too much oestrogen, for example, encourages fat storage, and, in excess, can antagonize thyroid hormone.[30] To optimize the balance of your sex hormones, see Chapter 9.

▶ Amazing as it may sound, an imbalance the gut's microflora can prevent you from losing weight. Animal studies have found that certain types of gut bacteria (those called *Firmicutes*) can cause more calories to be extracted from your diet than if the gut were better populated with another type of bacteria (called *Bacteroidetes*).[31] See the symptoms on page 43 to find out if you might have an imbalance of gut bacteria. This very common condition is called dysbiosis and there is a step-by-step programme in Chapter 3 to help get your digestion back to optimum health.

▶ Some experts believe that our weight-control systems can be disrupted by excessive exposure to toxins[32] and that this may explain why some people find it hard to lose weight even when they are eating a better diet and taking more exercise.[33] We all gradually accumulate hundreds of chemicals as we go through life, from sources such as traffic pollution, bacteria, alcohol, cleaning solutions and cigarette smoke, to name but a few. Toxins are generally stored in fat cells. On a weight-loss programme, these fat cells start to break down. As they do so, they release their stored toxins into the bloodstream, where they can affect cells and make us feel tired, irritable, headachy, nauseous – in a word, hungover. If you think you may be carrying a high toxic load, our advice is to support your detoxification systems before you start embarking on a weight-loss programme. Chapter 6 gives you some tips for doing this.

BOX 4.3 WHITE STARCH: THE ENEMY OF STAYING SLIM
WHITE STARCH: WHAT IS IT?

Basically, it's sugar – simple strings of glucose molecules. These strings split apart in the gut, allowing the glucose to speedily absorb into the bloodstream, causing surges in blood sugar levels.

White starch is everywhere – in every café, deli, supermarket, corner shop, bar and coffee house. To steer clear of it, you need to make a conscious decision to identify it and reject it – because it has become such a ubiquitous staple. Common examples are:

- White bread, including more rustic-looking loaves such as baguettes, focaccia and ciabatta
- Cornflakes, puffed rice and other processed breakfast cereals
- Bagels
- Pastry
- Brioche
- Rice
- Couscous
- Pasta
- Muffins
- Polenta
- Pizza bases
- Danish pastries
- Noodles
- Gnocchi
- Pancakes and blinis
- Crisps and crisp-like snacks
- Rice cakes
- Crackers and water biscuits
- Waffles
- Cakes
- Scones
- Biscuits

As far as your body is concerned, there is really no difference between eating any of these products and guzzling a bag of white sugar. And it's worth knowing that gluten-free versions of these starchy goods can be just as highly processed and therefore equally as fattening – it's just that you don't get the problems associated with the gluten.

WHAT'S THE PROBLEM WITH IT?

There are four key problems with treating white starch as a staple food:

- No nutrients: First, apart from the glucose, most white starch is devoid of essential nutrients. This is because, in order to make it, carbohydrate whole foods (such as wheat, rice and other whole grains) are stripped of their fibre, phytochemicals, vitamins and minerals. So, the more of your diet that is made up of white starch, the less opportunity you have to get those vitality-giving micronutrients from your food intake alone.

But, given that nowadays it is possible to supplement the micronutrients you're not getting from food, perhaps a more pressing problem with white starch is its catastrophic effect on your blood sugar levels and your weight.

▶ Weight gain: Excess sugar in the diet, including white starch (which quickly turns into sugar in the gut), is the number one dietary cause of weight gain. Every time you eat more starch or sugar than you can burn off, a limited amount is stored in the liver (as glycogen) and the rest is pushed inside fat cells, where it is converted into, and stored as, saturated fat.[34]

▶ Blood sugar rollercoaster: Every time you eat white starch, your blood is flooded with glucose. This gives you a short-term energy boost but within an hour or two your blood sugar levels will come crashing down and you'll be left in a state of 'hypoglycaemia' (see page 71). This is where the level of sugar in the blood is so low that you can't function properly. You feel irritable, moody, tired, perhaps even a bit shaky. And you get cravings for pick-me-ups such as tea, coffee and, of course, sugary and starchy foods.

▶ Addiction: Finally, we need to mention the highly addictive nature of these white starchy foods. You'll see in Chapter 10 that sugar is so overwhelmingly addictive that in animal research it has been found to surpass cocaine reward. White starch is sugar and is therefore difficult to moderate, once you are hooked. The more you eat, the more you end up craving it. And the blood sugar crashes it causes simply exacerbate these cravings, making it even harder to control the amount you are eating.

WHAT TO DO?

You need to kick the habit. Everything that is currently white in your diet needs to be swapped to a wholegrain version. And unless you are very physically active, you probably need to reduce your overall intake of grains by about 50 per cent.

To help combat the cravings while you are making these changes, follow these tips:

▸ Eat a low-GL diet – see Chapter 2 for more on this. In particular, increase the amount of animal protein you are eating. Eat fish, eggs, lean meat or dairy products at every meal. Don't make the mistake of thinking a protein powder will have the same effect. Whey, hemp, rice and pea protein powders are great for topping up on amino acids but they won't help you to manage cravings that are related to blood sugar problems. That's because they don't require the lengthy digestion that protein foods do, so they don't have the same beneficial effect of slowing down the rate at which glucose is released into the bloodstream.

▸ Eat no less than three meals a day, each containing protein, fat and a low-GL starch, preferably beans, pulses or non-potato root vegetables (see Chapter 2).

▸ Get eight hours of good-quality sleep a night.

▸ Keep busy and active, in order to keep your mind and body occupied.

▸ Take one of the following supplements about 30 minutes before breakfast, lunch and dinner: chromium, green coffee extract, L-glutamine or 5-HTP. See pages 63 and 90 for more information and dosages.

▸ Reduce the amount of stress in your life by following the recommendations in Chapter 6.

▸ Never go hungry, as this leads to overeating. Stock up on snacks that are healthy alternatives to white starch. Try any of the recipes for snacks in the recipe section later in the book – many can be batch-frozen. Other ideas are: oat cakes with hazelnut or almond butter; fresh or frozen berries with plain, live yogurt; yogurt made from coconut milk; a small handful of nuts and seeds; pumpernickel-like toast with hummus or a boiled egg.

▸ Once you are out the other side, you'll feel amazing. And you'll never look back.

HOW TO LOSE WEIGHT THE HEALTHY WAY
CONTROL YOUR CARBS

Booksellers and websites are flooded with weight-loss diets – Atkins, South Beach, Zone, Dukan, to name but a few. Do they work? We wouldn't advocate any of these diets as a long-term solution to weight control because they are so restrictive. This means that they are hard to stick to and also that you may end up getting too much or too little of certain nutrients. However, they do seem to enable people to shed the pounds in the short term, and the reason for this is that they control the type and the amount of carbohydrates eaten.

We looked at carbohydrate-controlled diets in Chapter 3, where we saw that restricting specific types of sugars and starches can help to improve gastrointestinal health. These gut health diets can also help to shed the pounds and control blood sugar levels, but if your gut health is already good, it's better to follow the carbohydrate advice in the current chapter and Chapter 2.

This advice centres on choosing meals that have a low glycaemic load. We explain all about low GL in Chapter 2. Essentially, it focuses on:

▶ whole foods high in protein such as lean meat, poultry, fish, eggs, beans, pulses, nuts, seeds and dairy products

▶ healthy fats and oils such as those found in avocados, olives, coconuts, nuts and seeds

▶ plenty of vegetables and some lower-sugar fruits such as berries.

The diet is very low in starchy and sugary foods (see Box 4.4 for how to recognise sugar on food labels). Whole grains and potatoes can be included in small amounts but aren't recommended if you have a lot of weight to lose. Instead, you should get your carbs from beans, pulses, root and other vegetables and a little fruit. Chapter 2 has more specific examples of how to swap high-GL starches to lower-GL versions.

This way of eating is helpful for general good health at any age, as well as for better control of blood sugar and insulin levels, and also for weight loss. It is a particularly effective way of helping to control those diet-busting cravings for sugary and starchy foods. A low-GL diet is not extreme in any way – you can eat as much as you want. It's about the quality of your food, rather than the quantity. You can adopt this way of eating for life, and it will help to keep you healthy, happy and energized.

Replacing some of the grains with deeply or brightly coloured vegetables also has another advantage: it increases your intake of antioxidants. If you have diabetes or have been told you are 'pre-diabetic', you are likely to be suffering from internal inflammation (see Chapter 8) and oxidative stress (see Chapter 5), making it important that you get antioxidants in your diet every day. Chapter 5 takes you through the different types of antioxidants and their benefits in ageing.

If you haven't already read Chapter 2, turn to it now to learn more about the low-GL diet and for some examples of low- and high-GL foods. Also see the low-GL meal plans and recipes in this chapter and Chapter 2.

KICK-START YOUR PROGRAMME WITH FASTING

If you want to go one step further, you may be interested in the emerging evidence for the dramatic results that can be gained from fasting, either on a daily basis or intermittently. (If you have blood sugar problems like those discussed above, it's best not to attempt fasting until you have these under control.)

Done properly, fasting is not only extremely effective in shifting those extra pounds but also has some promising evidence for improving longevity, as we saw in Chapter 2. If you are interested in this way of eating, read through the information in Chapter 2 to see whether it would be feasible for you to complement your low-GL diet with regular, short periods of fasting. That chapter includes information and meal plans on two different fasting schedules: the first is a short daily fast and the second involves choosing two days a week on which you stick to a very low calorie intake. Ideally, as this way of eating can become quite restrictive, you should enlist the help of a nutrition practitioner or other healthcare provider to ensure that you don't miss out on any vital nutrients in the long term.

Fasting is not for everyone, especially if you are on certain medications – see the contraindications listed in Chapter 2. If you fall into one of these categories, or if you suffer from regular low mood, intense cravings or binge-eating episodes, you'll probably do better on the low-GL diet without trying to incorporate fasting.

EAT FAT, BUT THE RIGHT FAT

It used to be thought that the way to lose weight and keep your heart and arteries healthy was to eat as little fat as possible. But, as you'll have seen in Chapter 2, we now know this way of eating can have a catastrophic effect on health, *promoting* degenerative conditions, rather than improving them, and causing hunger pangs that lead to weight gain. And indeed the most up-to-date evidence suggests that the risk of cardiovascular disease can be reduced by *changing* the type of fats that are eaten, rather than by *reducing* the overall level of fat in the diet.[35]

So-called 'healthy' low-fat products tend to have a far higher sugar content, in order to make them palatable. But the main problem with low-fat diets is that they lack the special types of fat that are crucial for good health and have to be eaten daily in order to increase your chances of ageing well. These are the omega 3 and omega 6 polyunsaturated fats (PUFAs), and also the omega 9 monounsaturated fats (MUFAs). The best food sources of PUFAs are oily fish, nuts and seeds (and their cold-pressed oils), and the best sources of MUFAs are avocados, nuts and olive oil.

Omega 3 PUFAs from herring, mackerel, salmon, trout, sardines and other oily fish help to reduce the elevated levels of blood fats and inflammation found in MetS.[36] They also increase levels of the hormone adiponectin that helps to prevent insulin resistance.[37] This is useful to know if you are overweight because those extra pounds hamper the secretion of this healthy ageing hormone.

All fats contain the same amount of calories (9 calories per gram, to be precise) but the fats to cut down on are saturated fats, found in lard, fatty cuts of meat, farmed fatty fish, intensively farmed eggs and full-fat dairy products. However, saturated fats are the safest for cooking with, so there is no need to avoid them altogether. We recommend coconut oil, a vegetarian and possibly healthier source of saturated fat.

Coconut contains a type of fat called medium-chain triglycerides (MCTs). MCTs are less likely than animal fats to be stored in your fat cells and are more likely to be burned for energy. Moreover, using MCTs as the main type of saturated fat in your diet may reduce your overall food intake and promote weight loss.[38] And while saturated fats are known for raising cholesterol levels, coconut fat appears to also increase the protective type of cholesterol, HDL-c.[39]

Do your best to avoid the toxic, man-made fats called trans- or partially hydrogenated fats. These promote insulin resistance and increase your risk of diabetes and cardiovascular disease (as well as inflammation and cancer).[40] You can do this by eschewing all processed foods.

Even if you are concerned about your weight or your blood sugar control, you should be consuming about a third of your calories every day as fat, as long as most of it comes from olives and olive oil, nuts, seeds and their cold-pressed oils, oily fish (especially wild-caught), avocados, coconut milk and oil, and organic eggs. Eat three 100g (4oz) servings of oily fish a week. Vegetable, seed and nut oils (apart from coconut) are delicate – to avoid damaging them, they should never be heated.

You can learn more about the different types of fats, healthy and unhealthy, and their food sources, in Chapter 8.

INCORPORATE SPECIAL FOODS AND SUPPLEMENTS

There is some evidence that certain foods and dietary supplements may help to improve both blood sugar control and weight loss.

Chromium

Chromium is an essential mineral that helps the body to use insulin, yet it is depleted from food during processing and refining. Supplementing chromium at 200–1000mcg a day may help to normalize blood sugar levels and improve insulin resistance,[41] including when used as an adjunct to medical therapies in diabetes.

It's worth knowing, however, that not all the human trials have reported benefits. It's not known exactly why, but it could be due to genetic differences. It may also be that people who already have insulin resistance with elevated levels of blood glucose and haemoglobin A1c get more improvements from chromium.[42] Although it's not possible to predict the extent to which you, as an individual, will benefit from taking chromium, if you want to give it a try, start with 200mcg per day and work with a nutrition practitioner or a doctor to increase the dose as necessary.

Food sources include romaine lettuce, raw onions, ripe tomatoes, brewer's yeast, liver, oysters and whole grains, especially barley. A good multivitamin and mineral supplement should include reasonable levels.

Magnesium

Magnesium is crucial for insulin to work properly to get glucose into cells. It's not surprising, then, that people who get more magnesium tend to have lower insulin levels in the blood[43] and a lower risk of developing insulin resistance and type 2 diabetes.[44] The risk was shown to be reduced by as much as 31 per cent in one 15-year study[45] and by up to 34 per cent in another large prospective piece of research.[46] What's more, if you already have diabetes, your risk of developing complications increases, the lower your magnesium status.[47]

The good news is that taking magnesium supplements may reduce insulin resistance[48] and may also improve the control of blood fats, blood sugar and blood pressure in people with diabetes.[49]

Food sources are Swiss chard, kelp, squash, pumpkin seeds, steamed broccoli, halibut and, to a lesser extent, other green vegetables, whole grains, nuts and seeds. A great many people in the UK are magnesium-deficient, for all the reasons explained in Chapter 6, so it is wise to supplement this mineral if you have blood sugar issues. We recommend 300–450mg a day, in a form called magnesium citrate, as this is one of the most readily absorbed. Other good forms of magnesium supplements are listed in Chapter 6.

Green tea

The health-promoting ingredient in green tea is a flavonoid (a type of plant chemical) called epigallocatechin gallate (EGCG). EGCG has powerful effects on human health, mainly because of its ability to switch genes on and off (it's what is known as an 'epigenetic' nutrient, as we saw in Chapter 1). We each carry around 24,000 genes but only about 3 per cent of them are ever switched on and working ('expressed') at any one time.

EGCG is a consideration for any weight-loss programme because it has been found to speed up fat metabolism.[50] A number of human trials have also found it to lower total cholesterol and LDL-c.[51]

One of the problems associated with diabetes is that the liver starts to release too much glucose. This is then dumped into the bloodstream, further disrupting your sugar levels. In healthy people, insulin stops the liver from going into this sugar production overdrive. In diabetes, however, the pancreas can't produce enough insulin to have this inhibitory effect.

Amazingly, EGCG from green tea may be able to mimic insulin's effects in slowing the release of newly made glucose into the bloodstream.[52] It does this by stopping a particular gene from activating an enzyme called glucose-6-phosphatase (G-6-P). (G-6-P is a powerful glucose-producing enzyme in the liver.)

People who drink 5–6 cups of green tea or more a day tend to be at a lower risk of developing diabetes.[53] If you are caffeine-sensitive, you should drink decaff or look to supplementation: 200–300mg EGCG per day in supplement form has been found to improve insulin sensitivity.[54]

Cinnamon

It was ten years ago that cinnamon (1–6g powder per day for six weeks) was first found to help normalize blood levels of glucose, fats and cholesterol in humans.[55] Since then, a good number of trials have found diabetes patients to benefit from reduced hyperglycaemia and blood pressure when supplementing their diet with this tasty spice.[56] It also helps people with pre-diabetes to control their blood sugar levels.[57]

Dosages of between 1g and 6g have been used in studies. Considering that 6g is little more than a heaped teaspoonful, it is relatively easy to get a therapeutic dose of cinnamon daily by using it in smoothies and sprinkling it onto stewed fruit and porridge.

Cinnamon switches on genes that make the insulin receptors and the glucose transporters work better,[58] and, like EGCG above, it stops the liver from overproducing glucose and dumping it into the bloodstream.[59]

Green (unroasted) coffee

Although we are used to thinking of coffee drinking as detrimental to health because of the unpleasant side-effects of excessive caffeine, the plant chemicals in coffee (including chlorogenic and caffeic acids) may be useful if you are overweight because they appear to curb overeating and reduce body fat.[60] It has also been found that people who drink more coffee may have a lower risk of type 2 diabetes.[61] In a recent trial of healthy people, those who took a supplement of green coffee extract were better able to keep blood sugar levels stable when challenged with glucose drinks than were the participants who did not take the supplement.[62]

Laboratory experiments indicate that coffee works on human cells in a number of different ways. For example, it reduces the absorption of glucose into the bloodstream, it increases the helpful hormone adiponectin (see above)[63] and, like green tea and cinnamon, it prevents the liver enzyme G-6-P from dumping newly made glucose into the bloodstream.[64] And the benefits may also extend to black (roasted) coffee, especially if it has been enriched with the flavonoid chlorogenic acid.[65]

If you are sensitive to caffeine, decaffeinated (organic) varieties and/or supplements of the polyphenol extracts would be a better option to consider. If supplementing, we recommend 400mg of decaffeinated green coffee extract a day, as that dose has been used to good effect in many of the scientific studies.

Fish oil

We've seen in this chapter that obesity, insulin resistance and elevated levels of blood fats are all health problems that are linked to each other; and that they all lead to premature ageing and disability. We've also seen that preventing or managing these problems is *not* about eating a very low-fat diet but about eating the right type of fat.

There is evidence that supplementing EPA and DHA may help with weight loss.[66] EPA and DHA are two omega 3 fatty acids found in fish and krill oils. These fats antagonize an omega 6 fat known as arachidonic acid (AA). AA may cause us to gain weight because it increases appetite.[67] (It does this by activating special 'cannabinoid' receptors on our cell membranes.) AA is found in intensively farmed animal foods such as fatty meat, eggs and dairy products.

There are literally hundreds of studies showing that EPA/DHA can help to prevent cardiovascular disease. Not only do these fatty acids dampen down inflammation in the arteries (helping to prevent the build-up of dangerous plaque), but they also reduce levels of blood fats (triglycerides),[68] they make LDL-cholesterol less harmful to arteries[69] and they reduce blood pressure.[70]

Because EPA and DHA are so effective at lowering triglycerides, they are particularly important to take if you are at the pre-diabetic stage. People with pre-diabetes (or MetS) are typically overweight and insulin-resistant, with high levels of blood fats and/or cholesterol. EPA and DHA improve the health of people with pre-diabetes and help to prevent the condition from progressing to full-blown diabetes.[71]

So, the overall message is to eat less of the intensively farmed animal foods, increase wild and organic oily fish, and supplement EPA and DHA (or fish oil). We recommend you take 1g a day of combined EPA and DHA. If you are specifically wanting to lower elevated levels of triglycerides, however, you're likely to need 3–4g a day.[72]

5-hydroxytryptophan (5-HTP)

As we saw in Box 4.2, some people find that taking 5-HTP can help to control appetite. Two recent studies have found an oral 5-HTP spray to be effective in controlling appetite during weight-loss programmes;[73] and there is plenty of anecdotal evidence that taking 5-HTP as a tablet or capsule curbs cravings and overeating if your serotonin levels are less than optimal. Take 100mg three times a day, half an hour before food.

Supplementing 5-HTP in combination with lecithin (a phospholipid we discuss in Chapter 7) and the amino acids tyrosine and L-glutamine has recently been reported to improve withdrawal and mood symptoms in detoxified heroin addicts.[74] This is relevant because sugar and starches are highly addictive (see Chapter 10). This study shows how helpful these types of natural substances can be in beating addictions.

Other dietary supplements that show promise for weight loss include fucoxanthin,[75] xanthigen,[76] mangosteen,[77] the mango-like fruit irvingia gabonensis,[78] saffron,[79] L-arabinose,[80] glucomannan[81] and white kidney bean extract.[82] You could consider adding one or more of these supplements to your programme, if you are not getting sufficient help from the food and supplement advice given above. But remember that everyone is different and that it is not possible to predict which of these, if any, may help you.

L-arabinose and white kidney bean extract may be more effective for those times when you want to eat carbohydrates, as they work by slowing the rate at which the carbs are digested and absorbed. Take them just before your carb-containing meal.

Other special foods for blood sugar health include the herb gymnema sylvestre (which is easily taken in a tea), fenugreek, apple cider vinegar and bitter melon.

Bitter melon, also known as bitter gourd, can be found in Asian stores and is available frozen in some supermarkets. It is commonly used in Thai dishes, stir fries and curries. Remove the seeds and stem. Salting the vegetable for a few minutes and then rinsing before using helps to reduce the bitterness.

Cider vinegar can be added to salad dressings and is a useful addition to the diet because vinegar lowers the levels of post-eating blood glucose and insulin in healthy individuals.[83]

LOOK TO YOUR LIFESTYLE

There is no escaping the fact that, for long-term weight loss and blood sugar and insulin control, you need to get regular physical activity. Weight loss from diet alone can cause you to lose valuable muscle mass, but adding in exercise helps to preserve this youth-promoting lean tissue, pushing you to lose fat instead.[84]

Exercise helps to keep blood sugar levels stable in healthy people as well as in people who have been diagnosed with insulin resistance or diabetes. But the activity must be regular and frequent,[85] and a combination of both aerobic exercise and resistance (weight) training is likely to be the most beneficial.[86] See Chapter 10 for exercise tips for healthy ageing.

Other lifestyle factors that affect weight gain and/or blood glucose control include:

▸ Chronic stress.[87] See Chapter 6 for some ideas for reducing the stress in your life.

▸ Poor sleep.[88] See Chapter 10 for advice on improving sleep.

▸ The regular use of stimulants, as they encourage the liver to inject the bloodstream with high quantities of glucose. Such stimulants include nicotine and caffeine (found in tea, coffee, colas, chocolate and some sports drinks). Paradoxically, drinking coffee and green tea may be helpful in weight loss and insulin sensitivity, as we've seen earlier in this chapter. But you should make sure you are only consuming the amount of caffeine that you can tolerate without side-effects (such as poor sleep, shakiness, rapid heart rate and hyperactivity). If your tolerance is low, stick to (organic) decaff.

BOX 4.4 KNOW YOUR SUGAR TERMINOLOGY

When checking food labels, it's worthwhile knowing how to recognize 'sugar'. All the terms listed below indicate that some type of sugar has been added to the food:

Agave nectar	Cane sugar
Barbados sugar	Caramel
Barley malt	Carob syrup
Beet sugar	Caster sugar
Blackstrap molasses	Confectioner's sugar
Brown sugar	Corn syrup
Buttered syrup	Corn sweetener
Cane crystals	Corn syrup solids
Cane juice crystals	Crystalline fructose

Date sugar

Demerara sugar

Dextrin

Dextran

Dextrose

Diastatic malt

Diatase

D-mannose

Evaporated cane juice

Ethyl maltol

Florida Crystals

Free flowing

Fructose

Fruit juice

Fruit juice concentrate

Galactose

Glucose

Glucose solids

Golden sugar

Golden syrup

Granulated sugar

Grape sugar

Grape juice concentrate

HFCS

High-fructose corn syrup

Honey

Icing sugar

Invert sugar

Lactose

Malt syrup

Maltodextrin

Maltose

Mannitol

Maple syrup

Molasses

Muscovado sugar

Organic raw sugar

Panocha

Powdered sugar

Raw sugar

Refiner's syrup

Rice syrup

Sorbitol

Sorghum syrup

Sucrose

Saccharose

Sugar

Syrup

Table sugar

Treacle

Turbinado sugar

Yellow sugar

Instead of the sugars listed above, you could try one of the lower-GL sweeteners, such as stevia, lo han, xylitol, bee pollen, maca, mesquite, yacon or coconut sugar. These are far better options if you are looking to keep the weight off and also keep your blood sugar levels steady throughout the day.

MEAL PLAN

Breakfast	*Tofu Vegetable Scramble*
Lunch	*Broccoli Pear Soup*
	Tomato Seeded Crackers
Dinner	*Pan-Fried Salmon with Sweet Soy*
	Kelp Noodles with mixed salad
Snack	*Salted Vinegar and Onion Kale Chips*
	Tropical Protein Smoothie

If you do nothing else, do this...

▸ Centre your diet on antioxidant-rich, low-GL meals/snacks, as explained in Chapter 2.

▸ Every meal should be based on deeply and brightly coloured vegetables, with some protein and fat.

▸ Up to a quarter of your plate can be starch (optional) but for best results replace potatoes and grains with fibre-rich beans, pulses, lentils, turnip, swede (rutabaga) and other root vegetables. There are two exceptions to this rule: one is if you are doing a lot of physical exercise and the other is if you find you suffer from debilitating cravings. In such cases, include a tablespoon of oats or brown rice with your meal, or a couple of oat cakes. Never eat a starch without a protein.

▸ Avoid sugar, alcohol and white starch. Box 4.4 lists some names of sugars to look out for on food labels, together with some lower-GL alternatives. Box 4.3 explains more about white starch and how to cut it out of your diet.

▸ Protein should come from lean meat, poultry, fish, shellfish, eggs, low-fat dairy, nuts and seeds, beans and pulses.

▸ Get your fat from olives and olive oil, nuts, seeds and their oils, oily fish, avocado and coconut.

▸ Eat 2–3 portions of fruit a day, preferably berries or citrus fruits, which tend to have a lower GL.

▸ Take time to eat, as this reduces the rate at which sugar gets into the bloodstream.

▸ Stop smoking and reduce caffeine to a level where it is not causing side-effects. Stop at three cups of coffee a day as a maximum – drink decaff if you want to add more to this quota.

▸ Reduce the stress in your life and get regular exercise and good-quality sleep (see Chapter 10).

▸ Incorporate the 'special' foods and supplements discussed above, especially magnesium, chromium, green tea, green coffee, fish oil, cinnamon and/or 5-HTP.

▸ Avoid fatty cuts of meat and processed foods containing trans-fats. Go easy on full-fat dairy foods such as cheese, cream and full-fat milk.

▸ Try sipping drinks throughout the day, as these can help you feel less of an urge to eat. Herbal teas, water, broths or coconut water are all good options.

CHAPTER 5

AGELESS BEAUTY FROM WITHIN

How much time, effort and money do you invest in potions, lotions and cosmetics in an attempt to keep the visible signs of ageing at bay? Such signs include the stealthy creep of thread veins, fine lines and wrinkles, and skin that is becoming more dry, flaky and fragile.

What results do you get from your diligent daily application of these wonder potions? Can you discern a noticeable difference? Are they really worth the money? In this chapter we show you another way to help your skin reach and maintain its full potential for radiance and resilience, despite the ageing process. This chapter is about supporting your skin (and your nails, gums, veins and capillaries) from the *inside*.

WHAT YOUR SKIN DOES FOR YOU

With a surface area of 1.5–2 square metres (16–22 square feet), your skin offers far more than barrier protection. It enables you to sense pleasure and pain, it helps to regulate your body temperature, it absorbs oil-based nutrients and drugs, and it excretes toxins. Your skin synthesizes vitamin D from sunlight and it produces melanin, the pigment (evident in freckles and moles) that provides protection from UV damage. The skin also contains immune system cells, which go into battle against potentially harmful invaders such as bacteria and parasites.

Officially classed as an organ, the skin is made up of two interdependent yet distinct layers: the dermis and the epidermis. The epidermis is the visible, outer layer of the skin (comprising five separate sub-layers), and it provides a flexible, waterproof barrier, which is entirely renewed every 45–75 days.

The dermis lies underneath the epidermis and is responsible for giving the skin its bulkiness – and so the effects of ageing are most commonly seen here. It is made mainly of the proteins collagen and elastin, which give the skin its powerful strength, extensibility (during pregnancy or weight gain) and elasticity.

Collagen and elastin synthesis are at their peak in childhood and, as you might expect, their production declines with age. We rely on dietary proteins to get the raw materials to produce them, as well as vitamin C and copper. Indeed, one of the best-known signs of vitamin C deficiency is the disease scurvy, in which lack of collagen leads to degenerative symptoms such as skin sores, wounds that won't heal, easy bruising and bleeding gums.

The dermis also contains blood vessels and other structures that help in the skin's many functions: nerves, sweat glands, oil-producing sebaceous glands and hair follicles.

Firm, radiant, clear skin requires balanced nutrition. A deficiency of nutrients, an overload of toxins, hormonal imbalances, stress or lack of sleep will soon show up in your skin. Symptoms can be as diverse as pimples, boils and other eruptions; dry, flaky skin; premature lines and wrinkles; rashes; saggy, grey skin; or various medical conditions such as eczema, urticaria (hives) and psoriasis.

If you're keen to safeguard your skin from daily attack, you need to learn about the key processes that drive skin damage and cause premature ageing. And these degenerative processes are not only confined to the skin; they also affect other types of connective tissue such as the blood vessels and the gums.

IS YOUR BODY GETTING RUSTY?

Start by answering the following short list of questions. Your score will give an idea of the extent to which you are suffering from a degenerative process called 'oxidation'. Oxidation is destructive to the skin and indeed to all body tissues. It is thought to be one of the main drivers of premature ageing in the skin, blood vessels and gums.

Tick the box for each statement that applies to you.

☐ Feel tired without any obvious reason (e.g. a late night)

☐ Frequent headaches

☐ Low mood

☐ Pigmented skin patches known as 'liver spots'

☐ More obvious skin lines and wrinkles than people of the same age

☐ Sagging, droopy skin

☐ Stretch marks

☐ Eat fewer than five portions fruit and veg a day

☐ Eat sugary foods or white starchy foods (white bread, bagels, rice, etc.) daily

☐ Spend a lot of time in the sun

☐ Have ever experienced sunburn

☐ Smoke cigarettes

☐ Eat processed foods

☐ Have sinusitis, bronchitis, arthritis or any other 'itis'

☐ Do prolonged periods of high-intensity exercise such as marathon running or sport at competitive level

☐ Eat barbecued, fried or griddled foods more than once a week

☐ Drink alcohol more than three times a week

Total score _____

If you scored 6 or above, it is likely that your body is burdened with oxidation. Oxidation is what happens to metal when it rusts, to a sliced apple when it turns brown and to the human body when it degenerates. Its most obvious signs are in the skin, in the form of pigmented patches, fine lines, wrinkles, loss of elasticity and sun damage. But it affects other body tissues just as much and is involved in many age-related diseases, such as cancer, cardiovascular disease and diabetes, Alzheimer's disease, Parkinson's disease, rheumatoid arthritis and neurodegeneration.[1]

What exactly is oxidation?

Oxidation is a chemical reaction that produces harmful molecules called 'free radicals'. These are so-called because they spin out of control, damaging cells and causing general havoc in the body.

It is perfectly normal for some oxidation to occur, even when we're in good health. Indeed, free radicals are produced inside the battery compartments of every cell as part of the perpetual process of converting food into energy. (These battery compartments are called the mitochondria and you'll learn more about them in Chapter 6.) A healthy body will extinguish the free radicals produced here by using special molecules called antioxidants (AOs).

AOs are knights in shining armour, saving us from the premature ageing and degenerative diseases brought on by elevated levels of oxidation. See Box 5.1 for the science stuff on how AOs work.

Problems arise if the level of free radical activity becomes so intense that it overwhelms the available supply of antioxidants. The free radicals can then run riot, unopposed, causing oxidative damage to nearby cells. The gradual accumulation of such damage eventually adds up to signs and symptoms of premature ageing and chronic disease.

But don't despair. Most people who find themselves in this situation can generally do something about it. The trick is to identify the sources of the excess free radicals in your life and then find ways of reducing or avoiding them. Next, you need to check you have enough antioxidant defences and, if these are lacking, boost them by consuming more antioxidant-rich foods and, in some cases, supplements. By the end of this chapter, you'll know how to do this.

BOX 5.1 THE MAGIC (AND SCIENCE) OF ANTIOXIDANTS

In all of our organs and tissues we produce spectacularly powerful agents called antioxidants. Antioxidants are vital to us as we age because they 'mop up' free radicals, preventing or slowing down the damage they cause to cells (known as 'oxidative damage').

The simplest way to understand how antioxidants work their magic is by looking at the way their electrons behave. Electrons are tiny pieces of electricity that are arranged in the outer layers, the shells, of all molecules. The electrons are usually arranged in pairs. This means that if an electron manages to escape, the other electron in its pair is left on its own, without a partner. The presence of this spare electron causes the molecule to spin out of control: it becomes a free radical.

The only way a free radical can become stable again is by stealing an electron from another molecule. This will provide a partner for the spare electron. Unfortunately, by doing this, the donor molecule is left with an incomplete electron pair, turning this molecule into a free radical. This is the beginning of a chain reaction of free radicals bumping into stable molecules in order to steal their electrons. As they do so, their aggression causes damage to local cells and tissues. This is one of the best-documented causes of cellular damage and premature ageing.

AOs are the only agents able to calm the rioting radicals, preventing further damage. They have a unique ability to do this because, unlike in other molecules, the electrons in their outer shells are *not* arranged in pairs. Rather, the electrons of AOs are equally spaced. This means they can donate electrons safely, without needing to split a pair, and therefore without themselves turning radical. In this way, AOs can disable any aggressive radicals that cross their path.

Such antioxidant behaviour is so vital for health and wellbeing that the human body manufactures a wide variety of AOs. They have names like glutathione, cysteine, alpha lipoic acid, coenzyme Q10 (CoQ10) and melatonin. However, we are also able to extract antioxidant molecules from some of the foods we eat and these help to keep our supply at good levels, ready to jump into action when required. See page 108 for the many different types of AOs found in food.

IS YOUR COLLAGEN COLLAPSING?

While free radicals are vehement enemies of healthy skin, there is another reason that our skin suffers as we age: it's because we're gradually losing collagen. Collagen is a crucial protein in all connective tissues – not just the skin but also in bone, the skeletal joints, blood vessels and in the mucous membranes like those of the gut and the vagina. It's what gives these tissues their strength and keeps skin supple, firm and elastic. Answer the following questions to see if your collagen levels may need some extra support.

Tick the box for each of the following signs that affect you.

☐ Thinning skin

☐ Wounds take an unusually long time to heal

☐ Varicose veins

☐ Broken capillaries or thread veins

☐ Haemorrhoids

☐ Anal fissure

☐ Water retention (swollen ankles)

☐ Swollen or bleeding gums

☐ Vaginal pain on intercourse (vaginal atrophy)

☐ Easy bruising

☐ Prone to injury in the muscles, tendons or ligaments

☐ Post- or perimenopausal

Total score _____

If you scored 4 or above, it is possible that you are lacking the nutrients to make adequate collagen. Alternatively, it could be that your collagen structures are being broken down too rapidly for the repair systems to keep up.

TOP TIPS FOR YOUTHFUL SKIN, GUMS, VEINS, HAIR AND NAILS

Your skin is a window on to the health and biological age of your body. If you take steps to look after your skin, you will also be doing a favour to the many other organs and tissues that need a little extra support as you get older. For example, Boxes 5.2, 5.4, 5.5, 5.6 and 5.7 give tips for healthy skin, gums, veins, hair and nails.

SLOW DOWN OXIDATIVE DAMAGE
Avoid free radicals

The more you can shield your skin cells from free radicals, the more clear, radiant and youthful it will appear. So, let's start by taking a look at where these free radicals come from.

THE SUN – FRIEND OR FOE?

The best-known enemy of the skin is strong sunlight. UV light damages skin cells by both oxidation and inflammation. To help counter this, special pigmentation cells in the skin produce a substance called melanin, producing a sun 'tan'. The real role of melanin, however, is not to give us a pleasing golden glow, but to absorb and neutralize the free radicals triggered by the sun's rays and to protect the nucleus of the cell from damage. (Nuclei that sustain damage can initiate the start of the cancer process.)

So it would seem that we need to be careful not to get so much sun that we burn or even turn too red. Getting some sun on your skin is important for vitamin D synthesis, and indeed there is currently some scientific debate about whether or not lack of vitamin D is a greater risk factor for cancer, including skin cancer, than is over-exposure to sunlight. Many experts now recommend exposing the skin daily, in the middle of the day, without sunscreen. Start with 2–3 minutes only and build up gradually to a maximum of 30 minutes, taking care not to burn. You can read more about vitamin D in Chapter 8.

But it's not all about the sun. Research shows that oxidative damage is greater when sun exposure is combined with urban pollutants such as cigarette smoke.[2] Air pollution is another oxidant, as is ionizing radiation from over-exposure to x-rays. So, try to avoid these as much as you can. For example, if you exercise outdoors, stay away from busy roads.

Allergies can also trigger free radical attack. If you have allergic symptoms such as runny or itchy nose or eyes, eczema or asthma, consider whether they may be caused by something in your surroundings. Common culprits include mould spores, animal hairs, harsh chemicals such as sodium lauryl sulphate (found in many personal care products), or allergens from the plant kingdom, such as certain pollens.

Dietary oxidants to watch out for

Changing your diet can help to reduce your free radical load.

▸ Smoked and overcooked foods: Reduce your intake of smoked and cured foods, such as kippers, smoked mackerel and smoked salmon, ham and bacon, and also browned or blackened foods such as meat, poultry and fish that have been barbecued, griddled, fried or grilled at high temperatures. All these foods contain cancer-causing chemicals such as heterocyclic amines (HCAs) and polycyclic aromatic hydrocarbons (PAHs).[3] High levels have even been found in foods as seemingly innocuous as grilled chicken breast.[4]

As luck would have it, there are safer ways to cook meat and fish, using methods that don't significantly increase the levels of these horribly carcinogenic chemicals. These alternative cooking methods include steaming, poaching, slow baking and pot roasting at lower temperatures. They can produce meat and fish dishes even more delicious than the barbecued, fried and grilled dishes you are used to. See, for example, our recipes for *Slow-Cooked Za'atar Lamb Shoulder* and *Moroccan Beef Tagine*.

▸ Damaged fats: Two categories of damaged fats are trans-fats and oxidised fats. Both tend to start life as healthy 'polyunsaturated' fats (PUFAs) from grains, nuts and seeds (e.g. corn, flax, walnut, rapeseed, sesame or sunflower oil). PUFAs become oxidised (that is, they deteriorate) if you heat them, as they are particularly fragile.

Trans-fats, as we saw in Chapter 2, are produced when PUFAs are processed ('partially hydrogenated') in a factory to make them easier to use in commercial baking systems and to extend their shelf life. If you eat processed foods, you will likely be consuming such trans-fats.

These are highly inflammatory, they hamper skin health and they also increase your risk of many age-related diseases, included insulin resistance, diabetes, cardiovascular disease and cancer.[5] Some countries have banned these man-made fats or have at least limited the amount that can be used in processed foods, while other countries stipulate that their levels have to be clearly stated on food labels, so that people can make healthier choices if they want to. Unfortunately, the UK has no such rules. But you can easily avoid these inflammatory fats by eschewing all processed foods, especially mass-produced margarines, bread, cakes, biscuits, pastries, ready meals, sauces, mayonnaise and salad dressings, and deep-fried foods. Box 5.2 has information on the types of fats to eat more of if you're concerned about ageing skin.

To slow down the ageing process caused by oxidation, you don't need to avoid these foods and cooking methods completely – just view them as an occasional part of your diet rather than a regular one. Remember that *no* food (unless you are truly allergic to it) need be completely off-limits. Of greater importance is the need for balance. As seen earlier, one way of achieving this is to adopt the 80–20 rule – do what you think is healthy for about 80 per cent of the time and then you can still indulge in unhealthier foods occasionally.

BOX 5.2 WHAT FATS FOR AGEING SKIN?

So, what fats should you be eating for youthful skin? Well, according to a recent population study of almost 3000 people, eating more omega 3 fatty acids is associated with a lower rate of sunlight-induced skin ageing.[6] Omega 3s in this study were from oily fish and plant oils. Flaxseed (linseed) is the most omega 3-rich plant source, although pumpkin seeds, hemp seeds and walnuts also contain some.

As you'll see in Chapter 8, omega 3 fats are converted into powerful anti-inflammatory agents in the body. It is therefore important to consume enough of them, especially if you are prone to inflammatory skin conditions such as eczema, contact dermatitis, hives or psoriasis.[7] If you want to supplement, we recommend 500–1000mg combined EPA/DHA a day, best taken in a fish oil.

Another fatty acid that is particularly important in skin health is gamma linolenic acid (GLA). This is an omega 6 fatty acid found in evening primrose oil, borage oil and starflower oil. In Chapter 8 there is a diagram of key beneficial omega 3 and omega 6 fatty acids and the best food sources. GLA is hard to get from the diet. Although a healthy body can synthesize it from other fatty acids, this process is often too slow for optimal health. This is where supplementing GLA can make a big difference to the structure and function of ageing skin, improving typical signs of ageing such as roughness and loss of moisture, elasticity and firmness.[8]

GLA helps to prevent water loss from skin cells,[9] but indeed both omega 3 and omega 6 fats are important to keep the membranes of skin cells supple and watertight – helping to prevent dry, flaky skin. Of course, you need to drink enough water as well – we recommend 1.5 litres (approximately 3 pints) a day of hydrating fluids such as water, coconut water, green juices or smoothies, meat broths or herbal teas.

GLA is also the first fatty acid you should consider increasing if you have atopic dermatitis or eczema. If you don't know whether your eczema is atopic, take a moment to consider whether you are also prone to asthma, hayfever or skin hives, and/or whether you have family members with the same. If the answer is yes, then you may well be 'atopic'. It's best to discuss the possibility with your doctor to make sure. And it is worth knowing if you are affected, not least because atopic people may not be able to make their own GLA. Although the evidence isn't conclusive, GLA is helpful to some people with atopic eczema.[10] We believe there is certainly enough evidence to give it a go for, say, three months and then review your symptoms. We recommend starting with 360–500mg of GLA a day.

Omega 6 and omega 3 polyunsaturated oils that come from vegetables, nuts and seeds are best eaten raw, such as in salad dressings. They can be easily damaged by heat and light. Make sure you buy them from a shop that has looked after them well by keeping them in the fridge, and make sure that the label says they have been 'mechanically pressed' or 'cold pressed'. These processes help to preserve the delicate fatty acids.

For cooking, you should use fats that are more stable. These are the saturated fats and include coconut oil and butter. Coconut oil may have some healthy ageing benefits, as we explain in Chapter 4. You can also use olive oil or avocado oil if you are cooking at lower temperatures, such as in casseroles and soups. This is because these oils comprise mainly monounsaturated fatty acids, which are not as fragile as polyunsaturated fatty acids. What's more, they are rich in vitamin E, meaning that their topical application to the skin may also be beneficial.

For more detailed information on the different types of dietary fats and their beneficial and harmful properties, see Chapter 8.

OXIDANTS FROM WITHIN

▶ Battery failure: Some free radicals do not come from things we eat or breathe in: they are produced within the body. We have already seen that it is the batteries within the cells (the mitochondria) that produce the most oxidants. They are normal by-products of the conversion of food into energy. The more physically active you are, the more the mitochondria have to speed up their energy production processes. So, while it's good to exercise daily, you'll be producing more free radicals if you're exercising intensively, such as when training for a competitive event.

Some people find that their mitochondria function less well as they age (we'll see more about this in Chapter 6). Ageing can cause the mitochondria to become leaky. This allows more free radicals to escape from these tiny organelles, causing more oxidative damage to surrounding cells. Chapter 6 shows you how to improve mitochondrial health.

- Inflammation: Another situation that is responsible for launching artilleries of free radicals is that of inflammation. If you suffer from hayfever, sinusitis, arthritis or any other 'itis', your immune system will be injecting powerful supplies of oxidants to the affected area, in an attempt to kill or clear whatever virus, bacteria, allergen or other invader has triggered your symptoms.

  So, it's wise to get to the bottom of what's causing the inflammation and eliminate or reduce this. Read the recommendations in Chapter 8 if you want to learn how to dampen down unwanted inflammation. Many of the anti-inflammatory nutrients we recommend in that chapter can be helpful in sunburn and other inflammatory skin conditions.

- Glycation: In Chapter 4 we saw how eating too much sugar or refined carbs can cause sugar in the blood to damage body proteins, in a process called glycation. Excessive glycation produces harmful 'AGE' products (advanced glycation end products). These are also found in certain foods, particularly those that have been browned or caramelized by heat. These are bad news for the skin, as they produce harmful free radicals and also damage collagen.

- Toxins: Don't forget that if you are overloaded with toxins, this will soon show up in your skin. If your liver and other detox organs are overburdened, toxins will build up in the skin and manifest as eruptions such as pimples and boils, excessively odorous perspiration and/or an unhealthy-looking yellowish pallor. Chapter 6 has plenty of advice on reducing your exposure to toxins and giving your detox processes the boost they need in order to take the pressure off the skin.

  The health of your gut is also important here, as so many toxins enter the body from the food we eat or from unwanted microbes in the gut and their potentially harmful metabolites. Refer to Chapter 3 for more information on how to get your gut into tip-top condition.

So, we've seen how reducing your exposure to free radicals is crucial for slowing down ageing processes that are caused by oxidation. The other important part of the equation is to make sure you have a good supply of antioxidants to quench these destructive radicals. The next section shows you how to do this.

Harness the amazing power of antioxidants

The AOs that have the most evidence for protecting human skin cells from sun damage are the vitamins A, C and E,[18] as well as two groups of plant chemicals known as carotenoids and flavonoids. Plants produce such chemicals to protect themselves from the sun. Research shows that if we ingest them, they become great scavengers of free radicals within our skin and elsewhere in the body.

What's more, these particular vitamins and phytochemicals are able to increase the amount of time we can safely spend in the sun, by providing a direct barrier from the sun's rays.[19] Carotenoids and flavonoids do this by colouring the skin: not only are they pigments that build up in the skin, but they may also increase melanin production. It's worth knowing, though, that these protective effects have mainly been seen when people have ingested doses far higher than are commonly found in the diet. So it is likely that you'll need to take a supplement of these phytochemicals, rather than rely on food sources alone.

VITAMINS

Vitamin C is found in fresh fruits and vegetables, especially bell peppers, papaya, guava, citrus, kiwi, strawberries, broccoli, Brussels sprouts and potatoes. Smokers use up to twice as much vitamin C as non-smokers every day,[20] so they need to make sure they are getting more in the diet or from supplements. Supplement 500–1000mg a day.

The best source of vitamin A is organic liver, but it is also present in eggs and dairy products. Vegans can eat orange and dark green fruits and vegetables for beta-carotene, which can be converted to vitamin A in most people. If you want to supplement vitamin A, try 2000 IU a day. Unfortunately, some people can't convert enough beta-carotene to make sufficient vitamin A. Sometimes this is due to a genetic variation, but it can also be due to undiagnosed/untreated low thyroid function.

Vitamin E is found in avocados, wheatgerm, sunflower seeds, hazelnuts, peanuts, almonds and their oils. Supplement at least 400 IU a day of *natural* vitamin E (which contains all eight tocopherols and tocotrienols).

CAROTENOIDS

The most photoprotective carotenoids are beta-carotene, found in orange and green leafy vegetables, tomato products, apricots and mangoes; lycopene, found in tomato products; and lutein and zeaxanthin, found in green leafy vegetables (mainly spinach and kale). They're better absorbed from food when they are cooked and eaten with oils or fats. And, interestingly, lutein absorption from a purified crystalline supplement appears to be almost twice that from food sources.[21] Take a supplement totaling about 15mg of the mixed carotenoids mentioned above.

FLAVONOIDS

The flavonoids that are the most important in skin, gum and blood vessel health are known as anthocyanins and oligomeric proanthocyanidins (OPCs). The best food sources of anthocyanins are dark red, blue and purple berries, sour cherries, cranberries and red wine, while OPCs are most concentrated in grape seeds/skins, apples, apricots, red wine, cherries, cocoa and dark chocolate.[22] The trouble is, eating enough of these foods for a therapeutic effect can be difficult. Take a supplement of 150–320mg OPCs.

Another phytochemical to top up daily is one called EGCG (or epigallocatechin gallate), found in green tea, as it reduces UV light-induced oxidative stress.[23] Take a supplement that provides 700mg of the catechin phytochemicals. Resveratrol (from grape skins and red wine) is another phytochemical to watch, as it is currently being researched for its potential anti-ageing effects in skin.[24] If you want to supplement it, we recommend 250–500mg daily.

As there are so many different types of AOs in plants, try to centre your diet on plant-based foods, of as wide a range of colours as possible – remember that most phytochemical AOs are pigments, so it is the deeply and brightly coloured plants that hold the most. And be sure to include the skins and outer leaves, as this is where the AOs are most concentrated. See Box 5.3 for a list of AO phytochemicals and where to find them in foods.

OTHER ANTIOXIDANTS

Earlier in this chapter we mentioned the antioxidants that our bodies produce when we need them – molecules such as glutathione, cysteine, alpha lipoic acid, CoQ10 and the hormone melatonin. People who are carrying a particularly high burden of oxidative stress sometimes find it helpful to take one or more of these AOs in supplement form. We recommend that if you want to do this, you should talk to a nutritionist or other healthcare practitioner. (Note that in the UK melatonin is only available on prescription.)

BOX 5.3 PLANT CHEMICALS AND WHAT THEY DO

Within the scientific community there is an explosion of interest in phytochemicals, many of which are potent antioxidants. These bioactives are abundantly available in fruit, vegetables, herbs, spices, edible fungi, nuts and seeds. Plants get their energy from the sun (via photosynthesis) – hence they need to produce natural sunscreens to protect them from the solar radiation. Here's a list of the main phytochemicals and their food sources. You'll see they are similar sources to the high-ORAC foods we explained in Chapter 2 – ORACs being a term used to designate a food that is rich in antioxidants.

► Carotenoids:

  ▷ Alpha-carotene: Carrots, squash, oranges, tangerines.

  ▷ Beta-carotene: Orange and green leafy vegetables, tomato products, apricots, mangoes.

  ▷ Lycopene: Tomatoes.

  ▷ Beta-cryptozanthin: Oranges.

  ▷ Lutein and zeaxanthin: Green leafy veg, especially kale and spinach.

- Flavonoids:

  - Flavonols (e.g. quercetin, kaempferol, myricetin): Onions, kale, broccoli, apples, tea, red wine, grapes, berries, cherries.

  - Anthocyanins: Dark red, blue and purple berries, sour cherries.

  - Flavan-3-ols:

    - Catechins (e.g. epigallocatechin gallate): Tea, especially green and white tea.

    - Proanthocyanidins: Apples, apricots, cherries, cocoa, dark chocolate.

  - Flavones: Parsley, thyme, celery.

  - Flavanones (e.g. hesperetin, naringenin): Citrus fruits.

- Other phenolic compounds:

  - Hydroxycinnamates: Caffeic acid (coffee and propolis).

  - Ferulic acid: Cereal brans.

  - Neochlorogenic and chlorogenic acids: Prunes.

  - Stilbenes: Resveratrol (red wine).

  - Vanillin, capsaicins, zingerone (vanilla, chilli, ginger).

- Phytoestrogens (isoflavones, lignans):

  - Soya, other pulses, seeds, grains, nuts.

- Plant sterols: Vegetable oils, cereals, nuts, seeds, avocados.

- Glucosinolates: Brassicas (Brussels sprouts, cabbage, broccoli, watercress, rocket/arugula) – key phytochemicals thought to be involved in reducing the damaging effects of reactive oxygen species in the development of cancer.[25]

- Terpenoids: Herbs and spices, such as mint, sage, coriander (cilantro), rosemary, ginger.[26]

Studies show that people who eat more plant foods have a lower risk of many age-related diseases, including high blood pressure, stroke, coronary heart disease, dementia and Alzheimer's disease, weight gain, osteoporosis and some cancers.[27] This is likely due to their antioxidant effects, but this is not the sole reason. These bioactive chemicals may also have other age-defying effects on our cells,[28] such as turning off genes that promote inflammation, helping to prevent blood from becoming too sticky (sticky blood is more liable to clot, causing heart attacks and strokes), keeping arteries flexible (helping to control blood pressure) and supporting detoxification processes (as you'll see in Chapter 6).

The government recommends five portions of fruit and vegetables a day. But if you're looking to optimize your health, rather than just to prevent malnutrition, you need to eat more like ten portions, ideally eight portions of vegetables and two or three portions of fruit. Refer to Chapter 2 for advice on what is a portion size. It's best to eat some of these foods raw, in order to preserve the micronutrients. However, beta-carotene and lycopene are better absorbed when the foods are cooked and eaten with fat. Glucosinolates may also be more useful to us when the cruciferous vegetables are lightly cooked, as the raw plant contains an enzyme that can stop the phytochemicals being converted to their active form.[29] (Note, however, that overcooking also reduces phytochemical absorption.)

BOX 5.4 THE BATTLE FOR HEALTHY GUMS

One of the biggest giveaways of your biological age is the state of your gums. Gum tissue should be pink and firm, with no swelling or tenderness, and it should fit tightly around the teeth. Your gums should not bleed when you brush or floss.

If you suffer from loose, swollen, tender, bleeding gums, and maybe the associated bad breath, you've got a condition known as gingivitis. If this is not swiftly addressed, it can lead to a more advanced condition called periodontal disease. You'll know if you have periodontal disease because space ('pockets') will start to develop between the teeth and the gums at the gum-line.

A recent government survey found that almost half of all adults had developed some periodontal 'pocketing'.[11]

And it turns out that gum disease isn't just a problem in the mouth. It also increases your risk of getting other age-related conditions, including type 2 diabetes,[12] cardiovascular disease[13] and osteoporosis.[14] What's more, there is evidence that if you reduce the inflammation in your gums, you can improve the health of your heart and arteries as you age.[15]

People get gum disease because of poor oral hygiene. This drives the disease by massively increasing free radical attack on the gums. Plaque from food remains builds up at the gum-line. This attracts harmful bacteria, which produce free radicals. The bacterial invasion also causes your gums to become inflamed. And then the inflammatory process itself starts to produce free radicals. Now you have free radicals generated from two different sources, and these in turn destroy gum tissue, making the disease even worse.

So, for healthy gums you need to floss and clean your teeth twice a day, and see a dental hygienist regularly. But you also need to reduce your intake of sugar, as this feeds the bacteria. Newer research has highlighted the importance of avoiding your exposure to free radicals generally (gum disease is worse in smokers, for instance) *and* increasing your supply of antioxidants.[16] The most important antioxidants for gum health turn out to be those that are also key to healthy skin, especially vitamins A, C and E, and the plant chemicals such as the anthocyanins. (And anthocyanins and vitamin C also help to preserve collagen – so they help stop gum tissue from degrading beyond repair.)

In particular, the anthocyanins isolated from cranberries have been found in laboratory studies to prevent harmful bacteria from sticking to the gum-line and also to reduce the amount of inflammatory chemicals produced by the gum tissue in response to the bacterial attack.[17] But for a therapeutic effect you'll probably need more than you can easily get from diet alone. We recommend taking a cranberry powder and a multivitamin and mineral formula that includes AOs and other nutrients that may be helpful in oral health, namely the B vitamins and vitamin D, the minerals calcium, magnesium and zinc, and the nutrient CoQ10.

BOOST COLLAGEN LEVELS

We've already talked about the importance of vitamins A and C as antioxidants and also for providing some photoprotection to skin.

Plant foods again...

VITAMINS A AND C

It just so happens that these amazing nutrients are also crucial for other aspects of skin health. Vitamin C, for example, is crucial for the synthesis of collagen fibres. Vitamin A, while not directly involved in collagen production, improves healthy cell turnover in the topmost layer of the skin (the epidermis), the nails and the hair. This is particularly important for keeping these tissues healthy because they have quite a fast turnover of cells. Skin cells, for example, are shed from the epidermis and renewed every few days. Vitamin A also nourishes and sustains the cells in the tiny blood vessels (capillaries) that feed the skin.[30] Capillaries tend to weaken as we age, causing 'thread veins'.

ANTHOCYANINS AND OLIGOMERIC PROANTHOCYANIDINS

One exciting research development is that anthocyanins and OPCs are now understood to be powerful collagen stabilizers. In other words, they help to preserve collagen, elastin and hyaluronic acid, and stop these important skin compounds from breaking down as we age.

In a trial of 60 healthy subjects, aged between 50 and 70 years, 12 weeks of supplementation with these flavonoids (total 320mg per day), together with the AOs lutein, zeaxanthin and green tea extract, was found to:

- improve skin elasticity by 12 per cent

- reduce the depth of wrinkles by 6 per cent

- protect the skin from UV sunlight damage to the level of a sun protection factor (SPF) of 10.[31]

Just how do anthocyanins and OPCs have such an effect? It turns out they work on a number of different levels. They improve blood flow to the epidermis, they reduce inflammation and redness, they mop up free radicals (as seen above), which reduces skin cell damage, and they also clamp down on aggressive enzymes that set out to destroy collagen. These enzymes are called matrix metalloproteinases (MMPs). By suppressing these enzymes, anthocyanins and OPCs keep collagen strong – they help shift the balance from collagen's destruction, towards its production, thus enabling skin to go into repair mode and heal damaged cells.[32]

Other collagen-boosting tips

▶ Protein: Make sure you eat high-quality protein every day and preferably at every meal. It is the amino acids in these protein foods that are used by the body to make collagen. The protein foods that are most easily digested, absorbed and used by the body are eggs, whey protein powder, fish and poultry.

   Vegans need to make sure they are eating combinations of whole grains and nuts, or whole grains and beans/pulses every day. You can also increase your amino acids by making a protein shake from hemp protein powder and coconut milk (see our recipe for *Tropical Protein Smoothie*).

▶ Supplementing collagen: New research indicates that taking collagen in supplement form may improve skin elasticity in elderly women[33] – 2.5–5g collagen hydrolysate has been shown to be effective. Evidence from animal studies also indicates collagen hydrolysate may have anti-inflammatory effects in the skin[34] and also help to prevent skin damage from the type of radiation produced by sunlight.[35]

▶ Sleep: Do your best to get 7.5–8 hours of good-quality sleep a night. Chapter 10 includes ideas for improving your sleep if you need some help. Sleep is vital for the release of growth hormone, which works hard during the night to repair and rejuvenate the skin (as well as the blood vessels, gums and other tissues).

▶ Hormones: And, talking of hormones, the adrenal hormone DHEA and the sex hormones oestrogen and testosterone are all fantastic collagen-boosters. That's one of the reasons that our skin ages faster post-menopause, and also if we are suffering from 'adrenal fatigue'.

Chapter 6 includes an action plan for supporting your adrenal function, improving DHEA levels, and Chapter 9 contains plenty of advice on improving and balancing your sex hormones.

BOX 5.5 AGEING VEINS AND WHAT TO DO ABOUT THEM

Tired, heavy, achy legs, ankle swelling (water retention), thread veins, haemorrhoids, varicose veins, even leg ulcers – all these problems of the venous system tend to increase with age. They arise when the lower leg veins become less efficient at carrying blood back to the heart.

Conventional treatments consist of compression stockings, medications for swelling and ultimately vascular surgery. But did you know that many of the nutritional and lifestyle recommendations for healthy skin also help to support veins and capillaries? This is because these tiny blood vessels rely so much on collagen for their strength, and also because free radicals attack the venous system just as much as they do the skin.

So, if you are suffering with these kinds of problems, follow the advice in this chapter on how to reduce exposure to free radicals, increase antioxidants and support collagen structures. The same anthocyanins recommended for skin health, for example, are widely used for venous disorders. They have been found to be effective in improving ankle and leg swelling and varicose veins, as well as lymphoedema from breast surgery.[36] Lymphoedema is a condition causing swelling and pain in the arms due to lymph node removal (during breast surgery) which inhibits the return flow of lymph fluid.

Another plant chemical with impressive effects on the venous system is aescin, which comes from horse chestnuts. It has been found to improve varicose veins, post-operative water retention and haemorrhoids.[37] A scientific review of 21 studies concluded that aescin at a dose of 50–150mg per day was as effective as compression stockings in reducing lower-leg swelling and the associated pain, itching and fatigue.[38]

BOX 5.6 KEEPING YOUR HAIR ON

Ageing is often associated with hair loss, not only in men but also in women. In men, this is a normal process due to testosterone, but in women it is usually a sign that something in their biochemistry is not quite right.

There are between 100,000 and 350,000 hairs on the human scalp and up to 100 of these are shed each day. If you are noticing that you are regularly losing more hair than this, perhaps in the shower when you wash it, or in your hairbrush, you may either have a genetic hair loss condition or, more commonly, you may have a condition called chronic telogen effluvium (CTE). Together, these two causes are estimated to be responsible for 95 per cent of unwanted hair loss in women.

So, which do you have? Genetic hair loss is easily recognizable because clear areas of the scalp tend to be exposed, usually from the front of the hairline across the top of the head. If you've noticed this, you should see your doctor for treatment options, which are likely to involve hormone therapy. CTE gives no noticeable bare patches, being more of a general overall thinning. By far the most common cause is low levels of iron, perhaps from heavy menstruation or from insufficient iron in your diet.

The best test for iron status is called a serum ferritin test and this can be ordered from your family doctor. What's interesting is that you don't have to be anaemic for low iron levels to affect your hair. There is evidence that excessive hair shedding can occur if your blood levels of ferritin are less than 70mcg per litre,[39] whereas to be classed as anaemic your levels have to be below 15mcg per litre.

You can increase your iron levels by eating red meat such as beef, lamb, venison and other game. Vegetarian sources include beans, pulses, dark leafy green vegetables and dried fruit. Note that iron from vegetarian sources is harder to absorb, but this can be helped by taking vitamin C at the same time. You could also take an iron supplement. Choose one that contains a highly absorbable form of iron and which also includes lysine and vitamin C to aid absorption. But you need to be patient – it can take six months of supplementation to see a noticeable effect.

Other causes of thinning hair include harsh treatments such as colourants and perms, changing the frequency with which you wash your hair, current or recent pregnancy, polycystic ovarian syndrome, menopause, protein deficiency and low thyroid function.

Take care not to towel-dry your hair too aggressively, and avoid harsh chemicals and hot hair dryers and heated rollers, as these can cause the hair to break, as well as causing dry, lifeless hair and split ends.

If you suffer from a dry, flaky scalp, follow the advice for skin health in this chapter. In addition, use only shampoos and conditioners based on natural ingredients and essential oils.

BOX 5.7 NUTRITION FOR NAILS

As we age, nails can become brittle, thin and weak, peeling and breaking easily. Some simple lifestyle changes may help, such as using gloves when washing dishes, and avoiding chemicals such as acetone (in nail varnish remover) which tend to dry the nails. You should also see your doctor to investigate possible medical causes such as poor thyroid function, poor circulation or a fungal nail infection.

There are two minerals particularly important for nail health: iron (it is thought that spoon-shaped nails may be linked to low levels)[40] and zinc (deficiency is anecdotally linked to excessive white patches). You can test your iron status by asking for a blood test for ferritin levels (see Box 5.6) and you can do a home 'taste test' for an indication of your zinc status (see Chapter 3).

Adequate protein intake is also important, as nails are made of the protein keratin. In addition, it has been reported that when people with brittle nails supplement the B vitamin biotin for several months, they get increased firmness, thickness and hardness of nails, with less nail splitting.[41]

We hope you'll agree that there is a great deal you can do to support your skin, gums, veins, hair and nails as you age. This chapter has focused on what you can do nutritionally. Many of these nutraceutical ingredients can now also be found in topical skincare products designed to help slow the ageing process. Antioxidants are popular additives – particularly vitamin A, vitamin C, tocopherols (vitamin E), alpha lipoic acid and CoQ10. You should also look out for creams or serums containing EGCG from green tea, resveratrol, OPCs (grape seed), curcumin, pomegranate and marine-based ingredients.[42]

Antioxidants applied topically have been shown to have anti-inflammatory skin benefits and to slow the rate of ageing from sun damage (photoageing).[43] And there is some preliminary evidence that topical resveratrol may also have some anti-cancer effects in the skin.[44]

Another popular natural ingredient is hyaluronic acid, used in topical formulations and in non-permanent dermal fillers. Peptide-based creams are also becoming more widely available. They may help to prevent the deterioration of collagen-producing cells in ageing skin, encourage collagen production and even visibly reduce the depth of wrinkles.[45] When reading labels, look for copper peptides or for palmitoyl pentapeptide (Matrixyl), which is one of the most popular. Neuropeptides are present in many products, but there seems to be relatively little scientific evidence for their value in preventing skin ageing.

MEAL PLAN

Breakfast	*Antioxidant Green Burst*
	Yogurt with mixed seeds
Lunch	*Vietnamese Chicken Salad with Chilli Lime Dressing*
	Tomato Seeded Crackers
	Bitter Greens with Grapefruit and Avocado
Dinner	*Thai Salmon Fishcakes*
	Mixed salad
Snack	*Beet Mint Dip* with carrot sticks
	Tropical Goji Sorbet

If you do nothing else, do this...

▶ Centre your diet on a wide range of brightly and deeply coloured fruit, vegetables, herbs and spices.

- Take antioxidant and collagen-supporting supplements at the dosages suggested in this chapter.

- For skin-healthy fats, eat nuts and seeds daily and eat oily fish three times a week. Alternatively, take a supplement of fish oil and GLA.

- Avoid sun damage to the skin.

- Eat high-quality protein at every meal.

- Get 7.5–8 hours of quality sleep a night.

- Support your levels of adrenal hormones (especially DHEA) and sex hormones (especially oestrogen and testosterone) by reading the advice in Chapters 6 and 9.

- Follow the advice in Chapter 6 on avoiding toxins.

- Do not smoke. (As nicotine is so addictive, many people find hypnotherapy useful.)

- Switch your brands of personal care products and cosmetics to those that are chemical-free.

- Cook meat and fish at lower temperatures.

- Stay clear of damaged fats, found mainly in processed foods, and take care not to heat vegetable, seed, nut or corn oils.

TIRED BUT WIRED
Tackling the Energy Crisis

Loss of vitality is an all-too-common feature of getting older. We hear in it in our clinics more regularly than any other complaint: 'I just don't have the energy I used to', 'It's a struggle to get up in the mornings', 'I could quite easily have a nap in the afternoon', 'If I drink alcohol I feel completely wiped out', 'My sleep isn't what it used to be' and so on.

All of the healthy ageing strategies described in this book – from losing weight and stabilizing blood sugar levels, to improving the functioning of your digestion, sex hormones, brain chemicals and immune responses – will give you more energy and render you better able to cope with the unexpected curve-balls that life throws your way.

In this chapter, we show you how to give a boost to two glands that are particularly responsible for energy, vitality and your ability to take stressful situations in your stride. These glands are the adrenals and the thyroid. And, to give you a third strategy for beating fatigue, we'll show you how to reduce your toxic load and support your liver in processing and excreting the toxins that bombard us on a daily basis.

THE ADRENAL GLANDS: SUPPLYING YOU WITH STRESS-BUSTING CHEMICALS
DO YOU HAVE ADRENAL FATIGUE?
You can take the following short questionnaire to gauge how well your adrenal glands are working.

Tick the box for each statement that applies to you.

- ☐ Tend to be a 'night person'
- ☐ Find it hard to get up in the morning
- ☐ Rarely wide awake within 30 minutes of rising
- ☐ Feeling tired even after eight hours' sleep
- ☐ Have a lot of day-to-day stress (e.g. a stressful job)
- ☐ Physical exercise makes you feel worse
- ☐ Have an inflammatory condition
- ☐ Apathy/lack of drive
- ☐ Clench or grind teeth
- ☐ Become dizzy when standing up suddenly
- ☐ Rely on tea, coffee or chocolate to get you through the day
- ☐ Low mood/anxiety
- ☐ Crave salty foods
- ☐ Unable to deal with stress
- ☐ Often tearful
- ☐ Chronic fatigue, or get drowsy often
- ☐ Everything seems like a chore
- ☐ Everyday tasks tire you out
- ☐ Not much seems to interest you
- ☐ Never do anything just for fun
- ☐ Feel run down or overwhelmed
- ☐ Afternoon headache
- ☐ Feel physically weak

☐ Low sex drive

☐ Often feel 'fuzzy-headed'

☐ Bad PMS

Total score _____

This set of questions is designed to give you an initial indication of how your adrenals are holding up. If you scored 8 or above, it is likely that your adrenals need some targeted support. It's a sign you may have adrenal dysfunction and/or adrenal fatigue. If this is the case and you ignore the signs, your adrenal function is likely to continue to worsen and you could end up with an adrenal 'crash', which can manifest as a 'nervous breakdown' or chronic fatigue syndrome.

You can find out how well your adrenals are functioning by doing a saliva test that measures the adrenal hormones. This is only available privately, so it's best to see a nutrition practitioner to support you. Typically, the only cortisol measurement done in a conventional medical setting will be to diagnose severe medical conditions of the adrenal glands. Adrenal fatigue does not come into this category; it is a more subtle decline of the hormones, rather than an absence of the hormones.

WHAT IS ADRENAL FATIGUE AND HOW DID I GET IT?
Your adrenal glands keep you feeling young

If you go to see your doctor because you are feeling exhausted, run-down, anxious and unable to deal with the stresses and strains of daily life, it's unlikely that your adrenal glands will come into the conversation. But it is your adrenal function that is largely responsible for your get-up-and-go and your ability to deal with stress.

The adrenals produce lots of hormones but the two we're most interested in here are cortisol – which gets us out of bed in the morning, gives us drive throughout the day and helps us to cope with stressful situations – and DHEA – which counteracts any negative side-effects of excess cortisol. Although cortisol is crucial for getting us through stressful periods, elevated levels can hamper the body's normal repair processes. DHEA is 'anabolic', ensuring that muscles, bones and other tissues don't break down under the influence of high cortisol levels. It's also worth noting that cortisol dampens down inflammation, so, as you will see in Chapter 8, good levels of cortisol during the day can help to curb any unwanted inflammation.

What's more, as you'll see in Chapter 9, it is the adrenal glands that your body relies on post-menopause for its supply of age-defying oestrogen and testosterone.

Your adrenals produce cortisol to a particular daily pattern: cortisol is at its highest between 6am and 7am, giving you the drive to get out of bed and start your day. (DHEA is not produced in such a 'diurnal rhythm' and its supply is more constant.) Cortisol levels gradually decline throughout the day, helping you to deal with whatever life throws at you, until it is time to go to bed. It is at its lowest point from about 11pm for the rest of the night.

When it starts to get dark, your sleep hormone melatonin is released and as this rises you begin to feel sleepy. Cortisol and melatonin are antagonistic, which means that if cortisol is following its normal rhythm and is low all night, melatonin can rise and remain high all night, giving you a good night's sleep.

When your adrenals are working well, you'll feel well. Unfortunately, however, their hormonal output can all too easily become disrupted, especially if you have been under stress for quite some time.

How adrenal fatigue develops

Say, for example, you're going along quite nicely when all of a sudden you get promoted at work. The new job is not what you expected and you find yourself working long hours in order to keep up with your new responsibilities. You begin to find it hard to 'switch off' in the evenings and this makes it hard for you to get to sleep. Increasingly, you find yourself relying on alcohol or starchy, sugary snacks. Although these may help you to relax, you find you are waking in the early hours, where you lie worrying about the stresses of the following day and find it hard to get back to sleep. You seem to catch every cold that's going round and you are becoming concerned about the number of headaches you are getting and your reliance on painkillers.

What's happening here is that your adrenal glands are working overtime to keep pumping out high levels of cortisol and DHEA. When cortisol rises in the morning, it stays high, to help you go into battle. This makes you feel 'wired' all day, and in the evening the high cortisol stops melatonin from rising and you find you can't settle or get to sleep.

Drinking alcohol or snacking on sugary, starchy foods just makes the situation worse because they severely disrupt the sugar levels in your bloodstream: a few hours later, your blood sugar levels plummet (see Chapter 4 for more information on this). Now, your brain and body are energy-starved. This is interpreted as a life-threatening stressor, and cortisol is activated yet again. This wakes you up and starts the cycle of anxiety, overactive mind and racing heart. No wonder you can't get back to sleep!

If this situation continues in the long term, your overworked adrenal glands start to become tired. They become less able to produce sufficient cortisol and DHEA for your excessive needs. What's more, the cortisol receptors, having been bombarded with so much cortisol for so long, can start to become *resistant* to the hormone.[1] This means that what little cortisol you are producing no longer has much of an effect.

With falling cortisol and DHEA, along with cortisol resistance, you begin to feel tired all the time. You can hardly drag yourself out of bed in the morning. Increasingly, you have to rely on coffee and tea to get you through the day. Your mood is low. You don't seem to be interested in anything much and your mind is full of anxiety. You find that even small problems leave you overwhelmed and that you can easily become tearful.

ADRENAL PROBLEMS AFFECT AGEING

Poor adrenal function, from these types of long-term stress situations, causes premature ageing and dramatically increases your risk of developing age-related degenerative illnesses. One of the first people to link adrenal problems with premature ageing was the Canadian doctor Hans Selye, who claimed that 'Every stress leaves an indelible scar.' He says that we pay for our survival after a stressful situation 'by becoming a little older.'[2]

There is plenty of scientific evidence that if you have long-term elevated cortisol levels (from stress), you are far more likely to become obese, insulin-resistant and diabetic,[3] as well as to suffer from depression,[4] age-related cognitive decline[5] and sexual dysfunction.[6] What's more, if your long-term stress tips you over into adrenal fatigue, you're at an increased risk of rheumatoid arthritis and other autoimmune inflammatory diseases,[7] chronic fatigue syndrome,[8] 'atypical' depression, including seasonal affective disorder,[9] and fibromyalgia.[10]

As we see time and time again throughout this book, chronic inflammation is at the root of premature ageing and degenerative diseases – hence the term 'inflamm-ageing'. In adrenal fatigue, you lack sufficient cortisol. Cortisol is your most powerful anti-inflammatory hormone. Thus, adrenal fatigue makes inflamm-ageing, including age-related illnesses, far more likely to affect you.

THE THYROID GLAND: MAINTAINING A YOUTHFUL METABOLISM

Your thyroid gland is a butterfly-shaped gland, situated at the throat, which keeps your metabolism at the right speed to enable you to get the most out of life. A healthy metabolic rate maintains your temperature, keeps you feeling energized and helps you detoxify the toxins that bombard you all day, every day.

MIGHT YOU HAVE A SLUGGISH THYROID?

When problems occur with your thyroid, you can end up either over-producing the thyroid hormones (this is called hyperthyroidism) or, conversely, not producing them in sufficient quantities for your day-to-day needs (hypothyroidism). By far the most common age-related thyroid problem is subclinical *hypo*thyroidism, estimated to affect as many as 20 per cent of women over the age of 60 years.[11] (Subclinical hypothyroidism does not affect all the thyroid hormones but can still cause low-thyroid symptoms and associated health problems.)

A sluggish thyroid will cause your metabolism to slow down and this can contribute to unwanted weight gain and a whole host of other debilitating symptoms that we often associate with 'getting older'. Such symptoms include:

- feeling tired all the time

- morning stiffness, Raynaud's-type symptoms

- slow thinking, poor memory, foggy head

- low mood

- sluggish bowels, constipation

- cold hands and feet

- low sex drive

- infertility

- hair loss

- dry skin.

THYROID PROBLEMS AFFECTING AGEING

Many people struggle on for years with low thyroid function, without a diagnosis. But this isn't a good idea because the longer it goes on, the more likely it will lead to other age-related illnesses. For example, it increases the risk of cardiovascular problems,[12] probably partly because it raises LDL-cholesterol (LDL-c) in the bloodstream (the 'bad' type of cholesterol). LDL-c often returns to normal levels following thyroid hormone treatment.[13]

WHAT YOUR DOCTOR CAN DO

You can easily get your thyroid function checked by your doctor. Levels of thyroid hormones (typically hormones called TSH and T4) are usually included in standard blood tests offered in health checks to people over 40 years of age. What you may not realize, however, is that the 'normal' range for the level of thyroid hormones is extremely wide, meaning that what constitutes an optimal level for one person may not be high enough for good health in another. So, when interpreting your blood results, it's worth also alerting your doctor to the pattern of your symptoms, so that these can help to inform any diagnosis.

Medical treatment of low thyroid function is to take thyroid hormones at a dose that will raise your blood levels to the point where you are not experiencing symptoms. Some people opt for 'bio-identical' thyroid hormones, rather than the licensed formulas offered by their doctor. Bio-identical hormones are available from some doctors practising privately. For more information on bio-identical hormones, see Chapter 9.

If you have symptoms of low thyroid function but your tests do not indicate an immediate need for hormone replacement, you have an opportunity to get your thyroid back on track using the action plan later in this chapter.

THE LIVER: YOUR CLEANSING POWERHOUSE

One of the very best ways to increase your energy and vitality is to reduce your toxic load. And before you make the assumption that you are relatively toxin-free, take a moment to consider the phenomenal amount of toxicants with which you are bombarded every minute of every day.

All of the food, drink and medications you consume need to be detoxified, as do the myriad of chemicals and other toxins you are exposed to in your daily life. These include toxic metals, traffic pollution, bacteria, alcohol, cleaning chemicals and cigarette smoke, to name but a few. To add to this load, your body's normal biological processes produce masses of compounds (such as hormones, brain chemicals and immune system messengers), all of which need to be safely deactivated and disposed of, once they have done their job. We are, each and every one of us, gradually accumulating hundreds of toxins as we go through life.[14]

ARE YOU SUFFERING FROM TOXIC OVERLOAD?

Are these toxins affecting your wellbeing? Well, this depends not only on your level of exposure but also on how well your liver and other organs are able to recognize and disable them. If you are taking in more toxins than your detox systems can cope with, you'll quickly lose your vitality. Some indicators of toxic overload include:

- headaches

- night sweats

- fatigue and sluggishness

- skin eruptions

- low mood and irritability

- slow thinking and poor memory

- sensitivities to chemicals, perfumes or pollution (e.g. sneezing, wheezing, nasal drip and/or skin rashes)

- adverse reactions to food additives, such as sulphites (found in wine, salad bar food, dried fruit and many processed foods – always read the label)

- needing an excessively long time to recover after a general anaesthetic

- bloating, excess wind and constipation

- chronic itching

- bad hangovers from alcohol consumption

- having been on regular medication for some weeks, months or years.

DETOX PROBLEMS AFFECTING AGEING

Far from simply making you *feel* old, a high toxic load can also increase your risk of getting age-related illnesses. Pollutants that disrupt the sex hormones, for example, may make you more susceptible to oestrogen-driven breast cancers.[15] What's more, unless your detox systems are in tip-top condition, they can actually make toxins become even more carcinogenic.[16]

Toxins may trigger certain autoimmune diseases.[17] Mercury may be a risk factor for autoimmune thyroid disease in some people,[18] for example, and you'll see in Chapters 3 and 8 that autoimmune diseases can be triggered by toxins getting into the bloodstream through a 'leaky' gut wall. Problems with detoxifying oestrogen may worsen symptoms of the autoimmune disease lupus.[19] A high toxic load has also been linked to the development of fibromyalgia, chronic fatigue syndrome, Parkinson's disease[20] and other diseases of nerve degeneration.[21]

Some scientists have even proposed that excessive toxicity may disrupt the body's ability to control weight gain and weight loss.[22] Could this help to explain why some people find it so much harder to lose weight than others?

HOW TO GET YOUR VITALITY BACK

Carrying a high toxic load and suffering from adrenal fatigue are both very real and debilitating situations. But the good news is that the right nutritional and lifestyle interventions can often get your adrenals and your detox systems functioning well again. In many cases, this will also take some pressure off your thyroid gland. This is because a flagging thyroid can be brought on by stress and adrenal issues[23] and also because toxic metals, especially mercury and cadmium, can hamper thyroid function.[24] There are also things you can do to directly support your thyroid function. So, read on to find out how you can reclaim your zest for life…

BECOME A STRESS DETECTIVE

The first and most obvious action is to take a long, hard look at all the different sources of stress in your life (mental, emotional and psychological stress) and come up with a plan to remove or reduce them.

Stress is at the centre of adrenal problems and often of thyroid disruption as well. And stress is cumulative, meaning that your adrenals can be suffering now because of stressful events that happened months or even years ago. If you suspect this may be part of your picture, try taking a good exploratory look over your life history, to identify some of your earlier stressors. Then you can consider whether, and how, to either address them – or, alternatively, come to terms with them.

You may need to enlist the help of someone else for this task – a psychotherapist, for example, or a trusted friend or family member.

If you've identified current sources of stress – working long hours, for example, or a difficult relationship – your adrenals are unlikely to recover unless you do something about these stressors. Ultimately, you have three options: change whatever it is that's causing the stress, walk away from it or change your own attitude towards it. Again, you may need to work with others in order to decide your best course of action.

GET THE RIGHT TYPE OF EXERCISE

There are many lifestyle changes you can make to reduce stress, including getting enough sleep, being part of a strong social support network and using relaxation techniques such as mindfulness. Regular physical activity is also important, not only to help reduce stress but also to normalize thyroid function.[25]

Remember, though, that if you are feeling particularly low in energy and vitality, a fast- paced exercise routine may do you more harm than good. In such cases, it's better to engage in low-intensity exercise, such as stretching and light walking, or some of the Eastern forms of exercise such as yoga, qigong and tai chi. These cultivate more energy than they expend, leaving you with enough energy to stimulate and fortify your own natural healing processes.[26] If you like to visit the gym, try adapting your usual routine so that you perform it slowly, with far lighter weights, making sure that you are breathing deeply and relaxing your mind. This combination of low-intensity movement and proper breathing, with a quiet mind, stimulates digestion and elimination, as well as normalizing cortisol if it is elevated and improving your levels of growth and repair hormones.[27]

Chapter 10 contains detailed information on a range of stress-busting activities, as well as advice on how to get a good night's sleep.

STABILIZE YOUR BLOOD SUGAR LEVELS

Stress is not only psychological or emotional in origin. Another common source of stress is erratic blood sugar levels.

It's hard to keep your blood levels of sugar and insulin steady if you are eating a typical modern diet of processed foods, caffeine (tea, coffee, cola, energy drinks and chocolate) and alcohol. As we saw in Chapter 4, all of these cause sharp rises of glucose in the bloodstream, leading to a surge in insulin followed by plummeting blood sugar levels. These episodes can add catastrophically high levels of stress to an already exhausted body. Also be aware that if you drink alcohol regularly, this may be reducing your ability to make the active thyroid hormone.[28]

Switch caffeinated drinks to decaff varieties or sip green tea, rich in calming theanine (see below), and focus on eating the low-GL, antioxidant-rich diet we describe in Chapter 2. Also follow the action plan in Chapter 4 to get your blood sugar levels back under control.

In Chapter 2 we suggested the practices of calorie restriction and fasting as options to consider, to improve your chances of ageing well. This is because there is some evidence for them improving insulin sensitivity and other signs of healthy ageing. However, if your adrenals or thyroid need support, you should not attempt these programmes because they may be too stressful for your adrenal glands and because they can also lower thyroid hormones.[29] If your thyroid is working well, this is rarely a problem, but if your thyroid is already struggling, these dietary regimes may do more harm than good.

Paradoxically, fasting is often promoted as being good for detoxification. The truth, however, is that any fast that lasts for longer than 48 hours can make you *more* toxic. This is because, without the regular intake of protein and other detox nutrients, you'll release toxins from your fat cells but they won't efficiently get through the liver's detox systems. Rather, they're more likely to hang around in the bloodstream, where they can trigger 'fasting' symptoms such as headaches, nausea, skin eruptions, fatigue, low mood, slow thinking and irritability.

TACKLE ANY ONGOING INFLAMMATION

Chronic inflammation puts a huge strain on the body. It can also hamper the activation of thyroid hormones. So, it's best to invest some time in considering whether inflammation could be affecting you.

Chapter 8 gives you an insight into the many different sources of inflammation. Allergies, food intolerances and bacterial infections (such as in the gums or the gut) are common undiagnosed sources. Do you think you may be reacting to any particular types of food? Do you suffer from allergic symptoms such as nasal stuffiness, sneezing or itchy eyes or skin? Do you notice red spots on the toothbrush when you brush your teeth? Read Chapter 8 for more information on dampening down unwanted, destructive inflammation.

STAY CLEAR OF TOXINS, WHERE YOU CAN

Reducing your exposure to toxins will start to relieve the burden on your detoxification systems not only in the liver but also in the gut lining, the skin, the lungs and the brain. There are many simple changes you can make to protect yourself from pollutants in the home, at work and when out of doors. Read the suggestions in Box 6.1 and see how many of them you can put into action within the next week.

BOX 6.1 REDUCING YOUR EXPOSURE TO TOXINS

If you follow these tips, you will be significantly reducing your exposure to toxins. Your liver, your adrenals and your thyroid will all breathe a huge sigh of relief.

YOUR ENVIRONMENT

- ▶ Don't use pesticides or herbicides in your garden.

- ▶ When choosing haircare and skincare products, look for those without added alcohol, sodium lauryl sulphate, parabens, phthalates or other petrochemicals.

- ▶ Avoid aluminium-containing antiperspirants and antacids.

- ▶ When carpeting your home, opt for natural fibres or hardwoods, rather than standard carpets, which are usually treated with chemicals.

- ▶ Think twice before you opt to waterproof and flameproof your furniture coverings and clothes.

- When painting your home or office, opt for paints labelled low- or no-VOC. Paints and finishes release low-level toxic emissions into the air for years after application.

- Take steps to control the levels of dust, bacteria and moulds in your home and office. Make use of indoor plants. Consider using an air filter and/or ionizer to reduce the debris in the air.

- Swap chemically based household cleaners for natural cleaners such as spirit vinegar and bicarbonate of soda.

- Reduce your exposure to low-level EMFs (electro-magnetic fields) by restricting your mobile phone use and removing all but the most essential electrical items from your bedroom. Do you really need a TV in the bedroom? Can you swap your alarm clock for a battery-operated version or, even better, one that runs by clockwork?

- If you are exercising out of doors, stick to traffic-free zones. Be mindful of spending long periods of time in heavy traffic. Is there another way you can get to work or school?

- Avoid passive smoking wherever possible.

YOUR FOOD AND DRINK

- Buy organic food where possible and affordable. In particular, use organic dairy products (milk, cheese, yogurt, etc.), meats and eggs. Wash all fruits and vegetables before eating.

- Avoid eating the larger oily fish such as swordfish, tuna, marlin and shark. These are higher in mercury and chemical pollutants, so switch to the small oily fish like sardines, mackerel, pilchards and anchovies.

- Keep cooking temperatures low, preferably below 200°C/400°F. Meat and fish that is well done or very browned (as in frying, grilling or barbecuing) contains carcinogenic chemicals. If you microwave meat before you cook it as you would normally, and if you eat high-fibre foods at the same time, you might prevent some of these toxic compounds being activated.[30]

- Drink less alcohol. During detoxification, the liver turns alcohol into a chemical called acetaldehyde (which causes hangover symptoms) which is far more toxic than alcohol itself and may increase your risk of cancer.[31] The authoritative World Cancer Research Fund recommends avoiding alcohol if you are keen to remain cancer-free as you age.[32]

- Avoid damaged fats: trans- and hydrogenated fats in processed foods, and vegetable and seed oils that have been heated. See Chapter 8 for more information on these toxic fats and how to avoid them. It's also worth knowing that the 'good' fats (those from oily fish, nuts, seeds and cold-pressed seed oils) help you to produce bile.[33] Good levels of bile ensure that the detoxified toxins are speedily excreted when you have a bowel movement.

- Avoid food additives such as colourings, preservatives, sweeteners and other flavour enhancers.

- Water can contain many toxins and in general it is better to filter tap water with a multi-stage carbon filter or a reverse osmosis filter.

- Try not to drink bottled water from soft plastic containers – chemicals from the plastic can leach into the water. Mineral waters in glass bottles are safer, or use your own steel or hard plastic bottle, filled with filtered tap water.

- Avoid sipping your take-away hot drink through the plastic lid.

- Don't use plastics in the microwave – use glass or ceramic containers instead.

- Make sure that any plastic containers you use for drinking, food storage or smoothie shakers are free from bisphenol A (BPA).

- Replace any Teflon cook- and bakeware with uncoated glass, clay, stone or enamel versions.

- Try not to use cling wraps or aluminium foil. Replace them with paper wraps such as baking parchment.

▶ If you need to lose weight, do it gradually. Toxins are stored in fat cells. Extreme weight loss programmes can cause fat cells to be broken down so quickly that stored toxins flood into the bloodstream. This can make you feel sluggish, headachy and irritable – and very likely to lose the motivation to continue eating healthily.

▶ Avoid recreational drugs. If you smoke, do your best to stop. As nicotine is so strongly addictive, many people find hypnotherapy and/or psychotherapy helpful. Chapter 7 has advice on kicking addictions.

▶ Try to avoid over-the-counter medications where possible, especially paracetamol, ibuprofen and other painkillers. Chapter 8 gives more insight into the problems with these drugs.

▶ If you are taking prescription medications, ask your doctor whether it might be possible to reduce any of them.

EAT SPECIAL DETOXING FOODS

Certain special foods help your detoxification systems to work better:[34]

▶ Pomegranate juice: Use it in smoothies such as our *Joint Repair Iced Shake*.

▶ Berries: In winter you can use frozen varieties. See our recipes for *Antioxidant Green Burst, Maca Stress-Busting Smoothie, Berry Muffins, Fruit Parfait* and *Tropical Goji Sorbet*.

▶ Green tea and coffee: Make them decaff if you are caffeine-sensitive. Try the recipes for *Tropical Protein Smoothie, Longevity Cashew Latte* and *Matcha Green Tea Chia Pudding*.

▶ Turmeric and ginger: These feature in our recipes for *Tofu Vegetable Scramble, Turmeric Glazed Fish with Cucumber Pickle, Anti-Inflammatory Turmeric Shake* and *Asian Chicken Noodle Soup*.

- Onions and garlic: Try our *Parchment-Baked Fish with Tamarind and Lime* and our *Tempeh Coconut Curry*.

- Citrus zest: You can use a fine cheese grater to zest the skins of oranges, lemons and limes. Make sure you use unwaxed fruits. A simple blitz of citrus zest, fresh root ginger, garlic and olive oil makes a lively dressing for fish, cooked vegetables or salads.

- Beetroot: See our recipes for *Energizing Beets Juice, Beet Mint Dip* and *Roasted Baby Beets with Tempeh and Walnut Dressing*.

- Various herbs including coriander (cilantro), dill, parsley, rosemary and mint: Add large handfuls to salads.

- Cruciferous vegetables such as cabbage, cauliflower, broccoli, Brussels sprouts, kale and rocket (arugula). Chapter 9 has more information on the age-defying powers of cruciferous vegetables. To get the best effects, eat them every day. You don't have to limit their use to lunch or dinner – see our tasty snack recipes for *Cauliflower Munchies, Salted Vinegar and Onion Kale Chips* and *Kale-onaise*.

Remember that if your detox systems are working well, your body will be far less damaged by the toxins you eat, drink, breathe in and touch. It is this ability to boost detox functions that makes certain plant chemicals good candidates for reducing your risk of cancer as you get older.[35]

Most of these nutrients are available in supplement form and are popular with healthy ageing enthusiasts. Many of the phytochemicals are also antioxidants (see Chapter 5) and anti-inflammatory (see Chapter 8), so they provide support in more ways than one.

GET ENOUGH OF THE MINERALS FOR ADRENAL, THYROID AND DETOX FUNCTIONS

These glands will not function well if you are deficient in essential minerals. Magnesium is one of the most important anti-stress nutrients. Deficiency hampers adrenal function and causes anxiety.[36] See Box 6.2 for more information on the importance of increasing magnesium.

There are four minerals that are absolutely crucial for keeping your thyroid working well. They are iodine, iron, zinc and selenium.[37] Iodine forms part of the thyroid hormones, while iron, zinc and selenium help thyroid enzymes to create the hormones and activate them. Iron is also needed to make your detoxification enzymes.[38]

Good food sources of iodine are sea fish, shellfish and seaweeds, and there is also some in eggs and milk. The best sources of zinc are red meat, crab, poultry and calf's liver, although there is also some in seeds (especially pumpkin seeds), seaweeds and whole grains. Selenium is found in Brazil nuts, meat, poultry, fish and whole grains.

If you are low in iron, by far the best source is 'haem iron' from lean red meat, liver and the darker meat from game, poultry and oily fish, as well as eggs. Vegetarian iron is found in beans, pulses, dark green leaves and dried fruit. Unfortunately, it is not nearly as well absorbed as haem iron, although this may be helped by eating foods rich in vitamin C foods at the same time, such as fruit and raw or lightly cooked vegetables.

A good multivitamin and mineral supplement should include useful levels of iodine, iron, zinc and selenium. It is unlikely to contain enough magnesium for adrenal support, so you should supplement this separately. Take 300–450mg of magnesium (ideally in the form of magnesium citrate), less if you are eating a lot of nuts, seeds and green leafy vegetables.

INCREASE THE THYROID-, ADRENAL- AND DETOX-BOOSTING VITAMINS

Vitamins are crucial for energy and vitality. This is hardly surprising, given their important role in producing adrenal and thyroid hormones. Vitamin B5, for example, is vital for adrenal hormone production.[39]

B12 and folate are two of the most important nutrients for keeping the process of methylation working well. In Chapter 7 we explain what methylation is and why it is so vital for keeping your mind, memory and mood in good working order as you age. It just so happens that this process of methylation is also crucial for detoxifying a huge array of different toxins. The better you are methylating, the less you will be affected by toxic build-up. And if you have a sluggish thyroid, it is worthwhile knowing that hypothyroid patients are more likely to be low in B12 and have higher homocysteine levels.[40] This makes B vitamin intake particularly important.

B vitamins are found in the protein foods mentioned above, as well as in nuts, seeds, whole grains and leafy greens. Look for a high-strength B vitamin complex or a multivitamin and mineral supplement that contains all the B vitamins, including B1, B2, B3 and B6 at 20–50mg of each and B5 (pantothenic acid) at 100mg. You want at least 400mcg of folate (in the active L-methylfolate form) and 300–400mcg of vitamin B12. Refer to Chapter 10 for more on supplements.

The adrenal glands hold a lot of vitamin C; and if your levels are low, this is hugely stressful to the body.[41] Good sources are salad greens, broccoli, bell peppers and fresh fruits, especially strawberries and citrus fruits such as oranges, lemons and grapefruit. If you are run-down and exhausted from adrenal fatigue, however, it can be hard to get a therapeutic dose of vitamin C from food alone. We recommend supplementing 1000–2000mg a day until you start feeling better. This is best done in two or more divided doses, or by taking a time-release supplement that provides you with vitamin C over a longer period.

The most important vitamin for the thyroid gland is vitamin A,[42] found in liver, eggs and dairy products. If you are vegetarian, eating lots of orange and dark green fruits and vegetables will give you beta-carotene. Most of us can convert beta-carotene to vitamin A. However, as we saw in Chapter 5, many people may be poor converters of beta-carotene to vitamin A, due to genetic variations. Because of this, supplementing vitamin A is probably wise if you are not eating foods rich in vitamin A. Look for a multivitamin and mineral supplement that includes pre-formed vitamin A.

LOOK AFTER YOUR BATTERIES

Inside each of our cells lie hundreds of tiny batteries called mitochondria. Their role is to turn the proteins, fats and carbohydrates from our food into energy that we can use to go about our daily lives. This energy is required for all body processes, including detoxification and the production of adrenal and thyroid hormones. As we age, our mitochondria become less efficient at producing energy. And, as you might expect, this can lead to persistent, debilitating fatigue, especially when under stress.

Problems with the mitochondria can also cause persistent muscular aches and pains and increase the risk of age-related diseases as diverse as chronic fatigue syndrome, migraine, fibromyalgia, depression, insulin resistance and diabetes, Parkinson's disease, Alzheimer's disease, periodontal disease (gum disease) and cardiovascular disease.[43]

We saw in Chapter 5 that the process of oxidation (the production of free radicals) is a key driver of premature ageing. It's worth knowing, then, that the greatest internal sources of free radicals are mitochondria that are malfunctioning. The mitochondria produce free radicals as normal by-products of their energy production processes. But if the mitochondria are not working properly, these free radicals can leak out and cause damage to surrounding tissues.

This is the reason that scientists now believe that damaged mitochondria are big players in the process of premature ageing. The American biochemist Bruce Ames proposes that if we can improve the functioning of these tiny batteries, we may be able to delay the ageing process.[44]

Identifying the most important nutrients to support the mitochondria is currently a popular area of research. As well as the vitamins and minerals already discussed in this chapter, nutrients that show promise for helping with fatigue and other mitochondrial illnesses include CoQ10, alpha lipoic acid, acetyl-L-carnitine and glycophospholipids. All of these have some evidence for making our batteries work better.[45] If you want to try supplementing them, we suggest starting with dosages of 100–200mg CoQ10, 1.5–3g acetyl-L-carnitine, 300–600mg alpha lipoic acid and 1–2g phospholipid mix (containing a broad range, such as phosphatidylcholine, phosphatidylethanolamine, phosphatidylserine, phosphatidylglycerol and phosphatidylinositol). Like most nutrients, each of these may be better absorbed and utilized if taken in two or more divided doses. And if you are taking statin medication, you should certainly be taking CoQ10 because statins prevent you from being able to produce CoQ10 yourself. Indeed, common side-effects of statin use include fatigue and muscular aches and pains, both symptoms of mitochondrial problems.

ADD STRESS-BUSTING PLANT COMPOUNDS

People living with adrenal fatigue often find that taking one or more of the botanicals listed below can provide a real boost:

- Maca (*Lepidium peruvianum*) is a Peruvian root that can be bought in powdered form from health food shops and online. It has long been used traditionally to support the body in times of stress and it has been found to reduce signs of stress in animals.[46] Maca can easily be added to smoothies and desserts and used in baking.

- *Rhodiola rosea* is a herb used in Asia and Russia for centuries to help enhance stamina and performance. It has an 'adaptogenic' effect on body systems involved in stress. This means that it is able to normalize factors such as stress hormone production, heart rate, mood and mental clarity in times of stress,[47] enabling you to better deal with whatever life throws at you, day to day. In human studies it has been found to reduce anxiety,[48] and also to alleviate fatigue, improving physical and mental performance.[49] Use a supplement of 300mg *Rhodiola rosea* that states on the label that it is standardized to 3 per cent rosavins. Take one capsule 1–3 times a day, depending on your particular need. It can be taken with or without food.

- Ashwaghanda (*Withania somnifera*) is a revered 'rejuvenating' herb of the Indian Ayurvedic system of medicine. It is used as a general nerve tonic and is thought to mimic the effects of the calming brain chemical gamma aminobutyric acid (GABA)[50] (see Chapter 7 for more information on GABA). Ashwaghanda has been found to help people with a history of chronic stress, reducing their raised cortisol levels and anxiety, and improving their general wellbeing.[51] It is used to improve stamina and may even be helpful in preventing stress-induced gastric ulcers.[52] The dose to try is 125–250mg of a standardized extract.

- Ginseng: *Panax ginseng* is another Eastern herb used to revitalize the mind and body. Its ability to increase resistance to stress and to improve general vigour has led to it being studied in stress-related conditions such as high blood pressure, pain, menopausal symptoms and suppressed immunity.[53] Another type of ginseng, Siberian ginseng (*Eleutherococcus senticosus*) also helps with stress and related problems such as ulcers and inflammation.[54] Take 250–500mg daily, standardized to 15 per cent ginsenosides.

▸ L-theanine is an amino acid found in tea leaves, but in such low concentrations that if you want to benefit from it, you should take it in supplement form. One of L-theanine's most common uses is to reduce anxiety and increase feelings of calm and relaxation,[55] and it may also help to curb sharp rises in blood pressure that occur when we are under stress.[56] L-theanine increases the activity of 'alpha-waves' in the brain, just like meditation does, and this leads to a relaxed yet alert state. We recommend 200mg of L-theanine on an empty stomach, twice a day, if you are under stress. At higher doses, L-theanine can cause drowsiness. This means that it can also be useful as an aid to sleep. Try 400mg on an empty stomach an hour before bedtime.[57]

▸ 5-hydroxytryptophan (5-HTP) is another amino acid, one that your body and brain make by using tryptophan from animal protein foods, especially chicken and turkey. You'll see in Chapter 7 that 5-HTP helps to improve levels of your 'happy' chemical serotonin, which improves mood. And you'll see in Chapter 8 that 5-HTP may also help with conditions of chronic pain. Both of these effects may help to reduce stress.

But 5-HTP may also reduce stress in another way: the serotonin it produces is then turned into the hormone melatonin, which helps you to feel sleepy and get a good night's sleep. If you think you may be low in serotonin (e.g. if you suffer from chronic pain, poor sleep and low mood, and you crave sugary or starchy foods), try taking 200mg 5-HTP on an empty stomach, about half an hour before bed. It can be taken together with L-theanine for an even greater therapeutic effect.

Many of our clients have been given renewed vigour from adding one or more of these tonics to their nutrition and lifestyle programme. We're all different in the way we respond to individual nutraceuticals:

a bioactive that may have amazing effects for one person may not do the same for another. The only way to find out what has the best effect for you is to try each one, individually. Give it at least four weeks to work before you make your mind up, and leave at least two weeks between trialling different supplements.

BOX 6.2 THE RESTORATIVE POWER OF MAGNESIUM

Magnesium is a mineral essential for life, as it is used in more than 300 biological reactions in the body.[58] Magnesium keeps your bones strong and helps to produce energy. It's important for keeping your blood sugar levels stable, for making vital proteins, for helping muscles and nerves work properly and for keeping inflamm-ageing (age-promoting, chronic inflammation) at bay.

Yet, most of us don't get enough of this age-defying mineral in our diets. According to government statistics, we get about 228mg a day from food.[59] This is considerably lower than the new recommended daily allowance (RDA) of 375mg.

WHY ARE WE LOW IN MAGNESIUM?

Magnesium is found in legumes, whole grains, vegetables, nuts and seeds. Because so much magnesium is lost during food processing, most people on a typical modern diet don't get enough. White rice and white bread, for example, contain only a fraction of the magnesium of their wholegrain varieties.

What's more, some magnesium-rich foods also contain compounds that hamper its absorption: some leafy greens such as spinach, beet greens, Swiss chard, okra and parsley contain oxalates that bind to magnesium before it can be absorbed. And phytates in soy and in whole grains such as wheat and rye have the same problematic effect. If you're going to eat these (healthful) greens, it's best to lightly boil or steam them to reduce the oxalate load.[60] Eating whole grains in the form of bread, especially sourdough bread, reduces the troublesome phytates.[61] If you want to further maximize the amount of magnesium you absorb from food, you may be interested to know that a particular type of soluble fibre, fructo-oligo-saccharides (FOS), can do just this.[62] You can take FOS in supplement form.

Another reason for so many of us being low in magnesium is that it is easily leached from the body under certain circumstances. Do you consume higher than average amounts of alcohol, fat, salt, phosphate (in carbonated drinks), caffeine or tannins (in tea)? Do you sweat a lot (in steam baths, for instance, or during intense exercise)? Do you experience prolonged periods of stress? Each of these factors can cause your magnesium stores to become depleted.[63]

It may be that, due to dietary and lifestyle factors, you have been living for many years with magnesium levels that are too low for healthy ageing. Addressing these same dietary and lifestyle factors is crucial to rectify the situation, but it may be worth also taking a daily magnesium supplement.

SIGNS AND SYMPTOMS OF LOW MAGNESIUM

Some typical signs of magnesium deficiency include fatigue and apathy, muscle cramps, muscle weakness or muscle twitching, pre-menstrual syndrome (PMS), blood sugar problems, asthma, poor sleep, mild depression, palpitations, high blood pressure and constipation. As we saw earlier in this chapter, many of these are also symptoms of adrenal fatigue. As low magnesium levels hamper adrenal function and cause anxiety,[64] you need to be especially sure to increase your intake if you are under stress.

SUPPLEMENTING MAGNESIUM: AN ESSENTIAL COMPONENT OF YOUR HEALTHY AGEING PLAN?

Magnesium has so many vital roles in the body that the range of illnesses caused by its deficiency has been described by scientists as 'staggering'.[65] Moreover, anyone who is looking to age well should consider supplementing it because it is anti-inflammatory[66] and it works as an antioxidant.[67] As we have seen throughout this book, both inflammation and oxidation are key drivers of premature ageing and degenerative diseases.[68]

Because it is so important for the process of energy production, magnesium is one of the first nutrients to consider if you are suffering from regular fatigue. It has even been used with some success in chronic fatigue syndrome and fibromyalgia – two debilitating illnesses of extreme tiredness.[69]

Magnesium is crucial for bone health and has been found helpful for improving signs of bone loss in postmenopausal women.[70] Bone loss and osteoporosis are real concerns during and after the menopause, as seen in Chapter 9.

Low magnesium levels are also something to consider if you are concerned about age-related gum disease and tooth loss. Magnesium is important for keeping the jaw bone strong, but it has also been found to reduce the probing depth between the teeth and gums in people with gum disease.[71] The probing[72] depth is the extent to which the gum tissue has started to pull away from the tooth as a result of inflammation caused by bacteria in the build-up of dental plaque.

People who get more magnesium tend to have lower insulin levels[73] and a lower risk of developing insulin resistance and type 2 diabetes. We saw in Chapter 4 that both these conditions are more prevalent as we get older, and having them also makes you age faster. If you already have diabetes, your risk of developing complications increases, the lower your magnesium status.[74]

The good news is that taking magnesium supplements may reduce insulin resistance[75] and may also improve the control of blood fats, blood sugar and blood pressure in diabetic patients.[76] Supplementing magnesium may be especially important if you are concerned about cardiovascular disease. Low levels of magnesium cause the arteries to constrict too much, leading to high blood pressure,[77] and there is some evidence that taking magnesium supplements may help to bring down elevated blood pressure.[78] What's more, magnesium may reduce angina attacks in people with coronary artery disease[79] and also help people with congestive heart failure.[80]

NOT ALL MAGNESIUM SUPPLEMENTS ARE EQUAL

Magnesium supplements come in many different forms. If you're going to use one, it is worth knowing that some are much better absorbed than others. The best forms are those that are either chelated (attached) to an amino acid (such as magnesium gluconate or magnesium taurate) or an organic acid (such as magnesium malate or magnesium citrate).[81] These are so well absorbed that you don't need to take them with food – you can take them between meals or at bedtime. This is useful because magnesium is also better absorbed when it doesn't have to compete with other minerals. A more commonly sold form is magnesium oxide but this may have an absorption rate as low as only 4 per cent.[82]

A dose of 300–450mg of elemental magnesium in one of the better forms listed above is a good level to supplement if you are suffering from stress or fatigue.

MEAL PLAN

Breakfast	*Grain-Free Breakfast Bowl*
Lunch	*Lemon Harissa Turkey Leaf Wraps* with mixed salad
Dinner	*Moroccan Beef Tagine*
	Chocolate Lime Mousse
Snack	*Maca Stress-Busting Smoothie*
	Blueberries with yogurt

If you do nothing else, do this...

▸ Identify the main sources of stress in your life and take action to reduce them – don't be afraid of enlisting the help of others to achieve this.

▸ Get enough (but not too much) physical activity every day.

▸ Eat a low-GL diet and optimize nutrients to stabilize your blood sugar levels (see Chapter 4).

▸ Tackle any ongoing inflammation (e.g. sinusitis, gum disease) (see Chapter 8).

▸ Reduce your exposure to toxins (see Box 6.1).

▸ Eat detoxifying foods every day, such as pomegranate, berries, green tea, onions, garlic, turmeric, ginger, beetroot, herbs and cruciferous vegetables (cauliflower, broccoli, etc.).

- Take a multivitamin and mineral supplement with good levels of vitamin A, B vitamins, selenium, zinc and iodine.

- Take extra vitamin C totalling 1–2g a day, and extra magnesium (see Box 6.2).

- Get your ferritin levels tested and take an iron supplement if this is indicated.

- Consider a trial of CoQ10, acetyl-L-carnitine and/or alpha lipoic acid at the doses recommended in this chapter.

- Consider trialling one of the stress-busting plant compounds outlined in this chapter, at the doses recommended: rhodiola, ashwaghanda, L-theanine, 5-HTP, ginseng (Siberian or Korean) and/or maca.

CHAPTER 7

MAKING THE MOST OF YOUR MIND, MEMORY AND MOOD

What's the point of old age if you can't enjoy it? This is a particularly pertinent question when considering the age-related changes that take place in the brain: your mood, your memory and your ability to think clearly are all very much dependent on the functioning of your brain cells and the balance of your brain chemicals.

WHAT BRAIN CHEMICALS DO

Brain chemicals are known technically as neurotransmitters. There are numerous types and their job is to transmit messages along and between neurons (the billions of nerve cells in the brain).

Some of the most frequently studied neurotransmitters are listed here:

▶ Serotonin is often described as the 'happy' neurotransmitter. Serotonin is further metabolized to melatonin, an important antioxidant hormone that promotes sleep. (See Chapter 5 for more on antioxidants.)

▶ Dopamine, adrenalin and noradrenalin (known as the 'catecholamines') help you feel energized and in control. They provide drive, energy, focus and an upbeat mood. Adrenalin is the first chemical released in response to stress. Dopamine gives us a profound feeling of reward from whatever it is that has triggered the dopamine release. Unsurprisingly, it is stimulated by addictive behaviours and substances, including smoking, recreational drugs and sugar. But it is also released in response to positive social interaction with the people around us.

- Glutamate is a potent stimulator of brain activity. Excessive levels can cause so much brain cell excitement that it can start to kill them off.

- Gamma aminobutyric acid (GABA) quietens brain activity, leading to a sense of relaxation and calm.

- Acetylcholine aids memory, mental alertness and skeletal muscle function.

- Endorphins promote a sense of euphoria and work in a similar way to opiate drugs, relieving pain.

THE PERPETUAL PROCESS OF NEUROTRANSMISSION

These neurotransmitters are phenomenally powerful, having the ability to change our entire outlook on life. Nevertheless, they can only be effective if they are able to latch on to, and activate, the special receptors on the neurons' membranes, and then transmit messages along these cells. (Nerve cells tend to be long and thin.) At times, the brain chemicals have to jump between synapses, which are bulb-like structures at the end of each long neuron. This helps one neuron to communicate with another. Once the neurotransmitter has fulfilled its message-delivery role, the brain needs to decide whether to break it down and get rid of it or, alternatively, recycle it for use again.

This entire process, known as neurotransmission, is extremely complex. These myriad message-carrying molecules have to convert themselves between chemical and electrical forms, many times over, in order to transmit emotions, thoughts and physical sensations. The importance of keeping neurotransmission on track as we age cannot be underestimated, as it so strongly influences how we think, feel and behave on a day-to-day basis.

THE NEED FOR BALANCE

The brain needs to manage the delicate *balance* of all the different types of brain chemicals. Problems can arise both from a lack of, and an over-abundance of, one or more of them.

Serotonin, for example, is a highly desirable chemical because it helps us to be happy – maintaining good mood, reducing our sensitivity to pain (both emotional and physical) and improving sleep (through its conversion to the sleep hormone melatonin). But did you know that if your serotonin levels become too elevated you can end up over-stimulating your nervous system? This can lead to symptoms such as muscle tremor, or you may feel agitated, restless and confused, or experience loose bowels. If left untreated, you can become delirious and seriously ill.

This situation can occur as a side-effect of using serotonin-enhancing drugs, such as the antidepressants known as selective serotonin reuptake inhibitors (SSRIs – Prozac and others), or by unforeseen drug interactions.[1] Where possible, it might be safer to enhance your mood and brain chemistry in a more natural way. Read on to find out how to do this…

How well balanced is your brain chemistry?
Take the following short questionnaire to gauge the extent to which your brain chemistry may need some support.

Do you experience the following symptoms? Tick the box for each statement that applies to you.

☐ Have found it impossible to give up smoking

☐ Feel a need to drink alcohol

☐ Starch and sugar cravings

☐ Binge eating

☐ Take recreational drugs

☐ Poor sleep

☐ Low pain threshold

☐ Inability to concentrate

☐ Hyperactivity/jittery/can't relax

☐ Low mood

☐ Irritability

☐ Anxiety

☐ Slow thinking

☐ Poor memory

☐ Feeling of not being connected with others

☐ Mental sluggishness and fatigue

☐ Apathy and lack of motivation

Total score _____

As we age, we need to work harder to keep these symptoms at bay. If you scored 5 or above, your brain chemistry may need some specific support. (Note that laboratory tests for neurotransmitter levels are also available through some qualified nutrition/health practitioners and may enable more targeted support.)

It's certainly worthwhile investigating and addressing the causes of such symptoms now, before they develop into something worse. Remember that when things are out of balance for too long, dysfunctions in body processes become so entrenched that they eventually become chronic diseases. You may have symptoms that you can just about live with at the moment, such as feeling generally low, irritable and apathetic, or suffering frustrating cravings for chocolate, cake and bread. These *may* be due to easily correctable imbalances. If so, do something about these *now*, before they progress into more serious symptoms that indicate disease. The body can put up with maltreatment for quite some time – but not forever.

To get an idea of the types of serious chronic illnesses that develop partly due to brain chemistry imbalances, see Box 7.1.

BOX 7.1 BRAIN CHEMISTRY IMBALANCES CAN LEAD TO CHRONIC ILLNESSES

The following very serious, debilitating chronic conditions all have their roots partly in brain chemistry imbalances. Many such imbalances, if caught early enough, may be resolved using drug-free methods.

▶ Depression: Major depressive disorders are thought to be due to a functional deficiency of serotonin and/or noradrenalin.[2]

▶ Alzheimer's disease: This condition arises partly because you lose your ability to convert the nutrient choline into acetylcholine within the brain.[3] (This conversion is undertaken by the process of methylation – see page 163.)

▶ Parkinson's disease: Here, the neurons responsible for producing dopamine are gradually destroyed.[4]

▶ Alcoholism: In alcoholics the dopamine, GABA and opioid systems are malfunctioning.[5] Similar patterns of compromised brain chemicals are found in drug abuse and other addictions.[6]

▶ Eating disorders, such as binge eating, anorexia nervosa and bulimia: These may be partly due to changes in the way that dopamine, acetylcholine and opioid systems behave in the brain.[7] These disorders have also been associated with abnormal levels of GABA.[8]

▶ Syndromes in which you have a heightened sense of physical pain, such as fibromyalgia and migraine (see Chapter 8).

As is the case with most degenerative diseases of ageing, many of the health problems listed here are either triggered or worsened by chronic, low-level, body-wide inflammation.

HOW TO OPTIMIZE YOUR BRAIN FUNCTION AND MOOD

As we've seen above, balanced brain chemistry requires that we produce the right neurotransmitters at the right times, that they latch on successfully to neurons, that they are transmitted smoothly along and between these cells, and are then broken down or recycled, according to need. In this section we give you the low-down on how to optimize these processes without the use of drugs.

PROTECT YOUR BRAIN CELLS FROM AN EARLY DEATH

Neurotransmitters are produced by specialized brain cells. So it makes sense to keep these brain cells healthy and preserve them from an early demise. Brain and nerve cells are known as post-mitotic cells. While other types of body cells are periodically renewed, sometimes in as short a time as a few days (e.g. skin cells and the cells of the gut lining), neuronal cells are rarely, or never, replaced during your lifetime. Some may even be as old as you are. Degenerative diseases such as Alzheimer's and Parkinson's are characterized by a progressive loss of neurons, and as the cells are rarely replaced, they are often lost forever.[9]

Keep them from rusting

One of the best-documented causes of brain cell death is the process of oxidation. This is where you become burdened with too many 'free radicals' and you don't have enough antioxidant power to calm them down and stop them from damaging cells . This destructive process can be likened to the gradual rusting of metal and it is explained in detail in Chapter 5. People suffering from neurodegeneration tend to have elevated levels of oxidation, and this has also been found in neurological diseases such as Alzheimer's disease[10] and Parkinson's disease.[11]

Reducing oxidation means changing your diet and lifestyle to avoid unnecessary exposure to free radicals. Chapter 5 has an action plan to help you achieve this. But, as you'll have seen in Chapter 6, one of the main sources of free radicals is your cells' batteries becoming faulty. All cells contain microscopic batteries – they're called the mitochondria and their role is to manufacture energy out of the raw materials that we get from food (these being sugars, proteins and fats).

Faulty batteries leak free radicals (causing oxidative damage to cells) and they also lead to a drop in energy production. It is for these two reasons that some scientists propose mitochondrial dysfunction to be the single most important factor causing premature ageing.[12]

In recent years, scientists have discovered that many disorders of the mind and mood are due partly to such a decline in battery power. They've found, for example, that mitochondria become sluggish and inefficient in Parkinson's disease patients years before these patients are diagnosed with the disease.[13] Other conditions of the mind, namely depression, seasonal affective disorder (SAD), chronic fatigue syndrome (CFS) and Alzheimer's disease, may also be partly due to battery failure.[14]

How can you reduce the damaging free radicals that leak from your mitochondria? One way is to increase your levels of antioxidants. In Chapter 6, we showed you that some specific antioxidants and other nutrients may be able to slow the decay of these microscopic batteries, and that this, in turn, may also help to delay the ageing process.[15] These key nutrients include the antioxidants CoQ10 and alpha lipoic acid, the amino acid acetyl-L-carnitine and certain phospholipids. Supplementing these 'energy' nutrients also seems to help patients suffering from the neurological conditions listed above, including depression, SAD, CFS and Alzheimer's disease.[16]

We suggest following the antioxidant recommendations in Chapter 5, including eating at least eight portions of brightly coloured vegetables and 2–3 portions of fruit a day. If you want to supplement the battery-supportive nutrients mentioned above, we suggest starting with dosages of 100–200mg CoQ10, 1.5–3g acetyl-L-carnitine, 300–600mg alpha lipoic acid and 1–2g phospholipid mix (containing a broad range, such as phosphatidylcholine, phosphatidylethanolamine, phosphatidylserine, phosphotidylglycerol and phosphatidylinositol). Like most nutrients, each of these may be better absorbed and utilized if taken in two or more divided doses.

Another excellent source of antioxidants is green tea. This super-beverage also offers another benefit: it contains an amino acid called L-theanine, which increases low levels of the brain chemicals serotonin, dopamine and GABA, enhances learning and memory, and also reduces anxiety.[17] Because of these effects, L-theanine is thought to reduce the potentially negative effects of excessive caffeine.[18] This may be why most people can drink 2–3 cups of caffeinated green tea a day, without feeling 'wired'. (Do monitor your own ability to tolerate caffeine, as we are all different.) Note that to get a truly therapeutic effect from L-theanine, you may need to supplement it, as explained in Chapter 6.

Protect their fuel supply

We've seen that brain cells need good battery power to remain healthy – they have a high need for energy. In order to produce this energy, the mitochondria rely on good and regular supplies of oxygen and glucose. If either of these is in short supply, brain cells are in trouble.

A sudden and extreme loss of oxygen to the brain is known medically as a stroke, which can cause temporary or permanent brain damage. More gradual, chronic problems with oxygen supply tend to cause dementia. An example of this is the memory decline associated with narrowing of the arteries in cardiovascular disease. Even a sedentary lifestyle can reduce the flow of blood and oxygen to the brain, leaving you feeling apathetic and depressed. Is it any wonder that aerobic exercise is one of the most effective pick-me-ups and has been found time and time again to help improve depressive symptoms?[19] See Box 7.2 for an action plan for improving mood.

Now, let's turn our attention to glucose. Dips in this fuel supply are well known for causing problems with memory and mood that are immediately noticeable. Such 'hypoglycaemic' symptoms can include irritability, fatigue, shakiness and dizziness, and can leave you feeling miserable, short-tempered, fuzzy-headed, with a sharp drop in memory function and the ability to concentrate.

These energy-sapping episodes of plummeting blood sugar levels tend to occur if you are eating a diet high in sugars, refined foods, caffeine or alcohol, or if you are under long-term stress or are not eating enough protein. The best way to prevent the 'hypos' is to adopt the low-GL diet introduced in Chapter 2. This will provide the brain with a steady supply of glucose. Remember, a low-GL diet is one that contains plenty of vegetables, pulses, nuts, seeds and their oils, lean meat, fish, eggs and poultry, as well as some optional whole grains and seasonal fruit. Processed foods should be reduced or, better still, avoided.

Prevent death by sugar

A low-GL diet will also help to prevent another cytotoxic process from damaging brain cells – the process of glycation. In Chapter 5, we saw that this occurs where there is so much sugar in the bloodstream that it attaches to proteins and cells in the body, damaging them and rendering them dysfunctional. As we saw in Chapter 4, people with insulin resistance and diabetes are particularly vulnerable, but anyone failing to control their blood sugar levels is at risk. Adopting a low-GL diet and getting some cardiovascular exercise every day are the best lifestyle choices to help prevent this situation.

The dietary practices of calorie restriction and intermittent fasting are currently being studied for their potential role in helping to slow brain ageing and the onset of disorders such as Alzheimer's and Parkinson's diseases.[20] Chapters 2 and 4 contain details on these ways of eating and how you can incorporate them into your healthy ageing programme.

BOX 7.2 DRUG-FREE MOOD BOOSTERS

Depression is a very real and very debilitating illness, and there is no doubt that some people with clinical depression gain significant benefits from antidepressant drugs, especially when combined with psychotherapy. But prescriptions for such drugs are now phenomenally high. A recent study found that antidepressant drug use in Europe has increased by an average of almost 20 per cent a year over the last 15 years.[21] Are all the patients taking these medications really clinically depressed?

Maybe you feel low in mood or occasionally depressed, but this does not mean you have a major depressive disorder. And it would be a lot more effective to identify and address all the factors that may be contributing to your low mood rather than artificially cause a massive increase in the levels of your 'happy' brain chemicals. Because this is what antidepressant drugs do: they prevent the 'reuptake' of serotonin, and sometimes dopamine and noradrenalin, leaving more of them available to have an effect on brain cells. Flooding the system with these chemicals may indeed have a mood-lifting effect, but it doesn't treat the *cause* of your depressive-like symptoms (unless the cause happens to be confined to abnormally low serotonin production).

And it's also worth remembering that all drugs carry the risk of side-effects. You only have to read the patient leaflets accompanying the medications to see the vast range of them. One particular aspect we want to stress is that the action of these drugs is not restricted to the brain alone: it also causes neurotransmitters to rise elsewhere in the body. Where the levels in certain tissues are already optimal, artificially pushing them higher will produce a new imbalance in the body and is likely to cause harm. For example, if noradrenalin becomes too elevated, this can lead to unwanted rises in blood pressure.[22] And within the last few years it has been seen that artificially raising serotonin (through the use of 'SSRI' drugs) may cause bone loss in women.[23] Many women are prescribed SSRIs to help them through a difficult menopause transition.

If you want to explore less risky ways of improving your mood, here are some factors to consider, in order to get to the bottom of what's going on:

▶ Are you stressed out? This can cause anxiety and low mood and can contribute to the development of depression.[24] Take the questionnaire in Chapter 6 to see if your stress responses need some support.

▶ How active are you? A sedentary lifestyle can lead to low mood, due to diminished blood flow to the brain, whereas regular exercise can help improve depression and mental health, as we've seen in this chapter. Aerobic exercise increases the feel-good endorphins, so try taking a half-hour brisk walk, twice a day. It's even better to exercise outside, in natural daylight.

▶ Do you have medical conditions that may reduce blood and oxygen flow to the brain, such as anaemia, narrowing arteries (atherosclerosis) or hypothyroidism? You can ask your doctor to test for these.

- Do you have hypoglycaemic episodes – sudden dips in blood sugar levels? If so, cut down on sugar, white starch and caffeine. See Chapter 4 for further advice on this.

- Are you addicted to drugs, nicotine, alcohol, caffeine or sugar? See Chapter 10.

- Can you attribute your low mood to a particular life event, such as a bereavement, a relationship breakdown or the loss of a job? Consider getting some specialist counselling to help you through. You can make a start today by looking at some relevant websites, such as:

  ▷ psychotherapy: www.bacp.co.uk

  ▷ cognitive behavioural therapy: http://babcp.co.uk

  ▷ psychoanalysis: www.psychoanalysis-bpa.org or www.psychoanalysis.org.uk

- Do you have irritable bowel symptoms, such as excessive gas, bloating, constipation or diarrhoea? The brain and the gut are directly connected to each other by what is referred to as the 'enteric nervous system', or the 'gut–brain axis', meaning that the health and function of one directly affects the other. Thus, gut symptoms such as bloating can severely affect mood. In Chapter 2 we saw how microflora imbalances in the GI tract and increased leakiness in the gut membrane can contribute to inflammation, allergies and autoimmune diseases. Recent research indicates that these changes in the gut may also promote neurological conditions such as anxiety, 'brain fog', depression and eating disorders.[25] Refer to Chapter 3 for further information and advice.

- Are you getting enough sleep? Lack of sleep is a widespread problem. As you'll see in Chapter 10, the average number of hours' sleep per night reduced from 9 in the year 1910 to 6.8 in 2005. Research shows that regular, good-quality sleep is vital for emotional health, with poor sleep resulting in irritability, short-temperedness and low mood.[26] Aim for 7.5–8 hours a night. See Chapter 10 for tips on how to improve both the quantity and the quality of your sleep.

- If you are female, consider whether your mood swings happen around the same time every month. Alternatively, could you be starting the menopause transition (the 'peri-menopause')? Significant dips in oestrogen can lead to plummeting levels of serotonin, dopamine, adrenalin and noradrenalin, and an increase in the associated symptoms,[27] including low mood and lack of drive. Conversely, chronically elevated oestrogen can lead to anxiety and hyperactivity.[28] Chapter 9 contains advice on how to balance sex hormones.

- Are you lonely? While everyone needs private space and quiet time, humans are essentially social animals. People living in areas of the world with higher than average proportions of long-lived, healthy inhabitants have in common the fact that they are part of supportive communities of friends and acquaintances, and also that they spend regular time with family members and other loved ones.[29] When you're feeling low, you may naturally avoid social situations. But making the effort can literally do wonders for your mood. And did you know that science has proved that the mere act of smiling can help to cheer you up?[30]

- Do you suffer more in the winter months? If so, you could be one of an estimated two million people in the UK (12 million people across Northern Europe) with seasonal affective disorder (SAD).[31] The most effective thing you can do is ensure you get a good daily dose of 'full spectrum' light.[32] You can do this by being out in the sunshine or by using a full spectrum light box, specially designed for this purpose. (Normal light bulbs won't produce the desired effect.)

- Sunlight is also the best natural source of vitamin D. There are many vitamin D receptors throughout the brain (indicating that the brain uses a lot of this vitamin). Low vitamin D levels in the blood are likely to contribute to depression[33] and also to cognitive impairment[34] and Alzheimer's.[35] See Chapter 8 for more on vitamin D.

- Might your thyroid function be a little sluggish? Other typical symptoms of low thyroid function include feeling tired all the time, having a tendency towards constipation, finding it difficult to lose weight and being overly sensitive to cold weather. If this pattern of symptoms is familiar to you, follow the advice in Chapter 6 and ask your doctor to test your levels of thyroid hormones.

▶ Are you in pain? Chronic physical pain can really get you down, whatever its source. Pain that becomes more common as we get older includes that from arthritis, backache and headache. Depression and anxiety are more prevalent in people who suffer regularly from headaches and migraines.[36]

▶ Might you be exposed to toxic metals? Metals such as mercury, cadmium, lead and aluminium interfere with brain chemical function by competing with the brain-friendly minerals discussed on page 166.[37] Anxiety and depression were included in the mercury and lead toxicity symptoms experienced by individuals exposed to the air at Ground Zero following the 11 September attacks on the World Trade Centre.[38] See Chapter 6 for tips on reducing toxin exposure. If you are concerned about previous exposure, you should speak to your healthcare practitioner about the options for testing.

▶ Are you getting enough mood-enhancing nutrients? The most crucial nutrients are:

▷ protein, for the amino acids tryptophan, methionine, tyrosine and phenylalanine (see page 161)

▷ the omega 3 fatty acids EPA and DHA, found in oily fish

▷ B vitamins, especially B12, B6 and folate – see page 163 for food sources

▷ the minerals zinc, iron and magnesium – see page 167 for the best food sources

▷ CoQ10, which, although present in tiny amounts in many foods, may best be taken as a supplement to increase your levels initially.

PROVIDE THE RAW MATERIALS

Having taken action to preserve your brain cells, we now need to turn to the production of the neurotransmitters. These are made up of molecules called amino acids, which are found in protein foods. The amino acids tyrosine and phenylalanine are used to make the 'catecholamine' neurotransmitters dopamine, adrenalin and noradrenalin. To make serotonin, you need the amino acid tryptophan. Many other amino acids, such as methionine and glutamine, also help to make brain chemicals.

Rather than getting hung-up about eating foods that have particularly high levels of any one specific amino acid, the simplest and most effective recommendation is to ensure you eat a good portion of a high-quality, 'complete' protein food every day. Those in the table below are 'complete' proteins, meaning that they contain all the dietary amino acids that are essential for health. If you go for organic, grass-fed, wild and/or low-fat sources, you will likely be eating the higher-quality products.

Lean meat (beef, pork, lamb)	Dairy (milk, yogurt, cheese, cottage cheese, crème fraîche, kefir)	White fish (cod, haddock, halibut, sea bass, sea bream)
Poultry (chicken, turkey)	Soy (tempeh, tofu, natto)	Oily fish (trout, sardines, salmon, mackerel, anchovies, eel)
Eggs	A combination of beans/pulses and whole grains	Seafood (prawns, mussels, crab, oysters, clams, cockles, whelks, lobster, crayfish)
Game (venison, rabbit, pheasant, duck, partridge)	A combination of nuts/seeds and whole grains	Protein powders (whey, hemp, rice, pea, egg) Spirulina (1 tbsp contains 4g protein)

If, however, you believe you might be particularly low in one of the individual amino acids that make brain chemicals (nutrition practitioners can organize laboratory testing so you can check your levels), you could trial a course of supplementation. If you are feeling depressed, for example, despite following the advice in Box 7.2, you could consider taking a supplement of the precursor to serotonin, which is called 5-hydroxytryptophan (5-HTP), a metabolite of the amino acid tryptophan.

You may wonder why we are suggesting this, when we've already said that, food-wise, it's better to ensure you are getting good-quality proteins every day, rather than focusing on foods high in any one amino acid. The reason is that, contrary to popular belief, no food can provide your brain with a therapeutic dose of a particular, single amino acid. This is because foods contain lots of different amino acids, many of which compete with each other for absorption through the gut barrier into the bloodstream, and, again through the blood–brain barrier into the brain. If you take amino acids singly, however, on an empty stomach, you have a better chance of them reaching the brain at a dose that may have some positive effect. When you take the amino acids in this way, there is no competition for their absorption.

This is borne out in studies of supplemental amino acids. Supplementing 5-HTP, for example, increases serotonin levels. There is evidence from some small trials that 5-HTP can significantly improve mood in moderately depressed individuals.[39] But because of the explosion in the use of antidepressant pharmaceuticals, there is, unfortunately, little financial incentive for extensive clinical trials. The big money-spinners are the products that can be patented but, unlike SSRIs and other drugs, 5-HTP is a natural compound and cannot be patented.

If you suspect you may have low serotonin – perhaps, for example, you may also suffer from pain syndromes such as migraine or fibromyalgia, or perhaps you have very poor sleep, or suffer regularly from cravings for starchy or sugary foods – you could try a supplement of 100mg, three times a day, on an empty stomach. You should not try this, however, if you are on any antidepressant medication, as this combination could elevate your serotonin levels too much.

Another important raw material for neurotransmitter production is a molecule called choline. Choline is converted into acetylcholine (for good memory). It is also an essential component of the phospholipid phosphatidyl choline (PC). PC, as seen below, is required for the membranes surrounding each brain cell to work well, so that they are able to act upon the messages delivered by the neurotransmitters.

Choline is found naturally in egg yolk, fish roe, organ meats such as liver, and lecithin granules (made from soy or sunflower). Lecithin can be added to recipes, such as our *Whipped Coconut Cream, Classic Almond Milk* and *Dandelion Root 'Mocha' Ice Cream*.

PROVIDE THE RIGHT 'ACCESSORY' VITAMINS AND MINERALS

Once you have enough of your raw materials, you then need to set about converting them into brain chemicals. This is done by a process called 'methylation'. Rather handily, this process also converts other raw materials (such as choline and fats) into phospholipids.[40] (The phospholipids support the neurotransmitter receptors and the myelin sheath that protects the nerve cells – see below.)

B vitamins

You might think that such an important process as methylation would just happen, day in, day out, whenever we need it. And it does. But only in the presence of the right nutrients. In particular, you need the B vitamins, particularly B12 and folate (see Box 7.3).

B vitamins are found in whole foods (not in processed foods), especially the proteins in the table above, plus nuts, seeds and whole grains. Green leafy vegetables are a good source of folate. So eat lots of rocket (arugula), watercress, romaine lettuce, spinach and spring greens. Beans, pulses, beetroot, nuts and citrus fruit also contain folate. Try our *Watercress, Apple and Walnut Salad with Creamy Mustard Dressing* and our *Bitter Greens with Grapefruit and Avocado* or *Beet Mint Dip*. The only bioavailable source of B12 is animal protein such as meat, fish, eggs and dairy products, so if you are a vegan you will need to consider supplementing.

The simplest and cheapest way to find out how well your own methylation process (or 'methyl cycle') is working is to measure your blood levels of homocysteine. Homocysteine is an amino acid that your body produces during methylation. (Remember, it's methylation that converts nutrients into brain chemicals.) In the presence of sufficient B12 and folate, homocysteine is quickly converted into other amino acids, meaning that only low levels of homocysteine are in the blood. But if B vitamin levels are too low, the methyl cycle can't work properly and this causes homocysteine levels to get too high. (It also seriously disrupts the synthesis of brain chemicals.) This is why your homocysteine level is a good indicator of your B vitamin status.

It may come as no surprise to learn that scientists have found elevated homocysteine to be a predictor of future memory loss, cognitive decline and even Alzheimer's disease.[41] Low blood levels of folate and B12 have also been found in Alzheimer's.[42] And elevated homocysteine and/or vitamin B12 deficiency has been implicated in depression,[43] as has low folate.[44]

The good news is that supplementing B vitamins may slow the brain shrinkage that causes cognitive decline, probably because they lower homocysteine and improve the function of the methyl cycle.[45] So, if you have the early signs of cognitive impairment and you also have high levels of homocysteine, this strategy is certainly worth a try. Supplementing these key B vitamins may also help to improve certain mood disorders, again by lowering homocysteine.[46]

It's also worth knowing that people who drink alcohol every day become particularly vulnerable to poor methylation and elevated homocysteine, as alcohol leeches B vitamins from the body. As we saw in Chapter 2, if you want to drink alcohol, do it for pleasure rather than thinking of it as an aid to good health, and drink it in small quantities only. We recommend having at least three alcohol-free days a week and, on the days that you do drink, sticking to two units a day for women and three for men.

How much of these nutrients should you supplement? The studies that use them to lower homocysteine tend to supplement far higher doses than the government's recommended daily allowances (RDA). Testing your homocysteine levels will help you to decide whether you may benefit from higher doses, up to 800mcg folate (in the active L-methylfolate form) and 750mcg B12, depending on the extent to which homocysteine is elevated. As other B vitamins are also involved in converting amino acids into brain chemicals, it is best to supplement a B complex (containing all the B vitamins) when supplementing B12 and folate. After you have been supplementing for a couple of months, retest your homocysteine levels. You should be aiming for a level of 7–8 or under.

Just before we leave the subject of B vitamins, we should mention that B12 also has another important role in brain health. It is the most crucial micronutrient for keeping the myelin sheath healthy. The myelin sheath covers and protects each of the nerve cells. The neurological condition multiple sclerosis (MS) is characterized by lesions in the myelin sheath. This means that messages cannot be efficiently transmitted. Instead, they leak from the nerve cells before they have had a chance to deliver their information. This inefficient and faulty messaging leads to symptoms such as numbness, tingling and pain, blurred vision, muscle weakness and tightness, and problems with mobility and balance. High-dose B12 and folate are often prescribed to complement drug intervention in MS.

BOX 7.3 FOLIC ACID: FRIEND OR FOE?

Folate is a B vitamin that is essential for healthy ageing because it repairs DNA and supports the growth and division of every cell in the body. And, as you'll see in this chapter, folate helps to keep methylation working well. This, in turn, lowers harmful homocysteine, reducing your risk of Alzheimer's and cardiovascular diseases.

As your body can't make folate, you need to ingest it; and preferably daily, as it is readily excreted through urine. People who don't get enough folate appear to be at greater risk of many age-related diseases, including some cancers,[47] so it's important to ensure you're eating lots of folate-rich leafy greens (spinach, kale, watercress, rocket/arugula, asparagus and fresh herbs), citrus fruits, beans, peas and nuts.

Unfortunately, folate is easily destroyed by cooking. This means that many people don't get enough folate from diet alone and they may tend to rely on supplements to top up their intake. However, supplements and fortified foods (e.g. some breakfast cereals) typically use a synthetic version of the vitamin, which is called folic acid. Recently, there's been concern that, as we age, high intakes of synthetic folic acid may do us more harm than good. In animal studies, it's been found to drive the growth of pre-existing breast cancer tumours[48] and cause pre-cancerous lesions in the colon to progress to colorectal tumours.[49]

Human trials using synthetic folic acid have had mixed results, some finding a reduction in cancer growth, but others demonstrating the opposite effect.[50] A recent large review of the studies found that, although there was no significant influence, there was a small increase in cancer risk with supplementation.[51] The researchers concluded that this may have been due to 'chance'. But if, like us, you'd rather not take any risk, you can choose to avoid folic acid supplements. Indeed, the British Dietetic Association already advises that people over the age of 50, or those with a history or bowel cancer, should not take more than 200mcg folic acid a day.[52] This is less than the dose typically found in many multivitamin supplements.

Our advice is to get your daily dose of folate by eating eight or more portions of veg daily, including plenty of leafy greens, and 2–3 portions of fruit. Our recipes for green smoothies, *Broccoli Pear Soup*, *Roasted Baby Beets with Tempeh and Walnut Dressing* and *Bitter Greens with Grapefruit and Avocado* are rich in folate. And if you think you may not be able to get enough from food alone, the good news is that some vitamin producers are now using the active form of folate in their supplements. Look for the terms 'L-methylfolate' or 'L-5-MTHF' on the label, in place of 'folic acid'. Start with 200mcg a day and work up gradually to 4-800mcg, depending on your particular circumstances. (You can also get active forms of B12 and other B vitamins.) If you're keen to find out more about your folate and/or B12 status, a nutrition practitioner can arrange appropriate laboratory tests.

Minerals

A number of minerals are required for optimal brain function, but three of the most important are zinc, iron and magnesium. Unfortunately, these can become depleted if you are eating a typical Western diet of cereal or toast for breakfast, sandwiches for lunch and ready meals for dinner, with crisps, cereal bars and biscuits for snacks, and regular tea and coffee intake.

- Zinc is the most abundant trace mineral in the brain and without it we cannot manufacture serotonin nor other brain chemicals. People suffering from depression tend to have lower levels of zinc in their blood.[53] Supplementing zinc may reduce symptoms in people suffering from depression, according to initial trials.[54]

  The best sources of zinc are meat, fish, game and seafood. If you are a vegan, you should look to nuts, seeds and seaweeds. A good multivitamin and mineral formula should supply about 15mg a day, which is a sensible level for the medium to long term.

- Iron is crucial for the structure and function of the central nervous system, yet many of us, especially women of menstruating age, have insufficient stores of iron for optimal health. (Blood ferritin levels indicate your iron stores.) See Chapter 5 for more on this.

  By far the best sources of iron are lean red meat, especially liver, the darker meat from game, poultry and oily fish, and also eggs. The type of iron in these foods is 'haem iron', which is easier to absorb and utilize than the iron in vegetarian foods. If you are vegetarian, eat lots of beans, pulses, dark green leaves and dried fruit to get your iron. Getting some vitamin C at the same time (from fruit, for example) may help the iron's absorption. Most multivitamin and mineral supplements contain a basic level of iron, which is safe in the long term for most people. If your levels of stored iron are lower, you will need to supplement a higher dose, based on your current ferritin reading.

- Magnesium is at pretty low levels in many people's diets. It's vital for optimal mood, memory and thinking power because, together with the B vitamins, it pushes along the process of methylation, to make brain chemicals (see above). Magnesium is also involved in nerve signalling at the junctions between cells (the synapses).

  Good sources of magnesium are Swiss chard, kelp seaweed, squash, pumpkin seeds, steamed broccoli, halibut and, to a lesser extent, other green vegetables, nuts and seeds.

  See Chapter 6 for more information on this crucial yet often depleted mineral.

KEEP THE NEURON MEMBRANES AND
RECEPTOR SITES HEALTHY

In order for neurotransmitters to do their important job of communicating messages around the brain, they have to jump from one brain cell to another. A chemical such as serotonin, for example, is released by the bulb-like 'synapse' structure at the end of one brain cell, so that it can move to another cell. Once it has found the target cell, it needs to dock on to special receptor sites within the membrane of the target cell. If these receptors are not healthy, they won't function well, meaning that brain chemicals will be unable to dock and unable to transmit their messages.

So, it's important to keep the brain cell membranes and receptor sites healthy. This means ensuring that your diet and/or supplement programme includes enough brain-friendly fats and also the fatty molecules we call phospholipids.

Phospholipids

Phospholipids are important components of brain cell membranes, anchoring the receptors firmly in place. They are also crucial components of the protective sheath that covers each of the neurons. This sheath is called the myelin sheath and it helps to make sure that brain chemicals travel efficiently along the neuron, without any leakage, so that their messages are delivered intact.

There are many different types of phospholipids. The ones most important for memory, mood and cognitive function are called phosphatidyl serine (PS) and phoshatidyl choline (PC).

Scientific studies have found that inadequate levels of PS lead to age-associated memory impairment (AAMI). If you're over 50 years of age and you are noticing a gradual loss of memory, you may have AAMI. If so, it is important to do something about it now, not least because AAMI has recently been classified in the US as the precursor condition to Alzheimer's disease. Unsurprisingly, low PS is found in Alzheimer's patients.[55]

Supplementing PS has been found in human trials to improve memory function in older adults.[56] You probably need around 100–300mg a day, best taken in divided doses. PS may work even better when taken alongside the fatty acid DHA.[57] (See below for more on DHA.)

The UK Department of Health does not give recommendations for PS intake. But if you have low levels in your cell membranes, this means you are not consuming, or manufacturing, enough of it. And you could be heading for AAMI, which could lead to Alzheimer's disease.

The other all-important phospholipid, phosphatidyl choline, was introduced earlier on in this chapter. Egg yolk, liver, fish roe and lecithin granules are all good sources. There is also some in fish and milk.

Brain-friendly fats

For your body to make PS, PC and other phospholipids, the most important raw materials are certain types of fatty acids, especially a fatty acid called DHA.[58] DHA is one of two brain-supportive fats found in oily fish. The other is EPA. Oily fish include sardines, trout, anchovies, salmon and mackerel. You should either make sure you are eating these fish at least three times a week or take a fish oil supplement. Flax, chia and pumpkin seeds are good sources of other types of omega 3 fats for cell membrane health but they don't have such a marked effect on brain function as EPA and DHA. (See Chapter 8 for more on the essential fatty acids.)

Low levels of DHA in the blood are associated with cognitive decline in both healthy elderly people and Alzheimer's patients, and higher DHA intakes are associated with a lower risk of developing Alzheimer's. However, supplementing EPA and DHA (e.g. in fish oil) appears to improve learning and memory in cases of mild cognitive impairment but not in Alzheimer's.[59] This tells us that if we are to make a significant difference nutritionally, it is better to get started early on, before the imbalances have become entrenched diseases.

A lack of these important omega 3 fats has also been implicated in mood disorders. Improving their levels has frequently been found to improve symptoms.[60] There is increasing evidence, for example, that EPA may be helpful in depression.[61]

There is a third fatty acid that is crucial for brain structure and function. Its name is arachidonic acid (AA) but it is rarely deficient, because not only is it found in meat, poultry, eggs and dairy foods, but it is also produced in the body from the omega 6 fats found in seeds and seed oils.

BOX 7.4 MEMORY AND CONCENTRATION IN THE AGEING BRAIN

Are you worried about developing dementia in your later years? The most common form of dementia is Alzheimer's disease, followed by dementia associated with narrowing of the arteries to the brain (vascular dementia). Alzheimer's is characterized by the formation of two types of faulty proteins in the brain, which cause brain cell death. These faulty protein structures are known medically as beta-amyloid plaques and tau protein neurofibrillary tangles.

Whatever the type of dementia, it is typically preceded by years or even decades of gradually declining memory, concentration and the ability to think logically and clearly. This pre-dementia state is referred to as mild cognitive impairment. (This includes the age-associated memory impairment – AAMI – mentioned above.)

As with all age-related degenerative diseases, the possibility for halting or reversing the decline is greater the earlier you start, before dysfunctions in body systems have become so entrenched that a disease is diagnosed. If you're prepared to start early, here are some measures to consider taking:

▶ Get your blood levels of homocysteine tested. If it is too high, supplement a B complex with extra B12 and folate (see the main text for more detail).

▶ Check out your cardiovascular health – discuss your blood pressure and your levels of LDL- and HDL-cholesterol, triglycerides and fasting blood glucose with your GP. See Chapter 4 for improving your blood levels of sugar, insulin and fats.

▶ Get eight hours of good-quality sleep a night. Sleep is thought to be even more crucial for brain function than for body function.[62]

Memories are stored and learning is consolidated during the phases of rapid eye movement (REM) (or dreaming) sleep. Poor sleep causes problems with both of these functions,[63] and sleep deficit may play a role in the progression of Alzheimer's disease.[64]

▶ Reduce your exposure to toxic metals, especially aluminium, which may lead to age-related neurological problems resembling Alzheimer's.[65] Common sources of aluminium include cooking pans, tin foil, metal-lined food containers including some juice cartons, deodorants/antiperspirants and some antacid medications and toothpastes.

▶ Check your blood level of vitamin D. Its likely importance in brain function is highlighted by the high number of vitamin D receptor sites situated on brain cells. And there is evidence that it may help to remove the harmful protein amyloid beta from the brain.[66] (The build-up of plaques made of amyloid beta is a key part of the development of Alzheimer's disease.)

▶ Consider supplementing with pyrroloquinoline quinone (PQQ). This is an important nutrient that helps to protect and repair the batteries (mitochondria) of ageing cells. There is some initial evidence that supplementation may improve cognitive function in middle-aged and elderly people.[67]

▶ Keeping your brain active as you get older may help to reduce cognitive decline.[68] You can do this by reading books and newspapers, learning new skills, doing crosswords and puzzles, and regularly engaging in stimulating social interaction.

▶ Make sure you are getting good daily amounts of antioxidants, the fatty acids EPA and DHA, and the B vitamins in your diet (fish, eggs and green leafy vegetables are particularly important and should become staples in your diet. If you are concerned about your risk of dementia, it would be wise also to supplement these at the levels discussed on page 164.

AND FINALLY, BEWARE OF INFLAMM-AGEING

Consider all possible sources of chronic inflammation. A healthy brain needs to be kept free of 'inflamm-ageing' – the kind of insidious, low-level, chronic inflammation that leads to degeneration and premature ageing, wherever it is found in the body. Depression, Alzheimer's disease and multiple sclerosis are just three of the many neurological issues that have been linked to chronic, long-term inflammation.

As we saw in Chapter 1, addressing any of the imbalances discussed in this book will help to reduce your overall level of inflamm-ageing, as all of these imbalances eventually cause inflammation. Also refer to Chapter 8 for more on the process of inflammation, how to identify the possible causes in your life and how to control it. In particular, certain anti-inflammatory nutrients such as curcumin (from the turmeric root) are thought to have potential in reducing the risk of Alzheimer's disease.[69]

MEAL PLAN

Breakfast	*Super Greens Frittata*
Lunch	*Creamy Red Pepper Soup* with *Dairy-Free Macadamia Pesto Tomato Seeded Crackers*
Dinner	*Macadamia Dukkah-Crusted Sea Bass with Green Beans and Rocket*
	Fruit Parfait
Snack	*Beet Mint Dip* with vegetable sticks
	Dandelion Root 'Mocha' Ice Cream

If you do nothing else, do this...

▸ Reduce your exposure to free radicals from smoking, pollution, processed foods and overcooked or barbecued foods.

▸ Eat a rainbow of brightly coloured fruit and vegetables for antioxidants. Eat leafy greens daily for folate.

▸ Take a good multivitamin and mineral supplement because this will contain a range of antioxidant vitamins and minerals and also B vitamins for methylation.

- Consider taking CoQ10, alpha lipoic acid and acetyl-L-carnitine.

- Take an extra 150–300mg magnesium a day, as magnesium citrate.

- If you are concerned about memory loss, consider taking a supplement of phosphatidyl serine (PS) and phoshatidyl choline (PC).

- Get your blood levels of homocysteine tested and consider a supplement of extra vitamin B12 and folate if yours is elevated.

- Adopt a low-GL way of eating.

- Cut down your intake of sugar, caffeine and alcohol. If you are a smoker or a user of recreational drugs, take steps to give up.

- Address your stress levels and consider all the possible sources of your stress, including physical and emotional pain.

- Ensure you get eight hours of good-quality sleep a night.

- Reduce your exposure to toxic metals such as lead, mercury and aluminium.

- Keep your brain active by engaging in cognitive tasks.

- Enjoy social interaction daily.

- Take 30–60 minutes of aerobic activity a day.

- Eat good-quality, complete protein every day.

- Eat oily fish three time a week or take a fish oil supplement giving you 1g combined EPA/DHA a day.

CHAPTER 8

PAIN-FREE LIVING

One of the most common fears about getting older is having to deal with daily pain and possibly increasing immobility. We fear it because, whereas some age-related illnesses may not be apparent to others (e.g. high blood pressure or diabetes), many of us have witnessed elderly relatives or friends visibly battling with regular or constant, debilitating pain.

Pain can be either acute or chronic. Acute pain can be viewed as a protective mechanism that makes you aware of an injury and is often short-term. Chronic pain is persistent and can last for months or even years.

If we consider that the top-selling over-the-counter drugs are analgesics, it's clear that pain is a real and prevalent problem. According to the British Pain Society, about 10 million people in the UK suffer pain almost daily.[1] The most common causes, in descending order, are back pain, arthritis and headache, which are all conditions that typically get worse with age. Add to this the pain that comes with injuries from age-related falls, osteoporosis, dental conditions and nerve problems (after a shingles outbreak, for instance), and there is a lot to be concerned about. Box 8.1 gives a more comprehensive list of things that cause pain as we get older.

Chronic pain can affect almost every aspect of your daily life. It makes it harder to keep working and exercising and to maintain hobbies. Even day-to-day living activities such as unloading the dishwasher or vacuuming can become a trial. Being in pain can prevent you from getting a good night's sleep; lack of sleep can worsen any feelings of anger, frustration or depression brought on by living with daily pain. This can affect your relationships – you are less likely to feel like socializing; you may be irritable and short-tempered with others; you may start to lose your libido. And as if this weren't enough to be coping with, you may be faced with increasing healthcare costs and lost workdays, both of which can be a drain on your finances.

So, what do you do if you are in pain? Many of us reach for paracetamol, aspirin, ibuprofen or other pain killers. They can be effective in the short term. But these are not recommended for regular use because they carry significant side-effects, many of which promote the ageing process. Box 8.2 explains the problems with these drugs later in this chapter; and also why in many cases they don't work at all.

The crux of this chapter is about the changes that you can make to your diet and lifestyle that may help to reduce your risk of developing age-related painful conditions, and make any existing pain more manageable. In order to do this, however, we first need to understand what pain is and where it comes from.

WHAT IS PAIN AND WHERE DOES IT COME FROM?

There are two categories of pain – nociceptive and neuropathic.[2] Nociceptive pain is often initiated by inflammation. This can arise from tissue damage – for example, if you injure yourself (perhaps you pull a muscle or you suffer a burn) or if the protective cartilage has worn away in a joint, leading to the arthritic grinding of bone on bone. Both the tissue damage and inflammation activate pain receptors (known as nociceptors) in the nervous system. These nociceptors send messages to the brain, which are then interpreted as pain. As we'll see later in this chapter, long-term inflammation can eventually lead to an *exaggerated* response to pain signals, because inflammation that goes on and on tends to lead to adaptive changes within the nervous system.

Neuropathic pain occurs because of damage to the nervous system, through injury, perhaps, or illness, surgery, chemotherapy or radiotherapy. This type of pain can involve sensations such as burning, shooting, tingling, 'raw' skin, or deep and dull aching. It is notoriously difficult to treat and can persist for many years. Classic and common types of nerve pain include that from diabetic neuropathy or the pain left behind after a shingles attack.

Increasingly, scientists are finding that most pain conditions are caused by a combination of both mechanical *and* nervous system problems. Our brains are flexible and quick to adapt, laying down new connections and circuits in response to signals from the environment. This is how learning and memory take place. But sometimes this propensity to adapt (known as 'neuroplasticity') goes wrong: if the brain has been receiving pain signals for a long time, it can start to misinterpret them, becoming hypersensitive to external stimuli. When this happens, you begin to interpret normal stimuli (e.g. gentle touch) as painful, and to interpret normal pain signals as excruciating pain.[3] It is now thought that many people with fibromyalgia, osteoarthritis, rheumatoid arthritis and low back pain are suffering partly because their brains have become hypersensitive to pain signals in this way.

This is important to know because drugs that help with pain from inflammation and tissue damage don't tend to help with neuropathic pain at all. This is why, in this chapter, we give you some ideas for helping not only with inflammation but also with the neuropathic, or 'mind', element of your pain. This dual approach should give you the best chance of staying pain-free.

BOX 8.1 THINGS THAT CAUSE PAIN AS WE GET OLDER

Do you suffer from regular pain? There are a great many age-related conditions that can cause chronic pain and discomfort. Some of them are listed below:

- gingivitis or periodontitis (swollen, bleeding gums)

- osteoarthritis (degeneration of the musculoskeletal joints)

- bulging or 'herniated' disks in the spine, causing back pain

- headache and migraine, which are common at all ages but can be a particular problem during the menopause transition

- autoimmune conditions such as rheumatoid arthritis, multiple sclerosis and inflammatory bowel diseases – these can occur at any age but, as they are progressive diseases, their effects become more difficult to deal with the older you get

- injured muscles and tendons, which take longer to heal as you get older

- broken bones from age-related osteoporosis

- diabetic-related conditions, such as degenerative nerve pain ('neuropathies')

- ongoing nerve pain from a previous attack of shingles

- pain related to cancer or the treatment of cancer (radiotherapy, chemotherapy)

- pain from a previous stroke.

BOX 8.2 PAIN DRUGS – MORE HARM THAN GOOD?

The most common type of pain medication is a group of anti-inflammatories called non-steroidal anti-inflammatory drugs, or NSAIDs. These drugs include ibuprofen and aspirin. They reduce pain and inflammation, often very effectively in the short term, by blocking enzymes that convert omega 6 fatty acids into inflammatory chemicals called eicosanoids. See page 184 for more on the eicosanoids.

These drugs can be quite risky to take in the long term, however. The best-known side-effect is that they damage the delicate lining of the gut, leading to leaky gut (see Chapter 3) and in some cases to more immediately obvious problems such as gastritis, peptic or gastric ulcers and even life-threatening haemorrhage. They also affect kidney function, cause high blood pressure and oedema (swelling), and at higher doses can increase the risk of heart attack.[4]

Because of the well-known problems with these drugs, newer versions called COX-2 inhibitors were brought to market some years ago. But these also carry risks of cardiovascular events such as heart attacks. At least one of these drugs has been withdrawn from sale because of this.

In serious inflammatory diseases such as autoimmune diseases, you may be prescribed immune-suppressing drugs like methotrexate. These are extremely effective at keeping a lid on inflammatory chemicals but they carry even more serious side-effects than the NSAIDs and the COX-2 inhibitors. If the immune system is suppressed too much for too long, your risk of infections and cancer dramatically increases, as you have no defence.

Paracetamol (also known as acetaminophen) does not fall into the drugs categories above. It is classed as a non-opioid analgesic, reducing pain but not inflammation. It does not cause as much gastric irritation as the NSAIDs but it is highly toxic to the liver and relatively easy to overdose.

If your pain has a significant neuropathic element, rather than being inflammatory in nature, most of the drugs above will be useless. Two other groups of drugs are used here. The first group comprises the antiepileptic drugs (e.g. gabapentin, pregabalin), originally developed for seizure control. Side-effects include sedation, dizziness and blurred vision. The second group comprises antidepressants (serotonin-norepinephrine reuptake inhibitors – SNRIs – and tricyclics such as amitriptyline). Side-effects include sedation, dry mouth, fast heart rate and weight gain.

For very severe pain syndromes, such as cancer-related pain, opioid analgesics are typically prescribed, such as codeine, morphine and methadone. They can vary in the extent to which they provide relief and they carry the very real risk of being highly addictive. This makes it very easy to start relying on them and extremely difficult to get off them. Chapter 7 has information about addictions and how to recover from them. Opioids may also disrupt hormone balance, including luteinizing hormone, follicle stimulating hormone and potentially testosterone.[5]

Other treatments include muscle relaxants and topical analgesic agents.

If you are in pain, these drugs can literally provide you with a new lease of life, or at least the will the carry on living. But, given the common side-effects, we think it's worth exploring nutrition and lifestyle changes that may enable you to rely less on these medications. Even if you are able to reduce your dosage of these medications by, say, 50 per cent, you will be doing your long-term health a great favour. (If you do have to remain on some medication in the long term, take a look at the advice in Chapter 6 on how to support your detoxification processes.)

KEEPING YOURSELF PAIN-FREE

Given what we've said above, keeping yourself pain-free comes down to three areas of action:

- giving your body the *structural* support it needs

- keeping inflammation at bay

- controlling the way your brain *perceives* pain. (There's no pain without a brain.)

Let's look at each of these in turn.

PROVIDING STRUCTURAL SUPPORT AS YOU AGE

As we get older, our tissues start to get weaker. Our levels of anabolic hormones decline (see Chapter 9), our cells are renewed more slowly and our repair processes become gradually less efficient. We become more prone to destructive processes such as oxidation (see Chapter 5), glycation (see Chapter 4) and hypomethylation (see Chapter 7). As a result, the components of our scaffolding – our bones, muscles, joints, blood vessels and other connective tissues – start to break down.

The importance of GAGs

One of the most important groups of structural molecules comprises the glycosaminoglycans (GAGs). GAGs are crucial in keeping you moving in your later years because they attract water to produce gel-like substances (e.g. synovial fluid in joints). Such substances help to cushion the joints and prevent painful friction between bones, tendons and cartilage. Hyaluronic acid is an example of a GAG. You may have heard of it because it is commonly added to 'anti-ageing' skin creams to help hydrate the skin.

Osteoarthritis (OA) is a degenerative and painful condition that is all too commonly part of the ageing process. The pain is caused by the GAGs degrading more quickly than the rate at which your body can manufacture them. (As we've seen above, this lack of GAGs reduces the comfortable cushioning between the joints.) OA is said to be due to general 'wear and tear'. It most frequently occurs in joints that have suffered previous injury, or where there is overuse over many years, or where there may be some misalignment of the bones.

One of the most important ways to help yourself if you have OA, or you are worried about developing it, is to take steps to lose any excess weight, in order to relieve the joints of any unnecessary pressure (see Chapter 4). You should also engage in regular, gentle exercise to keep the joints moving and adopt an anti-inflammatory diet and supplement programme (see below). But you also need to support GAG production. One of the things you could try in this respect is to supplement glucosamine sulphate.

Improving your GAG levels

Technically an amino-sugar, glucosamine's main function is to stimulate the production of GAGs, and it has long been used for helping people with OA. As we age, the rate at which we make glucosamine slows down and this is a problem because, without sufficient glucosamine, the cushioning GAGs cannot be made.

There is evidence that taking glucosamine sulphate can help improve both pain and movement in people with OA, especially that which affects the knee.[6] One of the problems with glucosamine research, however, is that the results can vary between studies. A recent review of trials totalling 3159 OA patients concluded that glucosamine sulphate helps to improve the functioning of joints affected by OA if it is taken for more than six months. This study didn't find any improvement in pain levels, however.[7] Another problem is that most of the studies tend to involve only a small number of participants.

Because of these issues, you won't be offered this supplement on the NHS. Based on the results to date, however, we think it's worth a try if you have the initial signs and symptoms of arthritis, or if you are particularly concerned about your risk because of previous injury, for example, or a strong family history of arthritis. We recommend 1500mg per day in two or three divided doses. The sulphate form of glucosamine may be superior to other forms, since the mineral sulphur plays an essential role in maintaining healthy cartilage. Take it for at least a month before evaluating its effectiveness.

There is another way to supplement sulphur. Some people choose to take methylsulfonylmethane (MSM), an organic sulphur compound with anti-inflammatory and antioxidant properties.[8]

Supporting collagen and bone

Elsewhere in this book, we cover other recommendations for giving yourself some extra structural support.

For example, to support your skin, blood vessels, gums and bones, you need to boost your production of collagen. This means getting plenty of protein, vitamin C and phytochemicals called OPCs and anthocyanins, found in dark berries. It's also a good idea to reduce any sources of destructive 'free radicals' and to increase your intake of rejuvenating antioxidants. The best food sources are fruits and vegetables, the more brightly and deeply coloured the better. See Chapter 4 for explanations of how free radicals and antioxidants can influence your rate of ageing, as well as an action plan for supporting collagen production.

You should also read the action plan in Chapter 9 for keeping your bones strong. It includes some specific 'must dos' such as upping your intake of calcium, magnesium, vitamins C, D, B complex and a particular type of vitamin K2 known as MK-7. Regular, weight-bearing exercise is also essential.

But perhaps the most powerful game-changer to slow the weakening of your skeleton, blood vessels, gums and skin is to put a stop to any ongoing inflammation.

KEEPING INFLAMMATION AT BAY

Inflammation is a theme running throughout this book because it is chronic, low-grade, often unnoticed inflammation that drives premature ageing and age-related degenerative diseases.[9] It's precisely this type of inflammation, or 'inflamm-ageing', that is such a significant cause of ongoing pain. While acute inflammation is involved in injuries and post-surgical pain, inflamm-ageing promotes bone loss, leading to osteoporosis and the pain of broken bones, and it is very much part of the picture of chronic back pain and arthritis.

What is inflammation?

Inflammation is a process that is vital for survival. It is our initial healing response to trauma from an invader, such as an infection or injury, which damages tissues. Blood vessels dilate and become more leaky, in order to swiftly deliver white blood cells, antibodies and other immune system chemicals to the affected site. Here, they work together to engulf and destroy the invaders and to wall off the inflamed area, isolating it from the rest of the body and binding the edges of any wound to slow blood loss.

But once the invader has been dealt with, a healthy immune system will shut off the inflammatory response and you'll go back into your resting, anti-inflammatory state. Similarly, a healthy immune system won't react (it won't mount inflammation) to invaders that are harmless – pollen, for example, or cat dander – because it will recognize them as such. Although a healthy immune system will always be on surveillance, for most of the time it will decide *not* to respond to things.

As we saw in Chapter 3, when your immune system is working well like this – when it dampens down any inflammation once the threat has been dealt with, and when it allows through harmless invaders without putting up a fight – you are said to have good 'immune tolerance'.

If you lose this tolerance, you will find that your immune system becomes too reactive. It may keep the inflammation going so that you have inflamed sinuses long after your initial virus has gone or it may trigger asthma or eczema when you eat dairy products. There are hundreds of other examples. The key thing to know is this: if you want to reduce inflammation, you need to improve immune tolerance.

Promoting anti-inflammation

GET YOUR GUT INTO GOOD CONDITION

If you've read Chapter 3, you'll be familiar with the growing scientific view that the most effective way to get your immune system back into full working order (i.e. to return to a state of optimal immune tolerance) is to improve the health of your gut. If the balance of your gut microflora is out of sync, or if the lining of your gut becomes too leaky, you'll be pushed towards a state of inflamm-ageing. This, as you'll know by now, is the type of chronic, low-grade, whole-body inflammation that you can't see on the outside, but which is causing long-term damage and increasing your risk of premature ageing and chronic disease.

Again, we saw in Chapter 3 that some specialists in this area of science believe that everyone with a chronic health condition should be investigated for undiagnosed problems in the gastrointestinal tract. Look back at that chapter for some examples of links between gastrointestinal problems and whole-body inflammatory conditions. In particular, the best way to help painful inflammatory autoimmune diseases (e.g. rheumatoid arthritis) may be to heal a leaky gut.[11] Once the gut's barrier function is restored, potential invaders cannot get from the gut into the underlying immune system and no inflammation will occur.

So, to reiterate, if you want to age well, you need to have good immune tolerance. If you lose your immune tolerance, you will lay yourself open to chronic inflammation. Chronic inflammation leads to pain. And it also underlies most of the degenerative conditions that bring misery to our later years. The most common reason for losing immune tolerance is poor gut health.[12]

Chapter 3 has a detailed plan for assessing your gut health and for getting it back into tip-top condition. One of the most important things to do is to stop eating any foods that you think may be affecting you. Common foods that cause reactions are gluten grains (wheat, rye and barley), dairy products (made from cow's, goat's or sheep's milk) and foods that are high in lectins, such as beans (especially soy), pulses and peanuts. Some of these foods promote dysbiosis and some cause leaky gut.[13] (And remember, having a leaky gut increases your risk of inflammation elsewhere in the body.)

Chapter 3 also includes other tips for improving microbial imbalance and healing and nurturing the delicate lining of the gastrointestinal tract.

This strategy really does work. We have helped many people in our clinics to reduce their pain and inflammation by optimizing the balance of their gut microbes and by healing their leaky gut.

What things trigger an inflammatory response? Some triggers cause inflammation for everyone affected by them – an injury, for example. But other things may cause inflammation in some people but not in others. Some people are sensitive to pollen, for example, and experience the inflammatory symptoms that we call hayfever.

We've seen that some foods promote inflammatory dysbiosis and leaky gut. Other common inflammatory triggers include:

▸ Man-made environmental toxins: cleaning chemicals, pollution, cigarette smoke, food additives, trans-fats, pesticides and medications.

▸ Natural environmental toxins: toxic metals (e.g. lead, aluminium, mercury), chemicals in browned meats, radiation and microbes elsewhere in the body (bacteria, viruses, fungus, parasites). To avoid inflammatory gum disease, for example, you need to keep bacteria at bay by paying attention to oral hygiene, brushing and flossing correctly twice a day and having regular dental check-ups and professional cleans.

▸ Toxins produced within your body: gases from unfriendly gut bacteria (like the odorous hydrogen sulphide), homocysteine (see Chapter 7), excess acidity (see Chapter 2) and psychological stress.

▸ Allergies and sensitivities: allergies to inhalents such as pollen; skin contact allergies (e.g. to nickel); or, as we've seen, sensitivities to common foods such as gluten grains.[10]

GET ENOUGH OMEGA 3 FATS

The membranes of each of our cells contain special fats that are converted into chemicals that control inflammation in the body. These chemicals are called eicosanoids (pronounced 'eek-o-son-oids') and some of them promote inflammation, while others are anti-inflammatory. The type of eicosanoids you produce depends largely on the balance of the special precursor fats in your cell membranes.[14]

The fats we're referring to here are the omega 6 and omega 3 polyunsaturated fatty acids (PUFAs). The diagram below shows some of the fats in both of these groups and also their food sources.

Inflammation tends to increase in the body, the older we get. If you want to age well, you need to make sure you are getting a healthy balance of omega 6 and omega 3 fats – this will help to keep a lid on any tendency towards inflammation. What's more, eating a healthy balance of these fats also keeps the membranes of all our cells healthy, improves our levels of blood fats and cholesterol, and may reduce our risk of many chronic diseases, including diabetes, depression and certain cancers.

So, what do we mean by 'a healthy balance'? Scientific experts in this area say we should be consuming omega 6 and omega 3 fats in a ratio of about 3 to 1. In other words, we should be eating three times as much omega 6 as omega 3.[15] The UK government currently recommends a ratio of 5 to 1.[16] The problem with the typical diet today is that the ratio is more like 20 to 1. This is because we eat so many omega 6-rich vegetable and seed oils and spreads, and we very rarely eat omega 3 foods like flaxseeds and oily fish.

A quick look at the diagram that follows will show you that omega 6 fats area easily converted into inflammatory chemicals (such as the one shown here called prostaglandin E2, or PGE2). You can also see that if you eat a lot of omega 3 fats, you can make chemicals (like PGE3) that dampen down inflammation. Without sufficient omega 3 in the diet, your body will become gradually more inflamed the older you get.

Therefore, if you have been eating a typical modern diet of meat, dairy, eggs, vegetable oils and processed foods, with very little oily fish and flaxseeds, your body is likely to be in a pro-inflammatory state.

Fats and Inflammation

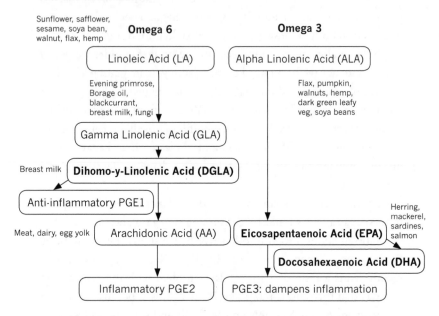

So, what should you do? By all means eat some omega 6 fats – in a healthy body they can also make anti-inflammatory chemicals like PGE1 (see diagram) and they also have other important roles. But make sure you are also eating three 100g (4oz) servings of oily fish a week, for their omega 3 fats. Oily fish includes fresh, tinned and smoked salmon, mackerel, trout, herring and sardines. It also includes fresh tuna but not tinned, as this is usually defatted before canning. (A word of caution, however: tuna, like other large fish, can contain contaminants such as mercury and dioxins. We recommend eating mainly the smaller fish, such as sardines, mackerel or anchovy, as these tend to be less contaminated.)

If you are a vegetarian or vegan, you can get some omega 3 fats from rapeseed oil, walnuts, flaxseeds and oil, chia seeds, hemp seeds, pumpkin seeds, tofu and green superfoods. But see Box 8.3 about the problems of relying on these alone for your omega 3 intake.

There is one type of omega 6 fat that has an important role in modulating inflammation: gamma linolenic acid (GLA). GLA comes from plants such as borage or evening primrose oil. Interestingly, GLA may also help to relieve neuropathic pain in some cases. Consider supplementing 300–600mg daily.[17]

BOX 8.3 FISH OIL SUPPLEMENTS: FAD OR FABULOUS?

Oily fish like those mentioned above contain very potent anti-inflammatory omega 3 fats called EPA and DHA. But, as you can see from the diagram on the previous page, the human body can also make its own EPA and DHA by using the omega 3 fats from certain nuts and seeds, such as flaxseeds. So, it you're a vegan, these are your best food sources.

Did you know, however, that some people are unable to make enough anti-inflammatory chemicals if they rely solely on nuts and seeds to get all their EPA and DHA? And, indeed, it is true that vegans tend to have lower levels of these anti-inflammatory fats in their cell membranes than people who eat animal products. The reason is that the conversion of omega 3 fats from seeds to those found in oily fish is very slow, even in healthy people and particularly in men. So, if you have a lot of inflammation in the body, you may not be able to manufacture enough EPA and DHA to counter this effectively.[18]

It's also worth knowing that most of the scientific studies showing benefits of omega 3 fats in inflammation and age-related illnesses have used supplemental EPA and DHA, rather than supplements of omega 3 from nuts and seeds.

Unless you have ethical reasons for avoiding it, therefore, it is important to consume fish oil regularly, either by eating oily fish or by taking a supplement, so that you do not have to rely on your body being able to make enough of its own EPA and DHA.

We've recommended eating three portions of oily fish. If you are pregnant or breastfeeding, however, you need to limit your intake to one to two portions a week because some oily fish is contaminated with mercury and toxic chemicals.[19] The most polluted fish are the larger varieties, such as shark, swordfish, marlin and tuna – all these should be avoided in pregnancy and breastfeeding. Smaller fish such as sprats, sardines, pilchards and trout may be relatively free of pollutants, as they don't live long enough to accumulate the toxins.[20] These fish are also in the most plentiful supply.

Due to very strict regulations in the UK, fish oil supplements manufactured in this country are free of the pollutants that can be present in the fish.

If you have *not* regularly been eating oily fish three times a week, we recommend you boost your levels of anti-inflammatory fats by taking a fish oil supplement. For general health, take one that provides 500mg a day of combined EPA and DHA. If you have an increased risk for cardiovascular disease (such as high blood pressure or a family history of heart attack, angina or stroke) increase this to 1000mg a day. And if you have an overt inflammatory condition, such as rheumatoid arthritis or another autoimmune disease, or if you have painful osteoarthritis, take 1800mg for three months, and then gradually reduce it to 500–1000mg, depending on your symptoms. EPA and DHA may also have a positive effect on neuropathic (nerve) pain.[21]

Nutritional therapists and other healthcare practitioners can organize blood tests for you to measure the levels and ratios of fats in your cell membranes. This will give you a more accurate idea of exactly how much of each type of fat you should be eating and supplementing daily, for optimal health.

And if you are a vegan for ethical reasons, you can still take EPA and DHA: in recent years, supplements of EPA and DHA sourced from algae have become available.

REDUCE INFLAMMATORY FATS

Be mindful not to buy *any* polyunsaturated (PUFA) oils unless they are in a bottle labelled 'cold-pressed' and are refrigerated at the point of sale. PUFA oils include those made from any of the foods listed in the diagram above and they are often labelled 'vegetable oil'. They should never be used in cooking and should be kept away from heat and light until you eat them, although they can be safely used in cold dressings for both warm and cold food.

Although you should not heat PUFA oils, it is safe to use seeds (whole or milled) in baking.[22] You'll see from the recipes that we use flaxseed in many of our baked goods recipes and this is because it makes muffins, breads and cakes more nutritious and also helps to keep them moist.

As well as getting your omega 6 fats down to healthier levels relative to omega 3 (as seen above), you should cut down on saturated fats, found in lard, fatty cuts of meat, farmed fatty fish, intensively farmed eggs and full-fat dairy products. However, saturated fats are the safest for cooking with, so there is no need to avoid them altogether. We recommend coconut oil, a vegetarian and possibly healthier source of saturated fat. Coconut oil may help to increase your levels of the good type of cholesterol, HDL.[23] It also contains a type of fat (called medium-chain triglycerides, or MCTs) that may help to promote weight loss.[24] MCTs are more easily burned for energy than other types of saturated fat. If you want to eat meat and dairy products, opt for organic, grass-fed varieties, as a greater proportion of their fat content is omega 3 PUFAs.[25]

Do your best to avoid the toxic, man-made fats called trans- or partially hydrogenated fats. These are highly inflammatory and also increase your risk of many age-related diseases, included insulin resistance, diabetes, cardiovascular disease and cancer.[26] Some countries limit the amount of man-made fats that can be used in processed foods, while other countries stipulate that their levels have to be clearly stated on food labels, so that people can make healthier choices if they want to. Unfortunately, the UK has no such rules. But you can easily avoid these inflammatory fats by eschewing all processed foods, especially margarines, baked goods, sauces, mayonnaise and salad dressings, and deep-fried foods.

GET YOUR VITAMIN D LEVELS CHECKED

Vitamin D is a powerful nutrient that improves immune tolerance, helping to reduce inflammation in the body.[27] Vitamin D has long been known to be crucial for keeping bones strong, but now scientists think that deficiency is associated with chronic pain of the joints and muscles,[28] and that getting levels back into the optimal range may also help people with inflammatory autoimmune conditions, such as rheumatoid arthritis, psoriasis, type 1 diabetes, Crohn's, multiple sclerosis and autoimmune hypothyroidism.[29] Vitamin D deficiency has also been linked to other conditions of chronic pain, including fibromyalgia.[30]

The main source of vitamin D is sunlight. But many people in the UK don't get enough year-round sun to make enough vitamin D for good health. This is because it can only be made from the type of sun rays that we get during the summer months. Even then, they can be blocked by cloud cover, clothing and sunscreen. In the summer, it is estimated that almost half of the English population may be deficient (have blood levels less than 40nmol/L) and that 75 per cent of us fail to reach the 'optimal' level of 75nmol/L.[31] Some experts are so concerned about this that they are calling for vitamin D deficiency to be classified as a major 'lifestyle' risk, along with smoking, alcohol, obesity and being sedentary.

The best food sources of vitamin D are cod liver oil, followed by oily fish. There is also a little in egg yolk, tinned tuna and fortified foods such as margarine. So, this is yet another reason to eat eggs and oily fish regularly. Vegans will be pleased to hear that some mushrooms also contain vitamin D.

It is also important to expose your skin to sunlight, in the middle of the day, every day from April to September, without sunscreen. Start with 2–3 minutes only and build up gradually to a maximum of 30 minutes, taking care not to burn.

How do you know if you are getting enough vitamin D? The best thing to do is to get your blood levels tested. You can either do this via your family doctor or you could get it done privately by talking to a nutrition practitioner. You want your level to be at least 75nmol/L. Some experts believe we should be aiming for levels as high as 100–150nmol/L if we are keen to reduce the risk of age-related chronic inflammation and the associated diseases.[32]

If your blood levels turn out to be low, you can take a supplement of between 2000 and 5000 IU a day. Retest your levels in 3–6 months' time, so you can see how quickly the dosage you are taking is having an effect. Once in the healthy range, many people continue to take a supplement of 1000–2000 IU a day in the winter and, if lifestyle does not permit regular sun exposure, all year round.

Stress appears to be a trigger for many conditions of pain – migraine, for example, or flare-ups in autoimmune conditions such as colitis. It's also worth knowing that adrenal stress hormones called glucocorticoids are anti-inflammatory,[33] perhaps the most potent group of anti-inflammatory chemicals produced by the human body. We need these hormones to keep inflammation under control. But long-term stress can hamper our ability to make enough glucocorticoids to keep inflammation at bay. This low-cortisol situation (termed 'adrenal fatigue – see Chapter 6) makes us more vulnerable to inflammatory and autoimmune diseases.[34]

So, if you want to better manage your pain, it's important to reduce the stress in your life and to support the glands that produce the glucocorticoids – the adrenal glands. Chapter 10 includes information on stress management, and Chapter 6 includes a step-by-step guide to restoring your adrenal function.

And, as we've said many times already throughout this book, one of the most powerful stress-busting actions you can take is to reduce or avoid the sugar and refined carbs in your diet. Eating these foods causes wide fluctuations in the level of sugar in your bloodstream. This puts a strain on your adrenal glands and it also leads to high insulin levels. Elevated insulin pushes your body into making inflammatory chemicals (eicosanoids – see above) from the omega 6 fatty acids in your diet.[35] So, all in all, if you are suffering from inflammatory pain, sugar and refined starches are going to make it a whole lot worse. Chapter 4 shows you how to swap sugary and starchy foods to healthier alternatives, and Chapter 2 outlines the low-GL diet to keep blood sugar levels steady.

LOSE WEIGHT IF YOU NEED TO
It's well acknowledged that carrying too much weight exacerbates many age-related health issues. But did you know that excess fat directly pushes the body into an inflammatory state? This increases your risk

for inflammatory pain and disease, and it keeps the fire of inflammation burning if you are already affected by an inflammatory condition.

Fatty tissue produces chemicals called 'adipokines' which are highly inflammatory.[36] They carry names such as tumour necrosis factor alpha (TNF-a) and interleukin 6 (IL-6).[37] These chemicals are involved in all sorts of inflammatory conditions, including autoimmune diseases and diabetes.

Eat an alkalizing diet

We saw in Chapter 2 that certain foods can alter the acidity of your body tissues and fluids. Some foods, such as meat, eggs, fish, dairy and refined grains, are acid-forming, while fruits and vegetables and some other plant foods have an alkalizing effect. Acidosis (acidic body fluids or tissues) tends to be a feature of many painful conditions, including arthritis, intermittent claudication and leg ulcers, leading some scientists to propose that a more alkaline diet may help to better manage pain.[38]

It's OK to eat some acid-forming foods – they are usually the best source of protein, for example – but the trick is to balance them with plenty of alkalizing foods, so that your overall diet is alkalizing. You can do this by ensuring you are eating 8–10 portions of vegetables a day and a couple of portions of fruit. See Chapter 2 for a guide to portion sizes.

Alkalizing fruits and vegetables are also the very best sources of a huge array of antioxidants. During the inflammatory process a barrage of toxic free radicals is pumped into the affected area, in order to engulf and destroy the bacteria, virus or other invaders. Antioxidants help to resolve inflammation by neutralizing these free radicals and reducing the oxidative damage that can be done to the surrounding tissues. Chapter 5 goes into detail on how free radicals cause premature ageing and damage to the body and how antioxidants work to reduce this.

Consider supplementing anti-inflammatory plant chemicals

What we hope to have shown you in this chapter so far is that there is a great deal you can do to help your body to better deal with pain and inflammation. By taking on board the advice above, you'll also improve your general health and your likelihood of a healthier old age.

To complement this, you could consider supplementing specific nutrients that have been demonstrated to reduce pain and inflammation.

▸ Bromelain: Bromelain is the umbrella name for a family of protein-digesting enzymes found in pineapple. You won't get much from eating pineapple, however, as it's found in the tough, woody stem. Used as a supplement, bromelain is anti-inflammatory and also acts as an analgesic, meaning that it blocks pain receptors.[39]

There is evidence from some human trials that it may reduce pain, swelling and stiffness in osteoarthritis[40] and in rheumatoid arthritis,[41] and also that it may help prevent injury and soreness from excessive exercise. Bromelain may also be helpful in reducing inflammation in the painful condition of ulcerative colitis.[42]

If you are keen to try bromelain, we recommend a dose of 1000 GDU (gelatin digesting units) 1–3 times a day. Take it on an empty stomach – for example, half an hour before food.

▸ Curcumin: Curcumin is a yellow pigment from the turmeric root, traditionally used in curries and other Asian dishes. It is a potent anti-inflammatory agent, reducing many pro-inflammatory chemicals in the body, including unwanted eicosanoids such as PGE2 (see above).[43]

Adding curcumin to conventional therapies for inflammatory bowel disease can improve symptoms and enable patients to reduce the dosage of their medications.[44] Small-scale studies also indicate that there may be some potential for curcumin to help with other painful inflammatory conditions. These include post-surgical fluid retention and pain, gastric ulcers, gum disease, multiple sclerosis, allergies, asthma, bronchitis, rheumatoid arthritis and inflammatory eye diseases.[45]

It's early days and many trials are ongoing but we believe there is enough evidence to give curcumin a try if you are suffering from inflammatory pain. We recommend starting with 500mg twice a day and increasing to 1000mg twice a day, if necessary. You need to be careful how you take it, however, because curcumin is notoriously hard to absorb. It's best taken 30–60 minutes before food on an empty stomach, preferably with an oil, such as a teaspoon of olive oil or with your fish oil supplement. Some manufacturers of dietary supplements are attaching curcumin to other molecules, in order to increase its absorbability.

Many other plant chemicals, such as quercetin (from apples and onions), anthocyanins (from berries) and those from green tea, sour cherries, ginger and rosemary, also have anti-inflammatory properties, as does honeybee resin (also known as propolis). Get as many of these foods as you can into your daily diet, or look for a combination supplement containing some of these.

LOOKING AFTER YOUR BRAIN MAY HELP REDUCE PAIN

If you are struggling to deal with daily instalments of pain, or if you are finding yourself taking regular painkillers but with little effect, it's worth remembering that tissue damage and inflammation aren't the only things that cause pain. Scientists now know that what goes on in the *brain* can often have more influence over how you feel pain than the severity of the damage (to skin, joints, bone, blood vessels, tendons, etc.) at the site of the pain. This is exciting news because it means there is another set of options you can try in your quest to reduce your pain. This involves looking at the balance of your brain chemicals.

We talked a lot about brain chemicals in Chapter 7 and we listed some of the most important ones and described their roles. In managing pain, we are interested in serotonin (your 'happy' chemical) and the catecholamines dopamine, noradrenalin and adrenalin (which give you drive and focus).

Increasing your catecholamine chemicals may reduce pain

A good example of how our brain chemicals affect how we perceive pain was shown in a study on osteoarthritis (OA). OA is by far the most common type of arthritis in the UK and its main symptom is pain. The charity Arthritis Research UK claims that one-third of people aged 45 years and over have sought medical treatment for osteoarthritis.[46]

When looking at the test results of a large group of patients with OA, researchers found that the level of pain people experienced did *not* correlate with the amount of cartilage destruction – damage to their joints. (The level of destruction was determined by way of medical MRI scans.)

Instead, they found that what correlated most with the level of pain experienced was the amount of certain brain chemicals in the patients' blood. They found that patients who had lower levels of dopamine, adrenalin and noradrenalin (due to a genetic variation) had three times the risk of hip pain than patients without such (genetically induced) lower levels.[47] The researchers concluded that lower levels of these brain chemicals caused these patients to become more sensitive to pain.

So, it's worth considering whether you may be able to reduce your own pain levels by improving the balance of your brain chemicals and, specifically, by increasing the catecholamines (dopamine, noradrenalin and adrenalin) if they are low. This way of thinking has led to certain types of antidepressant drugs being used in musculoskeletal pain disorders, with some success. These antidepressants are called tricyclics and serotonin-norepinephrine reuptake inhibitors (SNRIs) and they work by increasing dopamine, noradrenalin and adrenalin (see Box 7.2).

Chapter 7 shows you how you can improve the balance of your brain chemicals naturally. In particular, you need to eat protein, and foods rich in B vitamins and zinc. Take a good multivitamin and mineral supplement that includes these micronutrients and, if necessary, you can try supplementing the amino acid tyrosine (500–1000mg twice a day on an empty stomach), as the brain uses tyrosine to make dopamine, noradrenalin and adrenalin. Some people take L-phenylalanine instead, an amino acid that the body can convert to tyrosine.

Serotonin as a pain reliever

Another brain chemical – serotonin – also has a role in how we perceive pain. Both migraine and fibromyalgia are associated with lower levels of serotonin.

By increasing serotonin levels, it is sometimes possible to improve the pain experienced in both of these conditions. We saw in Chapter 7 how you can increase your serotonin levels without the use of drugs. In particular, taking a supplement of 5-hydroxytryptophan (5-HTP) can help with low mood and anxiety, by improving serotonin levels.

5-HTP (300mg a day) may also help with the pain from fibromyalgia.[48] People with this musculoskeletal disorder suffer from relentless widespread muscle pain, together with severe fatigue that doesn't tend to be relieved by sleep. 5-HTP can improve sleep quality and this in itself can reduce pain severity in fibromyalgia patients.[49]

What's more, there is some evidence that taking 5-HTP at the higher dose of 600mg a day may help with migraine.[50]

5-HTP should be taken in three divided doses, on an empty stomach (e.g. half an hour before food).

Melatonin

Melatonin is a naturally occurring hormone synthesized by the pineal gland, the part of the brain responsible for your sleep–wake cycle. Melatonin not only promotes sleep but is a potent antioxidant. It also has analgesic properties and has been reported in studies to reduce pain associated with fibromyalgia, migraine, irritable bowel syndrome (IBS) and other conditions.[51] Melatonin is available in the UK on prescription only. A dose of 0.3–3mg before bed is recommended.

Lifestyle alternatives to pain-relieving drugs

The examples of serotonin, melatonin and the catecholamines show that if you are suffering from debilitating, chronic pain, it's possible that you may find some relief by rebalancing brain chemicals. Doing this can also improve mood, sleep and the ability to cope with stress, all of which can independently aid your ability to manage pain.

Further evidence of the power of the mind to control pain comes from research on the practice of 'mindfulness'.[52] Mindfulness is thought of by some people as a type of meditation, and by others as more a type of mind training. It works by calming an anxious, stressed or hyperactive mind and body, by training the brain to focus exclusively on what is happening in the present. This might be, for example, the physical sensations felt by each part of the body, or the pattern of inhalation and exhalation, while attempting to slow the breath.

Other natural pain management approaches that have reportedly had some success include exercise and behavioural therapy,[53] acupuncture, biofeedback and electrical stimulation devices such as the Alpha-Stim (see Chapter 10). Everyone tends to respond slightly differently to natural therapies, meaning that it is impossible to predict how helpful any of these might be for you. We recommend trying them singly, so that you can gauge the extent to which each of them may be having an effect.

Micronutrients for neuropathic pain

Some micronutrients may be helpful in nerve pain, so it's worth ensuring you are getting sufficient of these in your diet and/or from supplements. B vitamins, particularly B1, B6 and B12, have been found helpful as an adjunct to medication in diabetic-related peripheral neuropathy.[54] And the antioxidant vitamins C and E may also help in various types of nerve pain.[55] Capsaicin, a compound found in chilli peppers, has been used topically as a pain reliever with some success.[56]

WHY IS ALL THIS WORTH CONSIDERING?

If you have a progressively worsening condition such as arthritis or chronic headaches, you'll probably be offered the standard 'treatment' of painkillers – aspirin or ibuprofen, for example. But, as we've seen in Box 8.2, these have well-documented serious side-effects, making it difficult for many people to take them long-term. What's more, they do nothing to treat the *cause* of the pain; they just suppress it. In some cases, they may make the underlying illness worse. There are many documented cases of rebound headaches caused by an over-reliance on these drugs, for example. And because they are notorious for causing leaky gut (see Chapter 3), they can theoretically increase the propensity to inflammation (and consequent pain) in the long term. (Remember, Chapter 3 provides a fuller explanation of how a leaky gut can cause inflammation almost anywhere in the body.)

MEAL PLAN

Breakfast	*Quick Mexican Baked Eggs*
Lunch	*Turmeric Glazed Fish with Cucumber Pickle* with mixed salad
Dinner	*Tempeh Coconut Curry* with wholegrain rice
	Lemon and Passionfruit Kefir Panna Cotta
Snack	*Joint Repair Iced Shake*
	Berries with yogurt

If you do nothing else, do this...

▸ Avoid toxins, allergens and trans-fats (processed foods).

▸ Get your gut into good condition and in particular address any microflora imbalance and/or leaky gut (see Chapter 3).

▸ Eat oily fish three times a week or supplement EPA, DHA and GLA.

▸ Check your vitamin D levels and supplement if necessary.

▸ Reduce the stress in your life and support the adrenal glands (see Chapter 6).

▸ Lose weight if you need to.

▸ If your pain is inflammatory, consider supplementing bromelain and/or curcumin.

▸ For long-term pain that may have a neuropathic element, consider supplementing L-tyrosine and/or 5-HTP.

▸ Take a multivitamin and mineral supplement with good levels of antioxidants and B vitamins.

▸ If you have osteoarthritis, consider taking glucosamine sulphate.

▸ Try some pain management activities such as mindfulness, acupuncture, biofeedback or the Alpha-Stim.

CHAPTER 9

BOOSTING SEX DRIVE AND BALANCING HORMONES NATURALLY

This chapter is about sex. It's about supporting healthy hormone levels as you age, which is key to maintaining your libido and keeping a youthful spring in your step.

One of the most significant drivers of age-related degeneration is the decline in sex hormones that occurs naturally as you get older. The deleterious effects are more immediately obvious in women than in men because women suffer a sharp drop in oestrogen around the age of 50 years, at the menopause, whereas men's hormones tend to decline more gradually.

In women, the key female sex hormones are the steroids oestrogen, testosterone and progesterone. Men also produce oestrogen, but it is testosterone that is produced in the greatest amount and has the most significant effect on health and wellbeing. The diagram below shows how these hormones are made in the body: they all require cholesterol, which is then converted into pregnenolone, progesterone, various androgens (male hormones) and then to the three types of oestrogen (oestrone, oestriol and oestradiol).

Sex hormone production

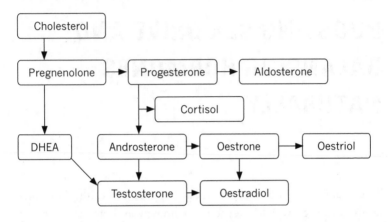

There are a great many other hormones that affect your wellbeing and rate of ageing. Some of these are covered in other chapters. For example, thyroid and adrenal hormones are covered in Chapter 6. Hormones involved in regulating appetite and blood sugar metabolism are discussed in Chapter 4. In this current chapter, we focus on the sex hormones.

SEX HORMONES AND AGEING

Sex hormones are thought of primarily for their role in sex drive and reproduction – erectile function and sperm production in men, ovulation and pregnancy in women.

But these hormones also have other, far-reaching effects on function and health. For example, they keep your skin and blood vessels supple and your bones and muscles strong, and they help with mood, memory and your ability to think clearly. This means that when these hormones decline with age, it is not only your sex drive and your fertility that suffers, but a great many other body systems as well.

A theme running through this book is the process of inflamm-ageing: that of chronic, insidious inflammation causing premature ageing and age-related diseases. We've also seen that there are many different drivers of such inflammation, such as carrying too much fat, high levels of sugar or insulin in the blood (see Chapter 4), excessive oxidation (see Chapter 5), elevated homocysteine levels (see Chapter 7), low cortisol levels (see Chapter 6) or problems in the GI tract with microflora imbalances or gut leakiness (see Chapter 3).

Now scientists are beginning to realize that age-related drop-offs in oestrogen can trigger inflammation in women. Thinning, weakened bones (osteoporosis), for example, is one of the degenerative risks after the menopause. Plummeting oestrogen levels at this stage in life trigger inflammatory chemicals and other immune system cells, including osteoclast cells, to quickly multiply within bone. Osteoclasts are responsible for breaking down bone. Hence, when they are forced to work overtime as part of the inflammatory response to low oestrogen levels, bone tissue gets thinner.[1]

The decline in sex hormones as you age, then, is yet another cause of inflamm-ageing to be aware of and, ultimately, to address if you want your middle years and beyond to be as healthy and fulfilling as those of your youth.

Another problem that can become more common as we get older is low mood or even depression. Levels of serotonin and noradrenalin (brain chemicals that help us to feel content and positive) are bolstered by good levels of oestrogen, as is the functioning of the serotonin receptors. So, it's hardly surprising that plummeting oestrogen levels during middle age can make us feel low, sad and even depressed.[2] See Box 9.4 below and also Chapter 7 for more on these brain chemicals.

AGE-RELATED HORMONAL IMBALANCES

Sex hormones are truly amazing chemicals, working wondrous effects on the body and keeping us looking and feeling great. But none of them works in isolation. They all need to work together, in hormonal harmony, in order to work their magic. Elevated or suppressed levels of one will affect the ability of the others to work well.

FOR WOMEN

One of the most common female sex hormone imbalances is that of 'oestrogen dominance', in which your oestrogen levels are too high, relative to your levels of progesterone. This situation can happen at any time of life but is particularly likely during the years leading up to the menopause, known as the peri-menopause.[3] (Read Box 9.1 to see if you may be going through the peri-menopause.) This is because, although your oestrogen levels may be on the wane, progesterone can be in even shorter supply, as it's only released if you are ovulating. As you head towards the menopause, more of your monthly cycles become 'anovulatory' – that is, they include no ovulation, meaning that progesterone isn't produced at all. You won't necessarily be aware of this, as lack of ovulation may not affect your menstruation.

Oestrogen dominance is more likely to occur if you are overweight. This is because, as we saw in Chapter 4, fatty tissue produces an enzyme (aromatase) that converts male hormones into oestrogen. This is one of the reasons that carrying too much fat can contribute to oestrogen-related problems such as endometriosis, fibroids and breast cancer.[4] Exposure to oestrogen-mimicking chemicals can also contribute to oestrogen dominance. These are found in herbicides and pesticides, as well as in some cosmetics, plastics and oily fish from polluted fisheries.

Although your levels of oestrogen relative to progesterone rise during peri-menopause, your *absolute* level of oestrogen declines, and this of course brings its own problems. At this time of life, not only might you experience the transient symptoms of fluctuating hormonal levels, such as mood swings, night sweats and hot flushes (see Box 9.1), but in the long term you are left with a greater risk of health problems from which you are protected by oestrogen in your younger years. These include vaginal dryness, urinary urgency and more serious conditions such as cardiovascular disease and osteoporosis. Box 9.6 provides tips for keeping your bones strong as you age.

FOR MEN

It is often said that men get it easy: they are not subjected to the wide hormonal fluctuations of the peri-menopause, nor do they have to cope with the sharp, sudden drop in overall hormone levels that occurs at the menopause. Nevertheless, men do suffer an age-related decline in beneficial sex hormones, and the resulting effects have been severe enough in some cases for the term 'andropause' to come into common parlance.

The male andropause refers to the gradual decline of testosterone, produced mainly in the testes, and also of DHEA, produced in the adrenal glands. Testosterone levels can begin to fall from the age of 30, at a rate of about 1 per cent a year; at the same time, your blood levels of a protein called sex hormone binding globulin (SHBG) begin to rise, making the testosterone that is left gradually less effective.[5] (See the information below on how SHBG can affect the activity of your hormones.)

To make matters worse, declining testosterone can lead to a type of oestrogen-dominance. Men have oestrogen in small amounts. It doesn't tend to fall at the same rate of testosterone, meaning that, as you age, your *relative* level of oestrogen can become too high.

These hormonal changes can leave you feeling irritable, depressed and tired all the time. It can affect your libido (see Box 9.7), your memory and ability to think clearly, and it can lead to erectile dysfunction, declining muscle strength, accumulating fat mass, sleep disturbances and a reduced sense of wellbeing, as well as an increased risk of cardiovascular disease.

SUPPORTING THE HORMONAL LIFECYCLE

Given that our sex hormones inevitably decline with age (and that in women oestrogen can plummet pretty sharply), it's important to give them extra support as we get older. This means supporting them at each stage of their life cycle: helping your body to manufacture them, transport them through the bloodstream to where they are needed, convert them to and from other hormones where necessary, latch on to their receptors so they can do their job, and, lastly, be effectively detoxified and eliminated.

In this chapter, you'll find out how to give your hormones the best support, at each of these stages, by using diet, lifestyle and nutritional supplements. We'll explain how making changes in these areas can make a huge difference to your hormonal balance and to any age-related 'hormonal' symptoms such as flagging energy levels and low sex drive (Boxes 9.4, 9.5, 9.6 and 9.7 provide recommendations for some specific 'hormonal' conditions). If you want to go one step further, you could also consider taking natural ('bio-identical') hormones to replenish your levels. For those of you who are interested in this, we've included some introductory information in Box 9.3. To do this safely, however, you should take the advice of a doctor who specializes in hormonal health – an endocrinologist.

BOX 9.1 ARE YOU PERI-MENOPAUSAL?

Complete the following short questionnaire to find out whether you may have started the menopause transition.

Tick the box for each statement that applies to you, if the symptom in the statement has become noticeably worse, or appeared for the first time, within the last year or two. If the symptom has existed for many years, do not tick the box. For example, only tick the box for 'Craving chocolate...' if this issue has only appeared, or got worse, within the last two years; leave the box blank if you have had chocolate cravings for most of your adult life or for at least ten years.

- ☐ Anxiety, irritability, tension or mood swings
- ☐ Craving chocolate, sugary or starchy foods
- ☐ Physical or mental fatigue
- ☐ Increased breast tenderness, bloating, water retention
- ☐ Unexplained weight gain
- ☐ Depression, crying, forgetfulness
- ☐ Excessively heavy or light menstrual flow
- ☐ Occasional skipped periods
- ☐ Variations in menstrual cycles
- ☐ Poor sleep
- ☐ Painful intercourse (dyspareunia)
- ☐ Vaginal dryness
- ☐ Hot flushes
- ☐ Night sweats
- ☐ Dry, thinning skin
- ☐ Skin itching, tingling, burning or crawling
- ☐ Headaches or migraine

☐   A racing heartbeat or palpitations

☐   Increased urinary frequency or urgency

☐   Back pain or pain in the joints or muscles

☐   Breast atrophy

☐   Low libido

Total score _____

If you are over 40 years of age and you scored 8 or above, it may be that you have started the menopause transition period, which is known as the peri-menopause. This is a period of time, which usually starts in your mid-40s and can last for a few years, during which your oestrogen and progesterone levels are declining, culminating in the menopause.

Officially, the menopause is defined as the day after your final menstrual flow, looking back from 12 months on. It marks the end of the reproductive stage of your life, and the average age in the UK is 52 years. Interestingly, the age of your ovaries (the number of eggs you have left) does not necessarily correlate with your chronological age, so the menopause may be earlier or later than 52 years for you. If you want to predict the likely age of your menopause, find out what age your mother experienced it, as there seems to be a hereditary element.[6] You can also test your levels of anti-Mullerian hormone (AMH) and antral follicle count (AFC), although this tends not to be offered on the NHS in the UK.

During the peri-menopause, not only are your hormone levels falling, but along the way they take a rollercoaster ride of sharp peaks and troughs – and this worsens the many debilitating symptoms that women can suffer during these years. To compensate for the dramatic fall in circulating oestrogen and progesterone, the pituitary gland in the brain tries desperately to stimulate the ovaries by producing very high levels of follicle stimulating hormone (FSH) and luteinizing hormone (LH). Elevated levels of these two hormones on a blood test can confirm that you are going through the menopause.

The good news is that even as your ovarian function declines, the ovaries can produce a little oestrogen, and oestrogen is also produced by your fat cells and by the adrenal glands. And, as long as you have good levels of the adrenal hormone DHEA, some oestrogen is produced in other tissues that need it, including the brain, the blood vessels and bones (see below). DHEA is also directly beneficial for healthy ageing: maintaining good levels can support your mood, cognition and memory, as well as your physical energy levels and your overall feelings of wellbeing.

This implies that, for an easier menopause transition, your adrenal glands need to be in tip-top condition. And, indeed, supporting your adrenal glands is one of the most effective things you can do to ease the journey through your 40s and 50s, while your ovarian function is declining.

For an even more complete hormonal picture, it can be useful to consider also your levels of pregnenolone and testosterone. Testosterone is needed for libido and bone and muscle mass, not only in men but also in women, while pregnenolone is a precursor to many of the sex hormones. Both these hormones decline with age (as does DHEA), although at a more gradual rate than oestrogen and progesterone.

TIPS FOR A TROUBLE-FREE ANDROPAUSE AND MENOPAUSE TRANSITION

If you want to minimize the chances of experiencing 'hormonal' symptoms as you get older, here's your lifestyle plan.

HELP YOUR BODY TO MAKE THE HORMONES

In women, as the ovaries move towards retirement, you rely increasingly on your adrenal glands to produce both testosterone and oestrogen, as seen in Box 9.1. So, for a smoother ride through the menopause, it makes sense to support the health of the adrenals.

Research shows that if you are under long-term stress (in other words, if you have chronically elevated levels of the adrenal hormone cortisol), you are more likely to experience severe menopausal symptoms.[7] What's more, as we saw in Chapter 6, long-term stress can eventually lead to a condition called adrenal fatigue. This is where the adrenal glands are exhausted and cannot produce enough cortisol and DHEA to keep you feeling healthy. Typical symptoms of adrenal fatigue include energy slumps, low mood, anxiety, tearfulness and an inability to deal with stressful situations – all symptoms commonly associated with the peri-menopause. So, you can see that flagging adrenals can make any peri-menopausal symptoms seem far worse.

It's also worth remembering that other body tissues use the adrenal hormone DHEA in order to make locally acting oestrogen. So, for example, bone-building cells (called osteoblasts) make oestrogen from DHEA for bone health.[8] This is particularly important post-menopause when the risk of osteoporosis dramatically increases.

Men also rely more on adrenally produced DHEA as the testicular production of testosterone declines with age. Hence adrenal health is equally as important as it is in women.

Refer to Chapter 6 to find out about how to assess your adrenal health. That chapter talks you through a plan for reversing adrenal fatigue and supporting your adrenal glands in the long term. Some of the most important actions are to identify and reduce the main sources of stress in your life, keep your blood sugar levels stable (see Chapter 4), get adequate, high-quality sleep (see Chapter 10) and ensure a good daily intake of vitamins and minerals, especially magnesium, vitamin C and the B vitamins. A particularly useful herbal supplement for flagging adrenal function is rhodiola, which you can read about in Chapter 6, along with other relevant nutraceuticals.

HELP NORMALIZE YOUR LEVELS WITH PLANT HORMONES
Phytoestrogens are plant hormones that have a very mild oestrogenic activity – many hundreds of times weaker than your own oestrogen. By latching on to the body's oestrogen receptor sites, phytoestrogens can increase oestrogen levels when your own levels are low. Conversely, because they are so much weaker than the oestrogen you produce yourself, they can lower your overall oestrogen if your levels are relatively too high.

Most of the research is on female (rather than male) health and has been undertaken on types of phytoestrogens called isoflavones. These are found in legumes, especially soy beans, and also in red clover. Many studies show that isoflavones can help with hormone-related hot flushes.[9] Regular soy consumption may also reduce the risk of postmenopausal illnesses such as cardiovascular disease and thinning bones.[10]

Other food sources of phytoestrogens are shown in the table below.

TABLE 9.1 SOURCES OF PHYTOESTROGENS

Food	Phytoestrogen content (μg/100g)	Food	Phytoestrogen content (μg/100g)
Flaxseed	379,380.0	Pistachios	382.5
Soy bean	103,920.0	Dried dates	329.5
Tofu	27,150.1	Sunflower seeds	216.0
Soy yogurt	10,275.0	Chestnuts	210.2
Multi grain bread	4,798.7	Dried prunes	183.5
Natto	5,893.0	Olive oil	180.7
Tempeh	4,352.0	Walnuts	139.5
Soy milk	2,957.2	Almonds	131.1
Hummus	993.0	Cashew nuts	121.9
Garlic	603.6	Winter squash	113.7
Mung bean sprouts	495.1	Green beans	105.8
Dried apricots	444.5	Onion	32.0
Alfalfa sprouts	441.4	Blueberries	17.5

In men, there is some preliminary evidence that isoflavones may be helpful in preventing and managing benign prostate disease (like the age-related enlargement of the prostate that is known as benign prostatic hyperplasia – BPH)[11] and even prostate cancer, although well-controlled clinical trials are still lacking. Relative to men in the UK, men in Japan and China have higher levels of phytoestrogens in their bloodstreams and also have a lower risk of prostate disease.[12]

To get a hormonal effect from phytoestrogens you probably need to eat 20–60g/¾–2½oz soy protein a day, or take a daily supplement of 35–120mg isoflavones.[13] However, before you start increasing your soy consumption, it's worth knowing that the effects vary markedly from person to person. This is evident from the trial results, which have not *consistently* shown benefits. This is probably because the effect you get depends on the make-up of your gut bacteria. (The gut microflora are responsible for metabolizing the phytoestrogens to make the active hormonal compounds.) For example, men who have the right balance of gut bacteria to metabolize daidzein (a phytoestrogen from soy) tend to have a lower incidence of prostate cancer.[14]

So, before you increase your phytoestrogens, take steps to get your gut into tip-top condition. Chapter 3 shows you how to do this.

Phytoestrogens may not be a good idea if you have a personal or family history of oestrogen-related cancer. This is because the results of studies on phytoestrogens in conditions such as breast cancer tend to be somewhat contradictory,[15] and so opinions are still divided on whether they may reduce the risk or increase it.

Some herbs can have helpful oestrogenic effects in women. As each of us is different, it is often a case of trying one at a time, for at least three months, before judging its effectiveness. If you supplement more than one simultaneously, it starts to become difficult to establish which of them is having the best effect. Herbs that have been shown in trials to reduce the frequency and/or severity of menopausal hot flushes include agnus castus (sometimes referred to as vitex),[16] St John's wort,[17] sage[18] and black cohosh.[19] Licorice phytochemicals may also have some mild oestrogenic activity in helping to maintain the mood-boosting brain chemical serotonin.[20]

HELP YOUR HORMONES TO BE MORE ACTIVE

Having good levels of hormones in the bloodstream is only one part of the hormonal harmony equation. Hormones are *in*active unless they can become 'free' from their protein carriers and unless they can latch on to the right receptor sites. With the right diet, supplements and lifestyle, you can promote both of these activities.

The main protein carrier for oestrogen and testosterone is SHBG. You can measure your levels with a simple blood test. When hormones are bound to SHBG they don't have any effect on the body at all. This means that if your SHBG levels are too high, you can suffer the ill-effects of oestrogen and/or testosterone deficiency, even if the levels of these hormones in the bloodstream are within range. Conversely, if SHBG levels are too low, you are at risk of having too much of a hormonal effect.

Your SHBG levels are determined by your weight and your levels of testosterone, oestrogen, insulin and thyroid hormones.[21] Broadly speaking:

▸ High levels of testosterone tend to lower your SHBG levels, whereas excessive oestrogen in the bloodstream causes the body to overproduce SHBG. Women on hormone replacement therapy (HRT), for example, have elevated SHBG because of the oestrogen they are taking.

▸ Insulin, as you may have seen in Chapter 4, is the hormone that gets sugar into cells. If your insulin levels are too high (which can happen if you have 'insulin resistance', for instance), this will suppress SHBG production. This means that too much of your oestrogen and testosterone becomes free and active. Indeed, this is one of the problems that comes with pre-diabetes. (See Chapter 4 for more about insulin resistance and pre-diabetes.)

▸ If you are overweight and/or have low thyroid function, you may find your SHBG dips too low, whereas people who are underweight and/or have an overactive thyroid tend to have excessively high SHBG readings on blood tests.

If SHBG is suppressed, women may experience symptoms of oestrogen dominance. However, if SHBG is too high, both men and women are at risk of hormonal deficiency symptoms. Such symptoms include the atrophic conditions that come with the menopause (thinning skin, urinary urgency, vaginal soreness, loss of bone density and failing blood vessel health) and the andropause (loss of muscle mass, bone density and skin suppleness).

To normalize your SHBG levels, the best advice is to get to a healthy weight, get your blood levels of insulin and glucose under control and check your thyroid function (see Chapters 4 and 6 for more on all these issues). And if you're female and your SHBG is too high, don't forget to check for low testosterone because this could be the cause. Women need testosterone just as much as men – it may help with sex drive and bone health, for example – but in far lower amounts.

So, for hormones to have an effect on cells, a great enough proportion of them needs to be free from their SHBG carrier. What's more, they need to bind to the receptor sites on the cell membrane. These receptors are seated in omega 3 fatty acids. Hence, these fats are likely the most important nutrients for hormone binding. You can get them from flaxseeds (linseeds), hemp seeds, chia seeds, pumpkin seeds and walnuts (and the oils of these). But the most important source is oily fish. Ideally, you should eat oily fish three times a week, or consider taking a fish oil supplement. A trial of 120 middle-aged women with hot flushes found that supplementing with EPA (one of the active omega 3 fats in oily fish) significantly reduced their frequency. The dose used was 500mg three times a day.[22]

CONTROL HOW YOUR BODY CONVERTS HORMONES INTO OTHER HORMONES

Sex hormones convert from one to another, depending on the body's needs. Testosterone, for example, can be converted to oestrogen by way of an enzyme called aromatase. Fatty tissue is very good at churning out high levels of aromatase. This means that if you are overweight, aromatase activity can massively increase, leading to oestrogen dominance. (Drugs that inhibit aromatase are sometimes used in the treatment of breast cancer.)

Excessive aromatase can cause problems for both men and women. It is perhaps more immediately obvious in men, in that if you are ageing and overweight your high-oestrogen-low-testosterone situation can cause you to develop 'man boobs' (or 'moobs').

Given the role that fat plays in producing oestrogen, it's equally important to avoid becoming *under*weight during the menopausal years. It's at this time of life that women rely more on fat cells to keep their oestrogen levels up (as well as on the adrenal glands, as seen).

So you need to make sure you are a healthy weight. Start off by measuring your waist-to-hip ratio (as detailed in Chapter 4) and follow the advice in that chapter.

Another conversion enzyme of note is 5 alpha-reductase. This converts testosterone to a more troublesome metabolite called dihydrotestosterone (DHT). In men, too much DHT (and oestrogen) can fuel the unwanted enlargement of the prostate that can come with ageing.[23]

DETOX YOUR HORMONES

Once they have done their job, hormones are detoxified in the liver, in two stages, called phases 1 and 2.

In phase 1, the hormones are converted ('metabolized') into toxic chemicals, which can play havoc with our health if they hang around for too long. Certain oestrogen metabolites, for example, may increase the risk of some oestrogenic cancers and autoimmune diseases such as rheumatoid arthritis and lupus in women.[24]

But there are things you can do to help your liver to produce more of the safer oestrogen metabolites and fewer of the disease-causing ones: avoid eating overcooked meats (or meats cooked at high temperatures, such as fried or barbecued) and increase your intake of oily fish (for the omega 3 fat EPA), flaxseeds and cruciferous vegetables (see Box 9.2).[25]

Once through the first stage of detox (phase 1), oestrogen and other sex hormone metabolites enter the phase 2 detox system. Various different detox processes are used, but the main one for hormones is called methylation. Chapter 7 goes into more detail on methylation, as this process is also used to manufacture brain chemicals.

If the methylation process if flagging, it won't be able to disable the toxic hormone metabolites. Luckily, there's a simple test you can do to find out how well you are methylating. The test measures blood levels of an amino acid called homocysteine. If this turns out to be too high, it's a good indicator that your methylation needs some support. As seen in Chapter 7, the best support is B vitamins, especially B12 and folate.

The other processes that help with detoxifying hormones also require specific nutrients to keep them working well. The most important ones are good-quality protein (from fish, meat and eggs), B vitamins (again) and the minerals magnesium, iron and molybdenum.[26] If you are low in iron, by far the best source is 'haem iron' from lean red meat, liver and the darker meat from game, poultry and oily fish, as well as eggs. Vegetarian iron is found in beans, pulses, dark green leaves and dried fruit. Unfortunately, it is not nearly as well absorbed as haem iron, although this may be helped by eating vitamin C-rich foods at the same time, such as fruit and raw or lightly cooked vegetables. Good sources of molybdenum are nuts, beans, lentils, peas and cruciferous vegetables. Magnesium is found in plant foods, but many people benefit from also supplementing this mineral, as it is so easy to become deficient. (See Chapter 6 for more on the importance of magnesium.)

EXCRETE THE SPENT HORMONES

Once detoxified, your hormones need to be safely excreted from the body. To speed this process along, they are attached to a molecule (called glucuronic acid) that is able to get them into the faeces. In this way, the hormones leave the body when you next have a bowel movement.

Unfortunately, if you have an overgrowth of unhealthy bacteria in the gut (a condition called dysbiosis), this hormonal excretion process can go wrong. Unfriendly bacteria can produce an enzyme (known as beta-glucuronidase) that breaks the attachment between oestrogen and glucuronic acid. This leaves lots of 'free' oestrogen in the gut. Free oestrogen can't easily be excreted and instead much of it is reabsorbed into the bloodstream. This can push blood levels too high – putting you into a state of oestrogen dominance, whether you are male or female.

To make sure this isn't happening in *your* gut, you need to look after the friendly microbes that reside there. Chapter 3 explains how to establish if you have an overgrowth of problematic bugs in the gut and, if so, what to do about it. In particular, your friendly microbes are likely to have taken a bashing if you have been under a lot of stress or have been taking antibiotics or medication for indigestion. If this is the case, consider supplementing some friendly bacteria (probiotics), as explained in Chapter 3.

It's also worth knowing that there is something that can help any 'free' oestrogen to be excreted rather than reabsorbed. This is soluble fibre and it is found in oats, brown rice, pulses (lentils, beans, chickpeas) and other vegetables, especially okra.

BOX 9.2 THE WONDERS OF CRUCIFEROUS VEGETABLES

Cruciferous vegetables include broccoli (and broccoli sprouts), cauliflower, kale, watercress, rocket (arugula), cabbage, turnips, Brussels sprouts, radish, pak choi, spring greens, collard greens, Chinese cabbage, diakon and kohlrabi.

These vegetables are good at helping the liver to detoxify hormones because they contain special phytochemicals called glucosinolates. These are converted in the body into wonder-molecules called isothiocyanates (including the anti-ageing molecule sulforaphane that we introduced in Chapter 1). Isothiocyanates slow down the phase 1 detox processes and this in turn reduces the production of toxic hormone metabolites. They also speed up the helpful phase 2 detox pathways,[27] ensuring that more of the toxic metabolites are swiftly disabled before they can do damage in the body.

These cruciferous chemicals are so effective in improving detoxification that they may even reduce our susceptibility to cancer-causing compounds[28] and help to cleanse the body of toxic metals such as arsenic[29] and mercury.[30] They may also offer some protection from cardiovascular and neurodegenerative diseases.[31]

Our advice is to eat at least one portion of these vegetables every day, preferably lightly steamed, rather than overcooked. You could try, for example, our Broccoli Pear Soup, Sauerkraut, Cauliflower Munchies, Asian Cauliflower 'Rice' Stir Fry, Watercress, Apple and Walnut Salad with Creamy Mustard Dressing, Salted Vinegar and Onion Kale Chips and the green smoothies.

There has been so much interest in the power of these phytochemicals that a new 'superbroccoli' was launched in 2011, containing far higher levels of glucosinolates and marketed as Beneforté.[32]

One word of caution: if you suffer from excessive gastrointestinal wind and bloating, please improve your gut health before you start eating cruciferous vegetables every day, as they can worsen these gut symptoms in some people. Chapter 3 shows you how to do this.

BOX 9.3 HORMONE REPLACEMENT THERAPY – IS IT RIGHT FOR YOU?

The practice of replacing hormones as your own production declines with age is called hormone replacement therapy, or HRT. HRT is an emotive topic and always has been: can it turn back the clock and give you a new lease of life, or is it so risky that it should be avoided like the plague? These are rather extreme views of HRT but they have nevertheless been widespread, and this can make it difficult for people to make decisions about whether or not to use hormones as part of a healthy ageing strategy.

If you're wondering about the pros and cons of using hormones, here are some things you should know.

First, it's not worth making any decisions without discussing your options with a doctor specializing in hormones (an endocrinologist). You can get a referral for a consultation, although some types of hormones (see below) are typically only available privately. Work with a doctor who will test your current levels of hormones and SHBG, and who will take a full and detailed history and family history, so that together you can calculate the likely risks and benefits of HRT for you as an individual.

HRT is known to help many people with menopausal symptoms such as hot flushes and also with bone density. But for the last 12 years, it has been treated with immense caution. And rightly so, given the results of a huge trial in 2002 (called the Women's Health Initiative – WHI), which reported that women taking HRT had a greater risk of thrombosis and breast cancer.[33]

Since then, however, the WHI trial has been criticized for using such an artificial form of HRT – women were given a combination of oestrogen from horses ('equine oestrogen') and an artificial type of progesterone called progestogen (or progestin). Critics also said that many of the women were offered the HRT too late, often not starting it until 12 years after the menopause, by which time some damage to arteries, from oestrogen deficiency, could already have been done. Some experts have proposed that giving HRT in a more natural way may provide more benefits and minimize the risks. Trials to test this idea are now underway.[34]

Although there are variations in design between these more recent studies, the overall trend is towards giving HRT earlier in the menopause, rather than starting many years later, and using forms of oestrogen and progesterone that are chemically exactly the same as those produced by humans. (Such hormones are known as 'bio-identical' hormones.) Some trials are also giving oestrogen by way of a skin patch, rather than a pill, which may reduce some of the risks associated with oral HRT.[35]

These more natural forms of hormones are available on medical prescription in the form of oestradiol patches, testosterone patches and creams, and oral micronized progesterone.

Meanwhile, there are many people all over the world, male and female, who are trying what is known as *compounded* bio-identical HRT (CBHRT). CBHRT uses bio-identical hormones at doses that are individualized to your unique needs. If you opt for this type of help, your hormone levels will first be tested by using blood or saliva samples. If they are low, you will then be prescribed oestrogen, progesterone, testosterone and/or other related hormones, including DHEA and/or pregnenolone, for example, at doses designed to complement your own production, to bring you up to a physiologically 'healthy' level.

This type of HRT is increasingly widely used, although it is only available privately. The benefit over conventional 'bio-identical' hormone replacement is that the dose is tailored to your particular individual needs. But critics of this approach say that, compared to standard HRT, we still have very little information on its effectiveness and safety. It has also been suggested that, because it is relatively unregulated, the purity and potency of the hormones may vary between batches – meaning that you don't always know the *exact* dose that you are getting.[36]

Whether you are male or female, our advice is that you initially try smoothing your age-related hormonal decline by using diet, nutritional supplements and lifestyle changes, of the kind outlined in this chapter. (And if you want to improve your levels of DHEA, you could consider taking a nutritional supplement called 7-keto-DHEA.[37] We recommend working with a health practitioner and starting with a dose of 5mg twice a day.)

You should give yourself a few months of a non-drug approach before you consider taking something as powerful as a hormone, even in its 'natural' (bio-identical) form. If, having done this, you believe your health is still compromised from your low hormone levels, go to see a hormone doctor with whom you can discuss your options and who will help you to assess your *individual* risk of developing osteoporosis, deep vein thrombosis, breast cancer and/or prostate cancer.

BOX 9.4 HOW TO KEEP HAPPY WHEN FEMALE HORMONES ARE FALLING

Oestrogen and progesterone have a huge impact on mood. It is normal to feel more emotionally stable when these hormones are at good, relatively steady levels in the bloodstream. Progesterone has calming and anti-anxiety effects on the brain. Oestrogen helps us to make and use the 'happy' chemical serotonin. It also helps to keep dopamine, adrenalin and noradrenalin in circulation, all of which help to give us energy, drive and a sense of motivation.[38]

It's hardly surprising, then, that as progesterone production ceases, and oestrogen levels rise and fall sharply during the peri-menopause, women can suffer terribly from mood swings, anxiety and depressive-like symptoms. Frequent yet unpredictable episodes of plummeting oestrogen during this time make serotonin and dopamine less available and also reduce activity within the regions of the brain responsible for emotional stability.[39]

If you're peri-menopausal and have been suffering from these types of symptoms, your doctor may well have suggested you take an antidepressant medication. This is becoming increasingly common, especially since HRT has fallen out of favour. One thing to be aware of, however, is that if you increase your serotonin levels too much, you could be harming your bones. As we saw in Chapter 7, taking antidepressants called serotonin reuptake inhibitors (SSRIs) may increase your risk of skeletal fracture.[40]

It may be safer to look at gentler ways of improving your balance of brain chemicals. Chapter 7 has an action plan for doing just this. Dietary and lifestyle factors are the crux of the plan, including keeping your blood sugar levels stable with regular exercise and the antioxidant-rich low-GL diet (see Chapter 2) and getting adequate amounts of good-quality sleep (see Chapter 10). In addition, you could try one of the following nutritional supplements, both of which are explained in more detail in Chapter 7:

▸ 5-hydroxytryptophan (5-HTP): 100mg three times a day on an empty stomach.

▸ L-theanine: 200mg once or twice a day on an empty stomach.

There are some simple steps you can take to keep your blood levels of glucose and cortisol steady overnight. (This will improve your sleep and help support your mood the following day.) Top tips are:

▸ Be physically active during the day.

▸ Avoid stimulants late in the day (caffeine, nicotine, sugar).

▸ Don't use alcohol to help you sleep.

▸ Don't go to bed hungry.

▸ Have a low-GL snack (e.g. kale crisps, roasted olives, or see our recipes for *Lime Guacamole* with vegetable sticks and *Tomato Seeded Crackers*).

▸ Experiment with teas made from chamomile, lime blossom, valerian, hops and passiflora.

BOX 9.5 TIPS FOR AGE-RELATED PROSTATE PROBLEMS

As you age and your hormones decline, you are more likely to be affected by low-testosterone issues such as erectile dysfunction, as well as prostate issues including prostatitis (inflamed prostate), benign prostatic hypertrophy (BPH) and prostate cancer. BPH is an age-related gradual enlargement of the prostate gland that can cause problems with urination, such as increased frequency, urgency and feeling that you are unable to properly empty the bladder.

Male hormonal problems are very much influenced by lifestyle. We know, for example, that testosterone levels fall earlier and faster in men with obesity[41] and type 2 diabetes,[42] in those who regularly drink too much alcohol[43] and in men who are under long-term stress.[44] Antioxidants, such as vitamins A and E, zinc and selenium, are also important for maintaining testosterone production.[45]

Scientists have found a heart-healthy lifestyle (taking exercise, reducing blood pressure and blood fats, eating a healthy diet, maintaining a healthy weight and controlling blood sugar levels) also reduces the risk of developing BPH.[46] Taking regular physical exercise may reduce the risk of erectile dysfunction, even if you only make this change in mid-life.[47] And lifestyle changes may make a real difference to your risk of getting prostate cancer and to its rate of progression if you already have it. Studies tend to focus on eating a low-fat, vegan diet, including regular exercise and adopting stress management techniques.[48]

To reduce the risk of these conditions, follow the advice given in this chapter on how to have a trouble-free menopause and andropause. Once you have done this, you could then consider increasing some of the following nutrients, depending on your circumstances. To get the most benefit from any such supplement programme, it would be best to work with a nutrition practitioner, who can tailor it to meet your particular needs.

- Men who consume more of the following nutrients tend to have a lower risk of prostate cancer:[49] zinc, selenium, carotenoids from tomatoes (beta-carotene, lycopene), green tea, soy phytoestrogens and omega 3 fats. Note that lycopene is better absorbed from the diet if is cooked and eaten with fat.

- These nutrients have been found helpful in BPH: lycopene,[50] soy isoflavones[51] and the herb saw palmetto.[52]

- These nutrients may help with erectile dysfunction: L-arginine[53] and red ginseng.[54]

BOX 9.6 KEEPING YOUR BONES STRONG

One of the problems of ageing is a gradual thinning and weakening of your bones, making you vulnerable to fractures. If the density of your bones falls below a certain threshold, you are said to have osteoporosis, while a diagnosis of osteopenia indicates a less severe loss of bone density. You can measure your bone density with a hospital test called a dual-energy x-ray absorptiometry, or DEXA test. If you have a family history of osteoporosis or you have other risk factors, you can often get this done through a referral from your family doctor.

Post-menopausal women are at particular risk of low bone density because of the sudden drop in oestrogen levels. Oestrogen stops the proliferation of bone-destroying cells called osteoclasts. Some experts believe that progesterone also supports bone health; this hormone also drops sharply during the peri-menopause. Testosterone and DHEA are also anabolic hormones and necessary for bone health, and they too decline as we get older, in both men and women.

If you are particularly concerned about the health of your bones, ask your doctor for a DEXA scan so that you can get a baseline measurement. Whatever your DEXA score, it is never too late to make a positive impact on your bone health and your risk of fracture. You may be prescribed drugs if are diagnosed with osteoporosis, but these can carry adverse side-effects, so it is worth looking at natural options too:

- Make sure you are neither overweight nor underweight, as both can increase your fracture risk.

- Reduce any sources of inflammation in your life. Chronic, low-grade inflammation drives bone loss, as already seen.[55] See Chapter 8 for a checklist of possible sources of inflammation so you can establish if any of them may be affecting you. Some of the sources – irritable bowel syndrome (IBS), for example, or gum disease – may not be immediately obvious.

- Make sure you are getting plenty of anti-inflammatory fats in the diet, by eating oily fish three times a week or, if you are a vegan, flaxseeds (linseeds), chia seeds, pumpkin seeds and hemp seeds and their cold-pressed oils.

- Cut down on inflammatory fats, namely saturated and trans-fats, as well as heated omega 6 fats. You can do this by reducing fatty cuts of meat and avoiding processed foods, including vegetable or seed oils sold in clear plastic bottles from supermarket shelves. In population studies and some (not all) trials, a higher intake of omega 3 fats has been associated with better bone health.[56] See Chapter 8 for more information on inflammatory and anti-inflammatory fats.

- Follow the recommendations in Chapter 2 for a wholefood diet that is also rich in antioxidants. Antioxidants are found in deeply and brightly coloured fruit and vegetables, so eat plenty of these every day.

- Your diet should also be rich in the bone-building nutrients calcium (whitebait, dairy products, tinned fish with bones, beans and pulses), magnesium (whole grains, beans and pulses, seeds), vitamin D (oily fish) and vitamin K2 (fermented cheeses, although the very best source is the fermented soy product natto). Lower rates of hip fracture among elderly women are found in eastern Japan, where natto is most widely eaten.[57]

- Get some sunshine for vitamin D. Expose as much of your skin as possible to the sun daily from late spring to early autumn, between 11am and 3pm, taking care not to burn.

- Get your levels of oestrogen, progesterone, testosterone, DHEA and SHBG tested and work with a hormone doctor to consider your options for improving levels if they are out of range.

- You should also check your thyroid function (see Chapter 6) as both an underactive and an overactive thyroid can contribute to poor bone health.

- Check your medications: certain antidepressants (called SSRIs), diabetes drugs (called thiazolidinediones), heartburn remedies (called PPIs) and steroids can promote bone loss. If you are taking any of these, discuss the pros and cons with your doctor.

- If you smoke, take steps to stop. Smoking causes bone loss and increases fracture risk. As nicotine is so highly addictive, you may find that hypnotherapy helps.

- Don't drink too much alcohol, as this reduces bone mass. See Chapter 2 for our recommended guidelines on drinking alcohol.

- Regular weight-bearing exercise is crucial for strengthening bones. Aim for at least half an hour a day of brisk walking, weight lifting, aerobics, dancing, jogging, rebounding (trampolining), or sports such as football, tennis or squash. (Swimming is good exercise but is not particularly beneficial for bone health.)

- Keep your blood sugar levels stable by following the low-GL diet outlined in Chapter 2 and following the advice in Chapter 4. Blood sugar problems can cause cortisol levels to get too high. Elevated cortisol is catabolic – it breaks down muscle and bone tissue.

- A low GL-diet includes protein at every meal. Protein is essential for bone health, since the bone matrix is made of protein (osteocalcin). Rather than eat too much animal protein, have some meals that include vegetable proteins instead, such as pulses, nuts and seeds.

- As all forms of stress can raise cortisol, take steps to assess and reduce the sources of stress in your life. See Chapter 6 for more on how to do this and on how to support the adrenal glands. Remember, keeping your adrenal glands healthy is important not only because this will help you to deal better with stressful situations, but also because the adrenals produce bone-supporting oestrogen, testosterone and DHEA.

▶ Reduce any sources of 'free radicals'. Chapter 5 explains how these cause oxidative damage in the body. Oxidation promotes bone loss. Common sources of free radicals are pollution, smoking, air travel, excess sunlight, processed foods and burnt, blackened or overcooked foods. This is another reason to eat antioxidant-rich fruits and vegetables, since antioxidants disable free radicals.

▶ Eat an alkaline-forming diet by including the alkalizing foods (mainly fruits and vegetables) discussed in Chapter 2. A more acid-forming diet, one that includes a lot of meat, grains, coffee and sugar, triggers the release of calcium from the bones to help re-alkalize the blood.

▶ Check your homocysteine levels, as elevated homocysteine in the blood has been associated with bone loss. See Chapter 7 for more information on homocysteine and how to get it down if it is too high.

▶ Consider supplementing micro-nutrients that have evidence for their important role in bone health:

▷ Calcium:[58] You need 800–1000mg of calcium a day, either from the diet, or from a combination of both diet and supplements. In older people or in people with digestive problems, calcium that is sold as calcium citrate, lactate or malate is often better absorbed than calcium carbonate. In recent years there has been concern that taking calcium supplements may increase the risk of cardiovascular disease in older women.[59] However, such studies have been criticized for supplementing calcium alone, without also giving equally potent levels of vitamin D, magnesium and vitamin K. These nutrients are crucial for getting the body to deposit calcium in the bone, rather than in blood vessels. Our view is that if you can get adequate calcium from your diet, that is all well and good. But if you are avoiding dairy (perhaps because it causes you digestive problems, a stuffy nose or sinusitis), you may find it hard to get all you need from diet alone. If this is the case, you should consider supplementation, but be sure also to take the 'accessory' nutrients that will encourage the body to use it properly.

▷ Magnesium: This mineral is crucial for bone health and has been found to be helpful for improving signs of bone loss in postmenopausal women.[60] As explained in Chapter 6, however, most of us don't get enough of it from diet alone. According to government statistics, we get about 228mg a day from food,[61] which is considerably lower than the recommended daily allowance (RDA) of 375 mg. Take 300–450mg a day of magnesium, more if you are also taking calcium. Chapter 6 tells you about the best types of magnesium supplements to buy.

▷ Vitamin D: There is a well-established link between vitamin D deficiency and osteoporosis, due to its effect on calcium metabolism: it controls the amount of calcium that you absorb from the gut and the amount that you excrete in the urine. Studies have shown that supplementing 700–800 IU vitamin D reduces the risk of hip fracture by about 26 per cent compared with supplementing calcium alone or a placebo.[62] You may need more than this dose, depending on your current blood levels. As we saw in Chapter 8, there is widespread vitamin D insufficiency in the UK, due to our lack of year-round strong sunlight. We recommend you get your blood levels tested, either through your family doctor or privately. Aim for a reading of at least 75nmol/L. If your levels are lower than this, take 2000–5000 IU a day and retest again in 3–6 months.

▷ Vitamin K2: Take 90–150mcg of a type of K2 called MK-7. Vitamin K2 activates a bone protein called osteocalcin. This enables osteocalcin to hang on to calcium, pack it away inside the bone and keep it there.[63] People who have better levels of vitamin K in their blood seem to have fewer fractures.[64] And increasing vitamin K intake has been shown to improve markers of bone health.[65] There are two types of K2 sold as supplements: MK-4 and MK-7. We recommend MK-7 because it seems to be better at increasing your blood levels of K2.[66]

▷ B vitamins, vitamin C, zinc, boron, copper, potassium: Since such a wide range of micronutrients is important for bone health,[67] you should complement the recommendation above with a good multivitamin and mineral supplement.

▷ Fish oil: Take 1000mg combined EPA and DHA a day. We're suggesting you take more than the government recommends for basic health (450mg a day) because fish oil is anti-inflammatory and inflammation promotes bone loss. If, however, you are eating oily fish three times a week, you can reduce your supplement to 500mg a day.

Now that you have gone through this checklist, you can see that calcium is only a very small part of the bone-health story. Keeping your bones strong involves looking at all aspects of your health, including those covered in other chapters of this book.

BOX 9.7 NATURAL PRODUCTS FOR SEXUAL FUNCTION

This chapter has focused on strategies for supporting healthy levels of testosterone, oestrogen and progesterone, all of which tend to decline as we age, potentially affecting our sex drive. If you want to go a step further, you could consider supplementing one of the natural foods that may (according to preliminary evidence) help to boost sexual function. Three of them are listed here. Remember, though, that there isn't a great deal of research, so it's really a question of trying each of them in turn and seeing which, if any, work for you:

► The Amazonian plant Muira Puama (*Ptychopetalum olacoides*) for male impotence/erectile dysfunction[68] and for female sex drive.[69]

► The sweet-tasting, powdered Peruvian root maca, as an aphrodisiac.[70] See our recipes for *Dandelion Root 'Mocha' Ice Cream*, *Maca Stress-Busting Smoothie* and *Grain-Free Breakfast Bowl*.

► *Tribulus terrestris*, also known as puncture vine, as an aphrodisiac.[71]

MEAL PLAN

Breakfast	*Tofu Vegetable Scramble*
Lunch	*Seared Beef Salad with Coriander Pesto*
	Mixed berries with yogurt
Dinner	*Chilli and Lime Spiced Sardines* with steamed vegetables
	(broccoli, pak choi and cauliflower)
Snacks	*Superfood Fudge*
	Antioxidant Green Burst

If you do nothing else, do this...

▸ If you feel that you are suffering the effects of declining hormones, ask your doctor to check your blood levels of FSH, LH, oestrogen, testosterone, DHEA (measured as its sulphated form DHEA-S), SHBG and thyroid hormones. Add to this progesterone if you are female.

▸ Eat the antioxidant-rich, low-GL diet outlined in Chapter 2.

▸ Support your adrenal function. See Chapter 6 for a detailed plan of how to do this.

▸ Unless you have a particular risk for oestrogen-related cancers, increase phytoestrogens either by eating soy protein or by supplementing isoflavones.

▸ Take steps to get your gut into tip-top condition (see Chapter 3).

▸ Consider trialling one or more of the hormone-balancing herbs, vitex agnus castus, St John's wort or sage. If you are feeling particularly low or anxious, you could consider supplementing either rhodiola, 5-HTP or L-theanine.

▸ Improve your detox pathways. Eat good protein foods daily but avoid overcooked meats. Eat flaxseeds and cruciferous vegetables, and take a magnesium citrate supplement. Measure your levels of homocysteine and supplement folate (as L-methylfolate) and vitamin B12 if your homocysteine level is high.

- Get plenty of soluble fibre, found in oats, brown rice, pulses (lentils, beans, chickpeas) and other vegetables, especially okra.

- Men concerned about the risk of developing prostate problems should also include tomatoes and green tea in their daily diet and consider supplementing zinc, selenium and lycopene. and, if appropriate, the more specific nutrients for BPH and erectile dysfunction listed in Box 9.5.

- If, having done this, you believe your health is still compromised from your low hormone levels, go to see a hormone doctor with whom you can discuss your options for hormone replacement therapy, in the context of your *individual* risk of osteoporosis, deep vein thrombosis, breast cancer and/or prostate cancer.

CHAPTER 10

LIVE TO GET YOUNGER

While your diet plays a major part in your health and longevity, the rate at which you age is also profoundly influenced by your mindset and by many different aspects of your lifestyle. Regular physical activity, for example, is a well-established life extender. Getting the right amount and quality of sleep is equally as important, as is your attitude to life, including the way you typically respond to stressful situations. Being part of a loving, supportive community can bolster your ability to deal with life's ups and downs, and indeed has been linked to living longer.[1]

Maintaining a generally positive and optimistic outlook appears to be particularly important for healthy ageing, as does the quality of resilience – the ability to take disappointments in your stride and to bounce back from them, perhaps having learnt something in the process. While you may not have the power to control every event in your life, you can determine your response, and this is thought to be more of a predictor of your health and happiness than the actual set of mishaps that may befall you.[2]

In this chapter you'll learn about some of the most important lifestyle habits to adopt for a healthier middle age and beyond.

HOW PHYSICALLY ACTIVE IS HEALTHY?
THE BENEFITS OF KEEPING ACTIVE
One of the unwelcome consequences of ageing is the gradual loss of physical strength. This can start as early as the age of 30. From here on, you lose muscular strength at a rate of about 1 per cent a year, accelerating with each passing decade. Loss of strength is due mainly to decreasing muscle mass. This, in turn, is due to factors such as reduced levels of physical activity, falling hormonal levels, insufficient protein intake and also the accumulation of inflammation that tends to occur with ageing.[3]

As muscle cells contain the greatest concentration of our energy-producing batteries (the mitochondria – see Chapters 6 and 7), declining muscle mass means that age-related loss of strength is usually accompanied by loss of energy. You're also likely to notice that if/when you get injured, it takes you longer to recover.

Chapter 6 has more information on the mitochondria and how to improve energy levels with diet and supplements. But it's also useful to know that loss of muscle and mitochondrial power can both be reversed by regular exercise, particularly strength training.[4] One study reported that just six months of strength training done twice weekly reversed muscle ageing by 15–20 years.[5] Another study demonstrated significant increases in muscle size and improved function following a strength programme in older men (aged 60–72 years).[6] This implies that, no matter how old you are, it is never too late to benefit from becoming more physically active.

Many other benefits of regular exercise have been documented, from thousands of clinical studies. There is no doubting the fact that not only does regular physical activity help to maintain strength, mobility, flexibility and, ultimately, independence as we age, but it also reduces the risk of unwanted weight gain, obesity and most age-related degenerative diseases.

As luck would have it, the most effective type of exercise for longevity appears to be moderate, regular activity, which is something that most people can achieve. The risk of developing chronic ill-health reduces significantly with as little as three hours a week of brisk walking,[7] and moderate, regular activity in general has been shown to increase life span by an average of 1–4 years.[8]

Regular exercise helps to stabilize blood sugar and insulin levels, both key markers of ageing, and can help prevent type 2 diabetes. We saw in Chapter 4 how insulin resistance and diabetes dramatically speed up the ageing process. Moderate exercise can also help control appetite and reduce cravings, making it easier to stave off any creeping middle-age spread. Weight-bearing exercise, such as walking, jogging, trampolining or racket sports, helps to improve your sense of balance and the density of your bones, both of which are crucially important in avoiding age-related skeletal fractures. And exercise is also a great way to reduce stress, boost your mood, improve your self-esteem and combat depression.

HOW TO EXERCISE

We've seen that regular, moderate exercise is best. But what type of physical activity should this include? A combination of both aerobic exercise and strength training (e.g. using weights) may confer the most benefit for longevity. Aerobic exercise (e.g. running, swimming, walking) helps improve respiration, blood sugar control, cardiovascular health and fat burning, while strength training helps build muscle mass, as seen above. It's also worth remembering that the greater your muscle mass, the easier it is for you to burn fat and maintain a healthy weight. This is because muscle tissue uses up far more calories than fatty tissue, even when you are resting.

How much is enough?

Ideally, you should aim for around 30–60 minutes each day. Depending on your level of fitness, you may not be able to manage this initially. That's OK: just work up to it gradually. If you are new to exercise, you may wish to seek advice from a fitness instructor. And if you have a medical condition, it's also best to check your plans with your doctor, before you begin.

What should it include?

One of the most effective ways to exercise is to include a combination of low-intensity aerobic exercise, strength training and some higher-intensity sessions. If you work up to this gradually, you will avoid putting your body under too much stress and your overall exercise level will be moderate. The exception to this rule is that if you are suffering from adrenal fatigue (see Chapter 6), you should stick to low-intensity programmes until your cortisol and DHEA levels return back to healthy levels.

For optimal health, you should build up a good base of low-intensity exercise for 30 minutes twice a day, before replacing some of this with intense activity. Low-intensity exercise usually means walking briskly, light jogging, moderate cycling, dancing or swimming. If you consider yourself significantly lacking in fitness, however, a slower walking or cycling pace would constitute low-intensity exercise for you. It's important that you do something you enjoy and that you can keep up comfortably for the 30 minutes – you should be able to hold a conversation while doing this level of exercise.

If you want to get technical, you might like to know that low-intensity exercise is generally considered to be around 55–75 per cent of your maximum heart rate. Your maximum heart rate can be estimated by subtracting your age from 220. If you are 40 years of age, for example, your heart should beat around 180 times per minute at its maximum rate. Multiply 180 by 0.55 and 0.75 to determine the target range of your heart rate during low-intensity exercise.

You can monitor your heart rate with a wireless heart rate monitor and chest strap. Alternatively, just pause during your workout and place your finger against the artery on the side of your neck and count how many beats occur in ten seconds. Multiply by six to get the heart rate per minute.

Exercising for too long at a higher heart rate than this can put too much stress on the body in the long term. One study published in the *British Journal of Sports Medicine* revealed that training at high intensity for 30 minutes or more can disrupt immune system function. In this study, it led to inflammation that lasted for up to 72 hours.[9] This implies that if you are exercising too intensively every three days or more, you will be in a permanent state of inflammation. Healthy ageing, as we've seen throughout this book, relies on keeping yourself as free of inflammation as possible.

There is, however, a place for high-intensity training sessions; the trick is to undertake them only for short durations, and to delay introducing them until your lower-intensity base has become well established.

How to safely include high-intensity interval training (HIIT)

HIIT can be done in many ways and you should find an approach that you enjoy. A commonly used method is to incorporate 'sprinting bouts' into your regular routine. Sprinting bouts are short periods of time during which you increase the pace of your exercise to the maximum speed possible. A typical session might involve a couple of minutes to warm up, followed by exercising as hard and as fast as possible for 15–30 seconds, then resting for 30–60 seconds, before repeating the cycle 6–8 times and finishing with a couple of minutes' cool-down.

You can do this with running, cycling or swimming sprints, or even sprints on gym equipment, such as the cross-trainer, the stair-climber or the humble skipping rope. You can also perform resistance training exercises in an interval fashion, using either free weights or weights machines. This would involve bouts of high-intensity movements with periods of rest. Try timed sets of 30–60 seconds for each exercise, with a rest of 15 seconds before performing the next exercise, and then repeating.

All types of HIIT, whether you are running sprints, undertaking circuits, using a stationary bike or even free weights, tend to increase your requirement for energy (calories). This speeds up your metabolism and leads to a more significant fat loss than steadier, lower-intensity aerobic exercise. HIIT also appears to burn more fat *after* the workout has finished.[10]

HIIT also brings other benefits for healthy ageing: it stimulates the release of growth hormone,[11] which signals the body to synthesize muscle tissue; and it improves endurance and aerobic performance. A practical benefit of HIIT sessions is that they take up far less time to complete than more steady-paced workouts. You can normally complete them within 20 minutes, making this way of exercising particularly convenient for people with limited time.

Strength training

Resistance workouts, such as weight lifting, stimulate the release of anabolic hormones, particularly testosterone and growth hormone, to help keep you lean and youthful. Strength sessions do not need to take longer than 30–45 minutes and are recommended at least twice a week.

Building in some form of progression increases the benefit you get from each session. But this doesn't mean you need to increase the time spent exercising. Instead, gradually increase the intensity (greater resistance) and at the same time reduce the length of time spent resting between sets. And if your goal is healthy ageing and longevity, rather than becoming a top-class professional athlete, more is not necessarily better. As we saw earlier, lengthy workouts can increase inflammation. They can also cause surges in the stress hormone cortisol. This isn't helpful: cortisol is catabolic and can lead to muscle breakdown and fatigue.

In summary, it shouldn't be difficult to undertake the right quantity and quality of exercise that is most beneficial for healthy ageing. Find something you enjoy, start slowly but aim for some moderate activity every day. Once you have established a basic level of fitness, incorporate resistance training twice a week and some short, high-intensity sessions.

THE RESTORATIVE POWER OF SLEEP

There is nothing quite so restoring and energizing as a good night's sleep. Yet what should come naturally tends to elude a surprising number of us. Whether it's too many late nights and early risings, or, alternatively, feeling unable to get to sleep or stay asleep, chronic sleep deficit can have a profound effect on your health and wellbeing – and on your rate of ageing.

In the short term, it can make you irritable, impatient and moody, and it impairs your memory and reduces your ability to concentrate. Longer-term, it affects your immune system, it increases the risk of overeating, unwanted weight gain, anxiety, insulin resistance, diabetes and cardiovascular disease, and it can shorten overall life span. The key mechanisms of relevance here may be that lack of sleep causes sharp elevations in levels of stress hormones such as cortisol, and it also disrupts leptin and other hormones that help to control appetite.[12]

Let's take a moment to see what happens when the quality and quantity of sleep are optimal. During a good night's sleep you experience two different sleep states, rapid eye movement sleep (REM) and non-rapid eye movement sleep (NREM). There are four progressive stages of NREM sleep. During the first stage you begin to drop off. (And it is during this stage that, as the muscles gradually relax, you can awaken suddenly, with the sensation that you are falling.) Then, during stages two and three, the heart rate progressively slows and your temperature falls. Stage four provides the deepest sleep and it is during this stage that the body repairs and regenerates tissues, builds bone and muscle, and helps to replenish the immune system.

Once you have completed all four stages, you are pulled out of the deep sleep by a phase of REM sleep, during which dreaming occurs. It's also during REM sleep that the brain stores the information it carries as memory. Taking pharmaceutical drugs to help you sleep can affect your memory because they tend to reduce your REM sleep, as does excess alcohol intake.

Completing all four NREM stages and the REM stage means you have completed a full sleep cycle. If you get a good 7.5–8 hours' sleep a night, you are likely to complete four or more sleep cycles. You can be woken very easily from the early stages of sleep but by the time you reach stage four, the deepest sleep, most people can sleep through noise and light quite easily.

Your total amount of sleep reduces with age at a rate of about ten minutes every decade. The quality of your sleep also changes: the periods of time spent in the deepest phases of sleep tend to get shorter and you spend relatively more time in stages one and two. Hence, as you age, you tend to sleep more lightly and awaken more frequently. We don't really know why this happens but it may be due to poorer regulation of sleep–wake-related hormones and brain chemicals. However, there's no real evidence that our *need* for sleep necessarily reduces.[13]

If you're suffering from lack of sleep, you are not alone. The average number of hours' sleep per night has reduced from 9 in the year 1910 to 6.8 in 2005.[14] Unfortunately, many conventional medications designed to aid sleep cause other health problems and some may even be associated with an increased risk of death.[15]

WHAT CAUSES POOR SLEEP?

Sleep problems occur for many different reasons. Insomnia can be a symptom of certain mental health problems, including anxiety and depression. As we mentioned above, lack of sleep can also contribute to these problems or make existing problems worse. A common culprit is stress-related 'racing thoughts' keeping you awake. This can heighten any existing anxiety, as you start to panic about your lack of sleep and what it will mean for your state of mind the following day.

Conditions of physical ill-health that can hamper your ability to sleep well include musculoskeletal problems such as arthritis or sports injuries, gastrointestinal and urinary problems, and any sort of pain, including headache and migraine. What's more, as you age, you become more likely to develop sleep-disordered breathing problems such as obstructive sleep apnoea (OSA). This is an extremely debilitating condition, as problems with breathing at night lead to regular short periods of low oxygen and consequently surges in stress hormones. This scenario wakes you up, often many times a night, although you may not be aware of this the next day, except that you feel very tired. The risk of OSA increases dramatically with both age and obesity. If you have it, or your partner does, you should discuss this with your doctor. Left untreated, it makes you more susceptible to many age-related degenerative diseases, including insulin resistance and type 2 diabetes, cognitive decline and cardiovascular disease.[16]

Men with lower levels of testosterone may be at increased risk of OSA. And falling levels of sex hormones can also affect sleep patterns in women, such as during the menopause transition, when many women find their sleep disrupted.

Dietary factors can play a role in poor sleep. Too high an intake of stimulants (caffeine, sugar and nicotine) can interfere with the brain's ability to relax. It can take between three and seven hours for your body to clear just 50 per cent of the caffeine you've consumed. This means caffeine consumption in the afternoon could easily interfere with sleep patterns.[17]

Although many people drink alcohol at night in the belief it can aid sleep, all too often it tends to have the opposite effect. Alcohol stimulates dopamine production, which is stimulatory. It can also disrupt blood sugar levels, resulting in nocturnal surges of cortisol and leading to night-time waking.

If you feel that you could benefit from improving your sleep patterns, take comfort from the fact that there is a great deal you can do to help the situation naturally.

HOW TO GET A GOOD NIGHT'S SLEEP

Making a few changes to your bedtime routine can bring significant improvements in your sleep:

- Make sure your bedroom is pitch-black. Use blackout blinds if necessary.

- Is your bedroom too noisy? If so, consider whether you can install double glazing, wear ear plugs or make other changes to reduce the noise levels.

- Pay attention to the temperature of your bedroom – too cold or too hot can interfere with sleep.

- Avoid eating large meals within 2–3 hours of going to bed – this can interfere with digestion and lead to bloating and pain.

- Don't go to bed hungry. Many people find that eating a low-GL snack (see Chapter 2) before bed can keep blood sugar levels steady overnight, helping to prevent night-time waking. As we saw in Chapter 6, if blood sugar levels plummet in the early hours, your adrenal glands will pump out the stress hormone cortisol. The cortisol will wake you up and shut off your production of the sleep hormone melatonin, making it hard for you to get back to sleep.

- Limit stimulants – cut out caffeine in the afternoon and evening. They keep cortisol high, which makes it difficult for the sleep hormone melatonin to rise sufficiently to help you nod off. See Box 10.1 for more on this.

- For the same reason, avoid vigorous exercise within two hours of bedtime. But do be sure to take some exercise during the day.

- Avoid alcohol late at night and try to make sure that any earlier intake accompanies a meal. Don't use alcohol to help yourself get to sleep, for the reasons mentioned above. Again, see Box 10.1.

- Clear your bedroom of as many electricals as you can bear to live without. Move the TV, radio and computer to other rooms of the house. Replace your digital alarm clock with a wind-up model. If you can't remove all of the electrical items, make sure you cover the digital displays to block out unwanted light.

▸ Aim to go to bed and get up in the morning at similar times each day, as this helps to establish a regular sleep pattern.

▸ Relax in a warm bath with chamomile or lavender essential oils added before you go to bed.

▸ Take steps to reduce the stress in your life, or at least to better manage your response to the stressful inputs that you face regularly.

▸ Does counting sheep help? It may do. Experts believe that calming imagery to distract you from the anxiety of not being able to sleep may help you to nod off.

SUPPLEMENTAL SUPPORT FOR SLEEP

If you're still struggling with sleep, you may wish to try some of the following natural supplements:

▸ 5-hydroxytryptophan (5-HTP): 5-HTP is an amino acid used by the brain to make the sleep hormone melatonin. Supplementing 5-HTP is often used to aid sleep, also because it can help to alleviate depression and anxiety by increasing serotonin. This is explained in greater detail in Chapters 6 and 7.

An alternative to 5-HTP is L-tryptophan, the amino acid that is used to make 5-HTP and which is also a precursor for serotonin and melatonin.[18] L-tryptophan levels can decline with age. Supplementation can help reduce the time needed to fall asleep.[19]

▸ Magnesium: Magnesium is commonly referred to as the calming mineral, as it helps to regulate muscle and nerve function, and is also involved in normalizing your circadian rhythms. Circadian rhythms are those of your biological processes that are driven by the 24-hour clock. They include the cortisol–melatonin (sleep–wake) cycle. Magnesium supplementation can be helpful in cases of insomnia associated with restless legs syndrome, and has also been found to improve sleep generally, when combined with melatonin (see below) and zinc.[20]

- ▸ Bioactive milk peptides: If stress is contributing to your sleep problems, you may wish to try bioactive milk peptides (casein formulas). These have been shown to promote sustained and restful sleep patterns, while also reducing the overall amount of sleep you need.[21]

- ▸ L-theanine: If you feel tired, yet 'wired' and anxious, try a supplement containing L-theanine. As we saw in Chapter 6, this is a naturally occurring amino acid (found in green tea), used successfully to enhance relaxation and improve concentration. It also reduces electrical brain activity associated with anxiety.[22] Chapter 6 has more information on L-theanine.

- ▸ Herbal support: Various herbs have been shown to support sleep quality. Valerian is probably the best-known herb for the treatment of insomnia.[23] It helps to calm down brain activity, reducing that 'wired' feeling. Some people find they need to take it consistently for two weeks before they notice a significant benefit.[24]

  Chamomile and lemon balm herbal teas are popular options for promoting relaxation and sleep, while some people find passion flower (passiflora) helpful in reducing anxiety. If stress is a contributing factor, ashwagandha may be useful. This herbal adaptogen improves your ability to handle stress and may increase GABA activity (see Chapter 7) to calm the brain.[25] Chapter 6 has more information on ashwagandha.

- ▸ Prescription options: If the dietary measures, lifestyle changes and supplements recommended above fail to make a significant difference, you may want to consider more powerful, prescription options for short-term relief. (We do not recommend that you rely on them long-term.) Rather than use more commonly prescribed sleeping pills, a healthier option is melatonin. (In the US and some other countries this is widely available, but in the UK you require a medical prescription.)

  Melatonin is a hormone made in the pineal gland important for sleep. Low levels have been linked to insomnia. Supplementing with melatonin has been shown to improve sleep quality and reduce the number of times people wake in the night.[26] Typically, dosages are around 3–5mg, to be taken before bed.

THE IMPORTANCE OF RELAXATION

In most of the chapters throughout the book we have highlighted the importance of managing your stress levels, if you want to age in a healthy way. One way to enhance resilience to stress is to practise relaxation techniques. These enable you to activate your parasympathetic nervous system, which is responsible for calming the mind and relaxing the body.

There are many different relaxation techniques to choose from. Some people reap great benefit from taking time out during the day to focus on deep, slow, nose-breathing, using the diaphragm. Did you know that all of us come into this world without the voluntary ability to breathe through our mouths? At birth, we are 'obligate nose-breathers'. Mouth breathing is a learned response triggered by stress.[27]

Nose-breathing is very much part of the therapeutic qualities of Eastern relaxation techniques such as yoga and meditation. Meditation can slow the heart rate, reduce high blood pressure, strengthen the immune system and reduce free radicals – this in itself can help slow down ageing.[28]

Very occasionally, people find it difficult to practise meditation, no matter how hard they try. In these situations, we often suggest that people invest in a bit of technological kit to get them started. One device that seems to get good feedback is the RESPeRATE (www. resperate.co.uk). By using a series of musical notes, it helps you to slow your breathing, which in turn reduces stress hormones. This machine has another advantage, in that it has also been found to help reduce high blood pressure.[29] This is because the reduction in stress hormones helps to relax constricted blood vessels.

You can practise nose-breathing, making full use of your diaphragm, during any type of exercise, with the benefit that it will prevent your heart rate and cortisol levels from soaring to unhealthy heights.[30]

If you suffer from anxiety, insomnia or low mood, you could try using a cranial electrotherapy stimulation device such as the Alpha-

Stim (www.alpha-stim.com). Such devices produce a microcurrent waveform that activates particular groups of nerve cells within the brainstem. By changing these nerve cells' electrical and chemical activity, these devices appear to increase alpha brain waves, which are associated with feelings of calmness, relaxation and increased mental focus. Using one of these devices for 20 minutes a day has been shown in clinical trials to boost mood, reduce anxiety and improve sleep.[31]

THE POWER OF OTHER PEOPLE

Feeling connected to others, being part of a mutually supportive community, is vitally important for our health and wellbeing.[32] Having loving relationships with your family and friends and being involved in the wider community provides a mutual sense of belonging, support and commitment to each other's goals. Becoming part of a positive social network can turn out to be a powerful force in evoking changes to your state of health, enabling you to feel more confident, resilient and optimistic.

So, surround yourself with people who care about your goals and will support your efforts to change. If you are making new plans to support your health, communicate your intentions to friends and family members who can encourage you in your efforts and help to keep you on track. Try to spend less time (or, even better, no time at all) with individuals who make you feel less than positive about what you are doing. We have had clients whose painstaking efforts to lose weight, for example, have been hampered by 'friends' who would encourage them to eat the wrong foods, as it made them feel less insecure about their own failed attempts to stick to a healthier lifestyle. Those who truly like and love you will want to see you take control of your health and lifestyle and will keep you motivated to see lasting, lifelong changes.

And it's not just about benefitting from the counsel of others: it is, of course, hugely rewarding to help and support others. If you feel your social life, family life or community life could do with a bit of a boost, you might find it helpful to start by focusing on what you could do for others. What support can you give? What kindness can you show, however small? What task could you do to help someone out?

Another way to keep motivated is to equip yourself with skills and knowledge, while also meeting like-minded people who share your goals. Why not come along to our *Eat to Get Younger* workshops? For more details visit our websites www.advancenutrition.co.uk, www.christinebailey.co.uk and www.lorrainenicollenutrition.co.uk.

And, finally, don't forget the power of thankfulness. Some people practise this through prayer, but you don't need to have religious faith in order to feel the benefit. Try, every evening, listing ten aspects of your day for which you are grateful. Don't stop at two or three – it's important to get to ten, however minor they may seem. It could be something as small as the fact that the bus driver waited for you as you were running to the stop, or something as significant as the enjoyment of being with your children, or that you feel grateful to have a particularly rewarding relationship or career. This practice of thankfulness doesn't sound like much but it is incredibly powerful. Just try it – and see for yourself…

BOX 10.1 WHAT'S YOUR ADDICTION?

Addictions are far more common than we think. Many of us tend to rely too heavily on some sort of stimulant or sedative, at certain points in our lives. For some, it may be recreational or prescription drugs, nicotine or alcohol. But for many of us, it is substances as seemingly innocuous as caffeine and sugar. All of these are highly addictive because of their ability to increase dopamine, endorphins and GABA, giving us feelings of warmth, joy, contentment and relaxation. Research on animals has found sugar to be so addictive that it can surpass cocaine reward.[33]

The problem is that, over time, regular use of these substances causes the brain to shut down some of its receptor sites for dopamine, endorphins and GABA. When that happens, we find we need more and more of the drug just to feel 'normal' *and* we experience horrible withdrawal symptoms if we try to kick the habit. This is a fast-track to debilitating mood swings, poor memory and fuzzy thinking.

So, is it safe to consume any of these addictive substances? We think it is. With the exception of cigarettes and recreational drugs, most people should be able to consume these pleasure-giving foods and drinks occasionally, in small amounts, without detrimental effects. It's when you are doing something day in, day out, that you need to question whether it is becoming a crutch.

However, it's generally a good idea to cut down your sugar intake. This means not only added sugar but also fruit juices and white starches (white rice, pasta, bread and pastry). Excess sugar in the diet causes chaos to blood sugar levels and also has the potential to kill brain cells. Adopt a low-GL way of eating, as described in Chapter 2.

When it comes to the amount of caffeine that we can safely consume, each of us is different. Some people naturally have a higher tolerance level. These individuals may benefit from enhanced mood and cognition[34] and, according to new research, a possible reduction in the risk of Alzheimer's disease[35] and Parkinson's disease[36] that appears to come with a higher caffeine intake. But if your threshold for tolerance is lower, you'll likely experience the negative effects of caffeine overdosing – disrupted sleep, gastric upset, jitters and shakes, and mental and physical 'crashes', not to mention a growing dependency and the risk of headaches if you fail to get your 'fix'.

If this is you, you should cut out all caffeinated fizzy drinks and reduce your coffee, tea and chocolate intake to a level at which you are no longer feeling dependent or experiencing these side-effects. You may want to reduce your intake very gradually, to minimize the likelihood of withdrawal symptoms.

Alcohol consumption should be kept well within government guidelines (see Chapter 2 for our specific recommendations).

OPTIMIZE YOUR HEALTH WITH NUTRITIONAL SUPPLEMENTS

It's often said that we can get all the nutrients we need from a 'healthy diet'. Unfortunately, there is plenty of evidence to the contrary. The UK government's National Diet and Nutrition Surveys consistently highlight shortfalls in the average British diet. In 2009, for example, the median intake for women was less than the recommended daily allowance (RDA) for vitamins B2, C and D, as well as for the minerals iron, calcium, magnesium, zinc and iodine.[37]

And the situation is likely to be even worse if you consider that the RDAs are not the amounts you need for *optimal* health, but the amounts considered necessary to prevent the classic deficiency diseases in the short term. (These include scurvy from vitamin C deficiency and rickets from lack of vitamin D.) What the RDAs fail to do is take into account the insidious health consequences of long-term (perhaps decades-long) nutrient insufficiencies of a more moderate order. In other words, even if you are getting enough vitamins and minerals to reach the RDA levels, you may still be vulnerable to age-related inflammation, elevated homocysteine, excessive oxidation and other biological problems. This is because your nutrient levels may be adequate enough to keep you alive, but not quite high enough to keep each and every one of your biological pathways in tip-top working order.[38] If healthy ageing is your goal, you need optimal, not merely adequate, levels of the nutrients that feed these body processes.

This is just one reason for complementing your diet with nutritional supplements. But there are many other reasons why it is hard to get everything you need from diet alone: intensive farming produces food with lower levels of nutrients, for example (such as the anti-inflammatory fats); and factory processing techniques deplete vital vitamins, minerals and phytochemicals from foods. Some of our most common foods contain anti-nutrients – molecules that hamper the absorption of essential minerals. These include phytates in soy and wheat and, to a lesser extent, in other legumes and whole grains; oxalates found in some green leaves (e.g. spinach and parsley), strawberries and rhubarb; tannins from tea; and caffeine in tea, coffee, chocolate and energy drinks. In addition, alcohol significantly depletes B vitamins.

There are also lifestyle factors that can prevent you from achieving optimal nutrient levels. Lack of sunlight exposure is responsible for a widespread vitamin D deficiency in the UK (see Chapter 7), and a seemingly common aversion to eating fish is leaving many people with insufficient levels of the omega 3 fats EPA and DHA.

You may face regular toxic exposure, from pollution, smoking and chemical-laden personal care and cleaning products. This increases your need for many micronutrients, as indeed do periods of chronic stress. To make matters worse, the absorption of vitamin B12 and some other nutrients becomes less efficient as you age. And you may find that as you get older your appetite starts to diminish, making it even less likely that you'll get a full daily quota of all the necessary nutrients. And, finally, ageing brings an increased likelihood of your being prescribed one or more prescription drugs, many of which increase your need for specific vitamins, minerals and other micronutrients.[39]

For these many reasons, nutritional supplements form an essential element of our *Eat to Get Younger* programme. At the very least, we recommend you take a high-quality vitamin and mineral formula, a supplement containing the anti-ageing epigenetic nutrients we discussed in Chapter 1; and a combined formula of EPA and DHA (either as fish or krill oil or, if you are vegan, in a supplement produced from algae). If you live in the northern hemisphere, are dark-skinned or have concerns about your bone health, you should get your vitamin D level checked, and supplement this vitamin if your result is below 75nmol/l. This may be particularly important during the winter months. A safe, regular dose is 2000 IU a day, retesting your blood levels in 3–6 months. You should aim to get to 80–100nmol/l. Some experts believe blood levels of 100–150nmol/L confer even more health benefits. Chapter 8 has more detailed information on vitamin D.

You should then add more specific nutrients to your basic supplement programme, depending on your unique combination of health concerns; and according to the recommendations in the preceding chapters. The lists below provide some suggestions to help you do this. (Remember, though, that it's best to seek support from a qualified healthcare practitioner before you start your supplement programme, and it is vital to do so if you are taking any prescribed medications or if you have a medical condition or any undiagnosed symptoms.) Each dosage represents the amount to supplement every day. All dosages for herbs are for the extracts.

BASIC EAT TO GET YOUNGER PROGRAMME

▸ A high-quality multivitamin and mineral formula.

▸ An omega 3 fatty acid supplement comprising a combined level of EPA and DHA of 500–1000mg.

- Vitamin D 2000 IU (after confirmation of need from a blood test).

- A phytochemical formula containing the 'epigenetic' antioxidants and anti-inflammatories curcumin, EGCG, sulforaphane and resveratrol. (See Chapter 1 for more on epigenetics.)

Here are some additional supplements to consider.

MIND AND MEMORY

- B vitamin complex and/or homocysteine-lowering formula. We recommend you get your homocysteine level checked and supplement if it is raised (above 7–8) with a specially designed formula, which includes B6, B12 (as methylcobalamin), folate (as L-methylfolate) and choline.

- Coenzyme Q10 (CoQ10) 100–300mg.

- Pyrroloquinoline quinone (PQQ) 10–20mg.

- Acetyl-L-carnitine 1000–3000mg.

- Magnesium citrate 150–300mg.

- Phospholipids – phosphatidylserine 100–300mg.

- Alpha lipoic acid 300–600mg.

SKIN, NAILS, GUMS AND HAIR

- For hair loss, check iron levels before supplementing with iron.

- Broad spectrum phytochemical antioxidant formula that includes the carotenoids beta carotene, lutein and zeaxanthin, resveratrol (250–500mg) and anthocyanins and OPCs (160–320mg combined) – or separate supplements if necessary to get the dosages required.

- CoQ10 100–200mg.

- Vitamin A 2000 IU.

- Collagen hydrolysate 2.5–10g.

- Use moisturizers and/or serums containing antioxidant vitamins and phytochemicals, and/or bioactive peptides. Use a sunscreen with dual protection against UVA and UVB with active plant ingredients.

DIGESTIVE SUPPORT

- Zinc and vitamin A should be present in the multivitamin.

- Glutamine 5g 2–3 times daily.

- Digestive enzymes with each meal.

- Broad-spectrum probiotic of at least 10 billion live organisms.

- Soluble fibre (e.g. psyllium), antimicrobials, herbal bitters and/or hydrochloric acid (HCl), as needed and agreed with a nutritionist or other healthcare practitioner.

SEX HORMONE BALANCE
Women

- For bio-identical hormones, including DHEA, seek support from a qualified practitioner.

- Vitex agnus castus 20–40mg.

- Black cohosh 40–80mg.

- Soy isoflavones 35–120mg (unless you have a history or family history of hormonal-driven cancer).

- Magnesium citrate 300–450mg.

- Adrenal support (see below).

- You could also consider gamma linolenic acid (GLA) 300–600mg if you suffer from painful, lumpy breasts.

Men

- For bio-identical hormones, including DHEA, seek support from a qualified practitioner.

- Tribulus fruit extract 150mg.

- A broad-spectrum antioxidant formula containing zinc 15–30mg, lycopene 20mg, selenium 200mcg and vitamin E 400 IU. (Note that dosages are the total amount that should be taken, including what is in the basic multivitamin and mineral formula.)

PAIN

- Cucurmin 1–2g.

- Bromelain 1000–3000 GDU (gelatin digesting units).

- GLA 300–600mg.

- Additional B vitamins so that your levels in total to start with are 400mcg methylfolate, 300–400mcg methylcobalamin and 20–50mg of the other B vitamins.

- 5-HTP 150–300mg in split doses.

- MSM 3–6g or glucosamine sulphate 1500mg.

- Antioxidant formula including vitamins C and E.

ADRENAL SUPPORT

- Pantothenic acid (vitamin B5) up to 500mg.

- Vitamin C 1–2g.

- L-theanine 200–400mg.

- Magnesium 300–500mg.

- Rhodiola 300mg 1–3 times a day.

- Ashwagandha 125–250mg.

THYROID SUPPORT

- A high-mineral formula that complements your basic multivitamin and mineral formula, so that you are taking in total: selenium 200–400mcg, iodine 150mcg, zinc 15–25mg and iron 15–60mg (test your ferritin levels before supplementing more than 15mg iron).

- ▸ Rhodiola 300mg 1–3 times a day.

- ▸ L-tyrosine 500–1000mg

SLEEP/INSOMNIA

- ▸ Melatonin (on prescription) 3–5mg at bedtime.

- ▸ L-tryptophan 500–1500mg, or 5-HTP 100mg up to three times daily.

- ▸ L-theanine 200–400mg.

- ▸ Magnesium 200–500mg as citrate.

- ▸ Zinc 15–30mg.

- ▸ Valerian 300–600mg half an hour before bedtime.

- ▸ Bioactive milk peptides 100mg.

- ▸ Ashwagandha 200mg.

RECIPES

In the preceding chapters, you'll have read about a wealth of different ideas for adapting your diet and lifestyle to optimize your health as you grow older. These ideas include some meal plans, designed to support particular body systems (particular areas of health) involved in the ageing process. Once you have decided which of these body systems to focus on initially, you'll probably be keen to get started – so we've developed recipes for all the dishes featured in the meal plans.

The recipes cover some staple foods (such as stocks and yogurts), as well as breakfasts, lunches, dinners, snacks, sweet treats, juices and smoothies. To add variety and nourishment, we've included a few unusual ingredients here and there, together with a short description the first time they appear.

To get the most from the recipes, we suggest you refer back to the meal plans in the relevant chapters, to see which will likely be the most helpful in your current situation. And don't forget to see the six days' worth of meal plans in Chapter 2, as this will help you to get used to the low-GL, antioxidant-rich, anti-inflammatory way of eating. Chapter 2 also gives example meal plans for intermittent fasting and lifestyle fasting, if you think either of these practices may benefit you.

STAPLES
BONE BROTH

Bone broth provides bio-available forms of calcium, magnesium, phosphorous and other minerals. It is rich in gelatine and collagen to support the health of the gut lining. As you will have seen in Chapter 3, a healthy gut lining is important for immune system health and for keeping inflammation in check. Any organic bones can be used. If chicken is easier to get hold of, follow our recipe for chicken stock. The addition of garlic not only adds flavour but is a valuable immune-supporting ingredient too.

Grain-Free, Gluten-Free, Dairy-Free, No Added Sugar, Nut-Free, Soy-Free

Ingredients

3–4 litres/5–7 pints filtered water

700g–1kg/1½–2½lbs of beef knuckle bones or marrow bones

1 whole head of fresh garlic, peeled but left whole

2 carrots, chopped

1 onion, quartered

2 tbsp apple cider vinegar

1 tsp sea salt or strip of kombu seaweed

Method

▶ Place all the ingredients in a large casserole dish or pan with a lid.

▶ Bring the stock to a boil, then reduce the heat to very low so that the stock is barely simmering.

▶ Ideally, cook the stock for at least 8 hours, but you can cook it for longer if you like – up to 24 hours. Top up with water if needed during cooking.

▶ Strain the stock through a sieve.

▶ Place the stock in the fridge – you can also freeze it in batches.

▶ Once completely cooled, you can skim off the fat that rises to the top. (You can store the fat and use it to cook with.)

▶ You can drink the stock at any time of day or use it as the base for soups and other recipes such as stews and casseroles.

CHICKEN STOCK

A nourishing stock, simple to prepare and very versatile. Use this as a base for soups, stews and casseroles or for cooking rice and vegetables.

Grain-Free, Gluten-Free, Dairy-Free, No Added Sugar, Nut-Free

Ingredients

1 organic chicken, about 1–1.3kg/ 2–3lbs

3 litres/5 pints of water

1 tsp black peppercorns

3cm piece of fresh root ginger, sliced

1 large onion, cut into wedges

2 garlic cloves, crushed

Method

▶ Put the chicken in a large pan and cover with the water. Add the peppercorns, ginger, onion and garlic, and bring to the boil. Reduce to a simmer. Cook for 1 hour until the meat is tender.

▶ Remove the chicken and take off all the meat. (Set aside to use in another recipe.)

▶ Place the bones back into the stock and simmer for a further 2–3 hours. Top up with water if needed.

▶ Strain the stock and reserve. Discard the vegetables and bones.

▶ When the stock is cool, you can refrigerate it or freeze it if not using it immediately. It will keep in the fridge for 2–3 days.

HOME-MADE YOGURT AND SOURED CREAM

When making your own yogurt, we recommend organic milk only. Soy yogurt can also be made in the same way. Goat's and soy yogurt tend to contain more liquid than cow's yogurt. To make your own yogurt, you will need to introduce bacteria into the milk. You can buy commercially available yogurt starter kits or empty a probiotic capsule containing *Lactobacillus*. You can also use a couple of tablespoons of 'live' yogurt as a starter. After making the first batch, you can use some of your yogurt to make the next batch.

Grain-Free, Gluten-Free, Nut-Free, No Added Sugar, Suitable for Vegetarians

Serves 6

Ingredients

1 litre/1¾ pints milk (goat's,
cow's, soy)

½ tsp probiotic powder, yogurt starter
kit or 3 tbsp live yogurt

Method

▶ In a pan bring the milk to just below boiling point. Do not boil.
Take off the heat and allow to cool down until the temperature is
around 38–40°C/100°F. This should feel warm on the skin. Either
add the starter kit to the milk according to packet instructions or
around 3 tbsp live yogurt. Stir well. You can put the mixture in a
yogurt maker or use a clean, dry thermos. Let the milk ferment for
24 hours. After fermentation, put the yogurt in a clean jug or bowl
and refrigerate.

▶ To thicken the yogurt, strain off some of the liquid. Place a piece
of muslin in a sieve set over a large bowl. Pour the yogurt into the
lined sieve and allow it to drip through for several hours. The longer
you leave it to drip, the thicker the yogurt. You can also create a soft
cottage-like cheese in this way.

HOME-MADE COCONUT YOGURT

To make your own coconut yogurt you will need to introduce bacteria
into the coconut milk. You can buy commercially available yogurt
starter kits or use ½ tsp probiotic powder as above or a small amount
of organic 'live' yogurt as a starter.

Grain-Free, Gluten-Free, Suitable for Vegetarians, No Added Sugar

Serves 6

Ingredients

2 cans full-fat coconut milk

2 tsp agar flakes

½ tsp probiotic powder, yogurt starter
kit or 3–4 tbsp live yogurt

Method

▶ In a pan bring the coconut milk and agar flakes to just below
boiling point. Stir well to dissolve the agar. Do not boil. Take off
the heat and allow to cool down until the temperature is around
38–40°C/100°F. This should feel warm on the skin. Add either

the probiotic powder, the starter kit or live yogurt. Blend well. You can put the mixture in a yogurt maker or use a clean, dry thermos. Ferment the yogurt for 24 hours. After fermentation, place the yogurt in a clean jug or bowl and refrigerate. As it chills it will thicken further.

Nutritional information per serving

Calories	Protein	Carbohydrates	Total fat
40kcal	1.2g	7.6g of which sugars 7.2g	0.8g of which saturates 0.5g

NUT YOGURT

Nut yogurt is a delicious nutritious alternative for vegans. Almost any nuts can be used but almonds, cashew nuts and macadamia nuts work particularly well.

Grain-Free, Gluten-Free, Dairy-Free, Suitable for Vegetarians

Serves 4

....

Ingredients

125g/4½oz cashew nuts, soaked for 2 hours and then drained

200ml/7fl oz water or coconut water

½ tsp probiotic powder (such as *Lactobacillus*)

1 tbsp honey or maple syrup (optional)

½ tsp lemon juice

....

Method

▸ Place the drained cashew nuts in a blender with the water and blend until smooth.

▸ Blend in the remaining ingredients and process for 2–3 minutes – this will warm up the mixture slightly and speed the fermentation process.

▸ Transfer to a bowl and ferment in a dehydrator at 40°C/105°F or a thermos, or simply place in warm place in the kitchen or use a yogurt maker. Place in the fridge to thicken.

Nutritional information per serving

Calories	Protein	Carbohydrates	Total fat
189kcal	5.5g	7.6g of which sugars 3.6g	15.1g of which saturates 3g

WHIPPED COCONUT CREAM

This is a delicious topping for pancakes, fruit, home-made granola or muesli.

Grain-Free, Gluten-Free, Dairy-Free, Suitable for Vegetarians

Serves 8

....

Ingredients

125g/4½oz cashews

250ml/8fl oz coconut milk

60g/2oz coconut butter, melted

2 tbsp honey

1 tbsp lemon juice

1 tbsp vanilla

Pinch of sea salt

1 tbsp lecithin

....

Method

▸ Simply process all the ingredients in a blender until smooth. Allow the cream to firm up in the fridge if necessary. This will keep in the fridge for 3–4 days and can be frozen too.

Nutritional information per serving

Calories	Protein	Carbohydrates	Total fat
187kcal	2.9g	8.3g of which sugars 6.5g	15.1g of which saturates 8g

CLASSIC ALMOND MILK

This is a basic recipe to make your own nut milk. Other nuts can be substituted, such as cashews, hazelnuts and Brazil nuts. For a creamier texture, try adding 1 tsp lecithin granules. For vanilla milk add 1 tsp vanilla extract.

Grain-Free, Gluten-Free, Dairy-Free, Suitable for Vegetarians, No Added Sugar

Serves 4

Ingredients

125g/4½oz almonds, soaked
overnight

3 pitted dates, optional

750ml/1½ pints water

Pinch of sea salt

Method

▸ Strain and rinse the almonds. Place them in a high-speed blender
with the remaining ingredients and blend until smooth and creamy.
Strain through a fine sieve or place in a nut bag (or use muslin for a
smoother texture).

Nutritional information per serving

Calories	Protein	Carbohydrates	Total fat
196kcal	6.7g	3.1g of which sugars 2.4g	17.4g of which saturates 1.4g

KEFIR

Kefir is a natural source of healthy bacteria to support our gut health,
digestion and immune system. An ancient cultured food, rich in amino
acids, enzymes, calcium, magnesium, phosphorus and B vitamins, it
contains several strains of friendly bacteria (*Lactobacillus caucasus,
Leuconostoc, Acetobacter* species and *Streptococcus* species) and yeasts
(*Saccharomyces* kefir, *Torula* kefir and others), which in combination
can dramatically improve digestive function and immunity (see
Chapter 3).

To get the full benefit of this delicious probiotic drink, ideally take
it every day. Kefir is made by using a mother culture, which is referred
to as kefir 'grains'. The grains digest sugar in a fermentation process.
Although cow's milk is typically used, kefir can be made with sheep's
milk, soy, coconut or nut milk.

Kefir grains can be purchased online. If you prefer, you can use
a kefir starter kit. Generally one starter kit will make about 1 litre of
kefir but the exact amount will vary according to the size of the starter
pack. It takes 24–30 hours to ferment the cultures in milk at room
temperature on colder days but less if it is warm. Once fermented,

store it in the fridge and consume within 4 days. You can take 200ml of your freshly made kefir to make another 1 litre portion of kefir, if you wish. This can be repeated about six more times before you need to purchase more starter powder.

In this recipe we have used UHT milk for ease. If you wish to use pasteurized milk it is best to heat it first and then allow to cool before using.

Grain-Free, Gluten-Free, Soy-Free, Nut-Free

Serves 8

....

Ingredients

1 kefir starter kit or 1–2 tbsp kefir grains

1 litre/2 pints organic UHT full-fat milk or milk alternative

....

Method

▶ You need a clean, sterilized jar big enough to hold 1 litre.

▶ Empty one starter culture sachet into a small glass and pour over a little of the milk and stir to make a smooth paste.

▶ Gradually add more milk and keep stirring to ensure no lumps, then pour all the milk and the culture into your prepared jar.

▶ Cover with a lid and leave to ferment in a warm place for at least 24 hours. The ideal temperature is 23°C/72°F.

▶ Place in the refrigerator and use within 4 days.

▶ If using kefir grains, simply place them in a clean jar and pour over the UHT organic milk. Cover and leave at room temperature for 24 hours away from sunlight. The milk will separate out to form the kefir liquid at the bottom. Strain through a nylon sieve (not metal), reserve the grains and start the process again. Do not use metal utensils with your grains.

Nutritional information per serving (for full-fat milk)

Calories	Protein	Carbohydrates	Total fat
83kcal	4.1g	5.8g of which sugars 5.5g	4.9g of which saturates 3.1g

WATER KEFIR

Water kefir is remarkably versatile. You can introduce various beneficial herbs or flavours to turn it into a wide array of probiotic beverages – for example, try adding a herbal tea bag or some dried fruit to the kefir for flavour.

Grain-Free, Gluten-Free, Dairy-Free, Nut-Free, Suitable for Vegetarians

Serves 8

....

Ingredients

65–70g/2½–3oz caster sugar

750ml–1 litre/1½–2 pints filtered, chlorine-free water (boil water and allow it to cool to warm temperature) or coconut water

1 sachet of water kefir grains

½ organic lemon

1 thin slice fresh ginger, peeled

....

Method

▶ Dissolve the sugar in the water. Add the water kefir grains, lemon and slice of ginger to the mixture of sugar water in a glass jar. Allow your water kefir to ferment in a lidded or covered glass jar at room temperature for 24–72 hours depending on the strength you prefer and the temperature of your home. Do not seal the lid as the gas can build up as it ferments.

▶ The warmer your home is, the faster water kefir will brew. Strain the water kefir grains, lemon and ginger from the water kefir and bottle the liquid in smaller containers. Allow the smaller bottles to sit out for another 24–48 hours to continue fermentation and produce natural carbonation.

Nutritional information per serving (for full-fat milk)

Calories	Protein	Carbohydrates	Total fat
35kcal	0g	9.2g of which sugars 8.8g	0g

SAUERKRAUT

Home-made pickled fermented vegetables make a delicious healthy addition to the diet. Unlike shop-bought versions, they are raw and therefore richer in beneficial enzymes. Commercially produced sauerkraut is pasteurized, which destroys these enzymes, and is also often high in salt and other additives. Sauerkraut is based on shredded cabbage but there are many other variations of pickled fermented vegetables (e.g. *Kimchi*). Pickled fermented vegetables can help populate the digestive tract with friendly bacteria and are traditionally thought to be alkalizing and cleansing. Aim to include them on a regular basis. To aid digestion we recommend having a few tablespoons 10–15 minutes before meals. The juice from the fermentation can also be used as a replacement for vinegar in salad dressings.

Use organic, fresh vegetables. Wash and dry them thoroughly. Vary the vegetables according to taste.

Grain-Free, Gluten-Free, Dairy-Free, Nut-Free, No Added Sugar, Suitable for Vegetarians

....

Ingredients

1 cabbage (e.g. savoy or napa, a type of Chinese cabbage, or a mixture of white and red cabbage), shredded in a food processor

3 carrots, grated or chopped finely

2 shallots, finely chopped

1–2 tbsp sea salt

125ml/4fl oz warm water

1 tbsp root ginger, peeled and grated

3 garlic cloves, peeled and chopped

2 tsp dill seeds

2 tsp fennel seeds

Handful of washed, soaked sea vegetables, chopped (optional)

....

Method

▸ Place the vegetables in a large mixing bowl.

▸ Place the salt and water in a separate small bowl and stir to dissolve. Pour over the vegetables and massage the mixture with your hands. Cover with cling film and set aside at room temperature overnight to soften.

▸ The following day, drain the cabbage mixture, reserving the salt water. Stir in the ginger, garlic, dill and fennel seeds, as well as the sea vegetables, if using. Mix well. Tightly pack the mixture into a large glass jar with a lid. Pour over the saved salt water and press it firmly so there is no trapped air and the cabbage is covered in its own juice. Tightly close the lid. Leave the jar in a warm, dark place for 3–4 days. It will take at least a week if left in a cool place.

▸ Refrigerate your sauerkraut after opening. It will keep for a couple of weeks in the fridge.

Nutritional information per heaped tbsp (30g)

Calories	Protein	Carbohydrates	Total fat
8kcal	0.4g	1.3g of which sugars 1.2g	0g

KIMCHI

Kimchi is a delicious Korean dish consisting of fermented chilli peppers and vegetables (usually cabbage). It is delicious as an accompaniment to meats and fish, or as a topping for salads.

Grain-Free, Gluten-Free, Dairy-Free, Nut-Free, No Added Sugar, Suitable for Vegetarians

Ingredients

1 napa or Chinese cabbage, cut into chunks

½ daikon radish, peeled and cut into chunks

1–2 tbsp sea salt

125ml/4fl oz water

3 garlic cloves, crushed

1 tbsp fresh grated ginger

1 tbsp Korean chilli powder or flakes

1 tbsp coconut sugar

Method

- ▶ Place the cabbage and daikon in a large bowl. Place the salt in the water and stir to dissolve. Pour over the salt water and mix well. Cover and leave overnight.
- ▶ Add the remaining ingredients and mix well. Tightly pack into glass jars pressing down the mixture so that some of water covers the top. Tightly close the lid. Leave in a cool place for 2–3 days before using. Once fermented, keep in the fridge.

Nutritional information per serving (30g)

Calories	Protein	Carbohydrates	Total fat
9kcal	0.5g	1.6g of which sugars 1.4g	0.1g of which saturates 0g

EASY PICKLED VEGETABLES

Slices of vegetables can be softened in vinegar and salt overnight. Vary the combination of vegetables according to taste.

Grain-Free, Gluten-Free, Dairy-Free, Nut-Free, No Added Sugar, Suitable for Vegetarians

Serves 8

....

Ingredients

200ml/7fl oz apple cider vinegar

1 tsp sea salt

2 tsp pickling spice

250ml/8fl oz water

½ cauliflower, cut into small florets

1 carrot, cut in thick rounds

½ cucumber, cut in half and then sliced thickly

1 shallot, cut into chunks

....

Method

▶ Place the vinegar, salt, pickling spice and water in a large mason jar. Add the vegetables and stir well. Make sure the liquid covers the vegetables. Cover and leave to marinate for a minimum of 6 hours. Keep in the fridge until required.

Nutritional information per serving

Calories	Protein	Carbohydrates	Total fat
19kcal	1.2g	1.7g of which sugars 1.6g	0.3g of which saturates 0.1g

JUICES AND SMOOTHIES

These drinks are packed full of highly bioavailable, energizing nutrients. Taking them once a day can significantly increase your intake of antioxidant vitamins and phytochemicals. It's better to opt for smoothies, rather than juices, if you have any signs or symptoms of blood sugar problems (see Chapter 4). And if you suffer from excessive gas or intestinal bloating, hold off the fruit juices and smoothies until your gut microflora have become more balanced, by following the guidelines in Chapter 3.

LIME MINT CLEANSER

This is a light hydrating juice – a perfect start to the day. If using pineapple, include the core of the fruit as this is higher in the digestive enzyme bromelain.

Grain-Free, Gluten-Free, Dairy-Free, Nut-Free, No Added Sugar, Suitable for Vegetarians

Serves 1

....

Ingredients

1 cucumber

2 celery sticks

Small handful of mint leaves

2 pears or ¼ fresh pineapple

1 lime, peeled

....

Method

▸ Juice all the ingredients and pour over ice to serve.

Nutritional information per serving

Calories	Protein	Carbohydrates	Total fat
89kcal	2.3g	18.3g of which sugars 18.3g	0g

CORIANDER DETOX JUICE

A stronger-tasting juice, coriander (cilantro) is a useful herb for promoting detoxification (see Chapter 6).

Grain-Free, Gluten-Free, Dairy-Free, No Added Sugar, Nut-Free, Suitable for Vegetarians

Serves 1

....

Ingredients

1 cucumber

2 apples

1 celery stick

Handful of coriander (cilantro)

Handful of kale or spinach

1 lemon, peeled

....

Method

▸ Juice all the ingredients together. Pour into a glass to serve.

Nutritional information per serving

Calories	Protein	Carbohydrates	Total fat
91kcal	2.9g	17.8g of which sugars 17.5g	0.9g of which saturates 0.1g

PERSIMMON CARROT GINGER-AID

Packed with beta-carotene and vitamin C. The addition of ginger helps support digestive health and gives this juice a real kick – perfect for an energizing morning drink.

Grain-Free, Gluten-Free, Dairy-Free, No Added Sugar, Nut-Free, Suitable for Vegetarians

Serves 2

Ingredients

2 persimmons	Small piece of root ginger, peeled
4 carrots	Water or coconut water to dilute if needed
1 apple	

Method

▸ Juice all the ingredients together. Dilute with water or coconut water if required.

Nutritional information per serving

Calories	Protein	Carbohydrates	Total fat
88kcal	1.1g	19.7g of which sugars 19.7g	0.3g of which saturates 0.1g

FENNEL DIGESTIVE CLEANSE

A light, refreshing juice. Fennel contains the phytonutrient anethole, which may support digestion and reduce inflammation.

Grain-Free, Gluten-Free, Dairy-Free, Nut-Free, No Added Sugar, Suitable for Vegetarians

Serves 2

Ingredients

1 fennel bulb	1 lemon, peeled
1 cucumber	2 apples
2 celery sticks	

Method

▸ Simply juice all the ingredients together.

Nutritional information per serving

Calories	Protein	Carbohydrates	Total fat
52kcal	1.7g	10.3g of which sugars 10.2g	0.4g of which saturates 0g

ENERGIZING BEETS JUICE

Beetroots contain phytonutrients called betalains, which have antioxidant, anti-inflammatory and detoxification properties. Beets are also a good source of nitrate, which can help to relax the arteries, reducing blood pressure if it is too high. They contain folate and iron, making them useful for supporting energy levels.

Grain-Free, Gluten-Free, Dairy-Free, No Added Sugar, Nut-Free, Suitable for Vegetarians

Serves 1

Ingredients

1 beetroot	2 apples
2 carrots	½ lemon, peeled

Method

▸ Juice all the ingredients together.

Nutritional information per serving

Calories	Protein	Carbohydrates	Total fat
118kcal	2.1g	25.9g of which sugars 25.9g	0.5g of which saturates 0.1g

GREEN SMOOTHIES

Green smoothies are an easy way to supercharge your diet. They are packed with antioxidants, vitamins and minerals, and are exceptionally alkalizing. Try adding a green smoothie in your diet daily for a real nutrient boost. They are also a great way to get children to include more greens in their diets. For additional protein, you can use nut milks and/or protein powders.

GREEN HYDRATOR

Grain-Free, Gluten-Free, Dairy-Free, No Added Sugar, Nut-Free, Suitable for Vegetarians

Serves 2

....

Ingredients

½ head of broccoli, separated into florets

Handful of spinach leaves or kale leaves

½ cucumber, peeled and chopped

2 small pears

1 lemon, peeled

1 banana, cut into slices and frozen

500ml/1 pint water or coconut water

....

Method

▶ Simply place all the ingredients in a food processor and blend until smooth.

Nutritional information per serving

Calories	Protein	Carbohydrates	Total fat
102kcal	4.8g	17.9g of which sugars 17.2g	1.1g of which saturates 0.2g

SUPERGREEN GUT HEALER

Grain-Free, Gluten-Free, Dairy-Free, No Added Sugar, Suitable for Vegetarians

Serves 2

....

Ingredients

300ml/10fl oz coconut water

1 small ripe avocado

¼ pineapple, cut into chunks

1 tsp green superfood powder

1tsp probiotic powder (optional)

1 tsp glutamine powder

Method

▶ Simply place all the ingredients in a food processor and blend until smooth.

Nutritional information per serving

Calories	Protein	Carbohydrates	Total fat
168kcal	5.1g	15.5 of which sugars 7.5g	10.2g of which saturates 2g

TROPICAL PROTEIN SMOOTHIE

Grain-Free, Gluten-Free, Dairy-Free, No Added Sugar, Suitable for Vegetarians

Serves 2

Ingredients

1 frozen banana, broken into chunks

30g/1 scoop protein powder (e.g. pea, hemp, rice)

1 tbsp ground chia seed

Large handful of green leaves (e.g. kale, spinach)

1 papaya

Juice of ½ lemon

400ml coconut water or cold green tea

Method

▶ Simply blend all the ingredients and serve. Add a little more water to blend if needed.

Nutritional information per serving

Calories	Protein	Carbohydrates	Total fat
154kcal	10.3g	18.4g of which sugars 8.4g	4.5g of which saturates 0.3g

ANTIOXIDANT GREEN BURST

Grain-Free, Gluten-Free, Dairy-Free, No Added Sugar, Suitable for Vegetarians

Serves 2

Ingredients

1 banana

300ml/10fl oz nut milk, e.g. coconut, almond, cashew (see *Classic Almond Milk* recipe)

Large handful of spinach leaves

1 tsp wheatgrass or other super green powder

Handful of blueberries

Handful of raspberries

Handful of strawberries

Method

▸ Simply blend all the ingredients and serve. Add a little more water to blend if needed.

Nutritional information per serving

Calories	Protein	Carbohydrates	Total fat
107kcal	3.5g	20.7g of which sugars 20.3g	0.9g of which saturates 0.4g

JOINT REPAIR ICED SHAKE

This healing smoothie is rich in anti-inflammatory phytochemicals. The herb *Cissus quadrangularis* is used in Ayurvedic medicine to support bone health. Collagen powder provides nutrients to help strengthen the lining of the gut, which in some cases can reduce discomfort in the musculoskeletal joints (see Chapter 8). Colostrum is a potent source of beneficial immune factors to help promote digestive health and reduce body-wide inflammation. Lucuma powder is a natural sweetener from the Peruvian lucuma fruit and contains B vitamins, beta-carotene, iron, potassium, calcium and phosphorous.

Grain-Free, Gluten-Free, Dairy-Free, No Added Sugar, Suitable for Vegetarians

Serves 2

Ingredients

2 cups of ice

150ml/5fl oz pomegranate or pure Montomercy cherry juice

2 tbsp colostrum powder

1 tbsp coconut oil

1 tbsp collagen powder

2 tbsp lucuma powder

1 tsp vanilla powder

1 tsp honey

1 tsp Cissus quadrangularis extract (optional)

Method

▶ Simply place all the ingredients into a high-speed blender and process until smooth and creamy.

Nutritional information per serving

Calories	Protein	Carbohydrates	Total fat
219kcal	12.2g	31.8g of which sugars 18.7g	5g of which saturates 3.9g

ANTI-INFLAMMATORY TURMERIC SHAKE

Turmeric contains curcumins, which have anti-inflammatory properties. Papaya contains several unique protein-digesting enzymes including papain and chymopapain. These enzymes have been shown to help lower inflammation.

Grain-Free, Gluten-Free, Dairy-Free, No Added Sugar, Suitable for Vegetarians

Serves 2

Ingredients

1 large banana

1 papaya

300ml/10fl oz *Classic Almond Milk* (see recipe) or coconut milk

1 tbsp ground flaxseed

2 tsp chia seeds

2 tsp turmeric powder

1 tsp probiotic powder (optional)

Dash of cinnamon powder

1 tbsp collagen powder (optional)

Method

▶ Simply blend all the ingredients and serve. Add a little more water to blend if needed.

Nutritional information per serving

Calories	Protein	Carbohydrates	Total fat
156kcal	4.1g	23.7g of which sugars 15.2g	5.7g of which saturates 0.9g

MACA STRESS-BUSTING SMOOTHIE

A wonderful smoothie when you feel stressed and tired. Maca is an adaptogen herb useful for supporting the adrenal glands, which produce stress hormones (see Chapter 6). Chaga is a tonic herb, rich in antioxidants and polysaccharides which may support the immune system. It is traditionally used in Siberia as a food to maintain overall health and wellbeing.

Grain-Free, Gluten-Free, Dairy-Free, Suitable for Vegetarians

Serves 2

Ingredients

1 tbsp acai berry powder or other superfruit powder

2 tsp maca powder

½ tsp chaga powder

2 tsp raw cacao powder

1 tbsp shelled hemp seeds

1 tsp almond nut butter

2 tsp Manuka honey (optional)

500ml/1 pint coconut water

250g/9oz strawberries or mixed berries, fresh or frozen

Method

▶ Simply blend all the ingredients together. Adjust the liquid according to taste.

Nutritional information per serving

Calories	Protein	Carbohydrates	Total fat
249kcal	7.7g	31.6g of which sugars 13g	9.8g of which saturates 0.6g

OMEGA VANILLA SHAKE

This is a great way to make use of over-ripe bananas. Simply slice and freeze them until firm. The bananas create a wonderful creamy texture for the shake, while the chia and hemp seeds provide omega 3 and 6 essential fats. Known as 'Food of the Gods', bee pollen has been used for centuries as a food source and to increase energy and stamina. It contains an array of vitamins, minerals and antioxidants, as well many essential amino acids.

Grain-Free, Gluten-Free, Dairy-Free, No Added Sugar, Suitable for Vegetarians

Serves 2

....

Ingredients

1 tbsp chia seeds	1 tsp bee pollen
500ml/1 pint coconut water	1 tbsp vanilla extract
2 tbsp shelled hemp seeds	1–2 tsp supergreen food powder
2 frozen bananas, cut into chunks	

....

Method

▸ Place the chia seeds in the coconut water and allow it to soak for at least 20 minutes. Process in a blender with the remaining ingredients until smooth.

Nutritional information per serving

Calories	Protein	Carbohydrates	Total fat
261kcal	11.1g	32g of which sugars 15.9g	10g of which saturates 0.8g

LONGEVITY CASHEW LATTE

A rich, creamy smoothie. *Gynostemma pentaphyllum* is considered an important anti-inflammatory and anti-ageing herb in Chinese herbalism. It is a very effective broad-spectrum anti-inflammatory. Ginseng or green tea could be used as an alternative in this recipe.

Grain-Free, Gluten-Free, Dairy-Free, Suitable for Vegetarians

Serves 2

....

Ingredients

60g/2½oz cashew nuts	½ tsp cinnamon
2 tsp Manuka honey	1 tbsp coconut oil
500ml/1 pint Gynostemma, Ginseng tea or green tea	1g MSM (methylsulfonylmethane) powder (see Chapter 8)
1 tsp vanilla powder	

....

Method

▸ Simply blend all the ingredients together until rich and creamy.

Nutritional information per serving

Calories	Protein	Carbohydrates	Total fat
236kcal	6.2g	11.2g of which sugars 7.1g	19g of which saturates 6.8g

BREAKFASTS
SOAKED CHIA MUESLI

This is a filling raw porridge that can be prepared the night before. Vary the ingredients according to taste.

Grain-Free, Gluten-Free, Dairy-Free, No Added Sugar, Suitable for Vegetarians

Serves 2

· ·

Ingredients

60g/2½oz sunflower seeds

30g/1oz pumpkin seeds

2 tbsp hemp seeds

30g/1oz dry coconut flakes

30g/1oz chopped nuts

60g/2½oz chia seeds

300ml/10fl oz *Classic Almond Milk* (see recipe) or coconut milk

60g/2½oz dried unsweetened cherries

30g/1oz goji berries

Citrus Vanilla Nut Cream (see recipe) to serve (optional)

· ·

Method

▶ Soak the sunflower, pumpkin and hemp seeds, coconut flakes and nuts in a bowl with water overnight. Drain and rinse well.

▶ Soak the chia seeds in the milk for 20 minutes.

▶ Place the chia seeds and milk in a food processor and process until smooth. Add the seeds and nuts and stir in the cherries and berries. Spoon into bowls and serve with *Citrus Vanilla Nut Cream* if you wish.

Nutritional information per serving (without *Citrus Vanilla Nut Cream*)

Calories	Protein	Carbohydrates	Total fat
352kcal	10.4g	24.6g of which sugars 20.1g	23.5g of which saturates 6.2g

CITRUS VANILLA NUT CREAM

Grain-Free, Gluten-Free, Dairy-Free, No Added Sugar, Suitable for Vegetarians

Serves 4

Ingredients

60g/2½oz cashew nuts, soaked in water for 1 hour and then drained

Juice and zest of 1 large orange

1 tbsp coconut butter

1 tbsp vanilla extract

Method

▸ Place all the ingredients in a blender and blend until smooth. Add a little water if needed to create a thick, smooth cream.

Nutritional information per tbsp

Calories	Protein	Carbohydrates	Total fat
50kcal	1.2g	1.8g of which sugars 0.9g	4.2g of which saturates 1.5g

MATCHA GREEN TEA CHIA PUDDING

High in antioxidants and omega 3 fats, this is a great anti-inflammatory recipe. The soluble fibre in the seeds can be helpful for constipation.

Grain-Free, Gluten-Free, Dairy-Free, Suitable for Vegetarians

Serves 4

Ingredients

500ml/1 pint *Classic Almond Milk* (see recipe) or coconut milk

1–2 tbsp maple syrup

60g/2½ vanilla protein powder

1 tbsp vanilla extract

Pinch of cinnamon

1 tsp matcha green tea powder

6 tbsp chia seeds

Pinch of sea salt

Handful of mixed berries to serve

Method

▸ Blend the milk, maple syrup, vanilla, cinnamon and matcha together in a blender till smooth. Add a pinch of sea salt.

▸ Pour the liquid over the chia seeds. Stir thoroughly. Stir again every few minutes for the next 15 minutes. You can allow the mixture to sit for 1 hour before serving or leave overnight. To serve spoon into bowls and top with the berries.

Nutritional information per serving

Calories	Protein	Carbohydrates	Total fat
232kcal	10.5g	27.9g of which sugars 14.8g	9.4g of which saturates 1.3g

GRAIN-FREE BREAKFAST BOWL

This is an easy-to-assemble grain-free breakfast option. As well as being wonderfully warming, it's perfect when time is short. Maca is an excellent tonic for stress and flagging energy levels.

Grain-Free, Gluten-Free, Dairy-Free, No Added Sugar, Suitable for Vegetarians

Serves 2

Ingredients

2 tsp almond butter

6 tbsp coconut milk or *Classic Almond Milk* (see recipe)

60g/2½oz goji berries, soaked for 20 minutes, then strained (reserve the liquid)

30g/1oz shelled hemp seeds

2 tbsp chia seeds

60g/2½oz unsweetened coconut flakes

1 tsp Maca

½ tsp ground cinnamon

Method

▶ Warm the almond butter and milk gently. Put all the remaining ingredients in the pan and stir. Spoon into bowls to serve.

Nutritional information per serving

Calories	Protein	Carbohydrates	Total fat
514kcal	12.1g	38.2g of which sugars 25.1g	35.8g of which saturates 17.2g

BUCKWHEAT GRANOLA

A crunchy gluten-free granola. To prepare the buckwheat, place in a jug and fill with water – soak for 30 minutes, then rinse well. Dehydrate until dry and crispy. You can do this in a low oven if you wish, around

120°C/250°F. You could also sprout the buckwheat for 2–3 days before dehydrating.

Gluten-Free, Dairy-Free, Suitable for Vegetarians

Serves 6

....

Ingredients

125g/4½oz soaked and dehydrated buckwheat (see above)	30g/1oz dried apples or pineapple, chopped
2 tbsp ground flaxseed	2 tbsp maple syrup
2 tbsp chia seeds	3 tbsp coconut oil
40g/1½oz sunflower seeds	1 tsp cinnamon
40g/1½oz pumpkin seeds	Dash nutmeg
50g/2oz raisins	Dash Himalayan salt

....

Method

- ▸ Put the buckwheat, flaxseed, chia, sunflower and pumpkin seeds, and the dried fruit in a food processor and process to chop up.
- ▸ Whisk together the maple syrup, coconut oil, cinnamon, nutmeg and salt. Pour over the dry ingredients and mix them well with your hands.
- ▸ Dehydrate at 115°C/240°F degrees for about 10–12 hours, or until the granola is sticky but adhering firmly.

Nutritional information per serving

Calories	Protein	Carbohydrates	Total fat
266kcal	6.4g	25.3g of which sugars 3.3g	15.9g of which saturates 6.1g

COCOA COCONUT WAFFLES

This is a delicious simple waffle recipe using coconut flour. The batter can also be used for pancakes or blinis if you don't have a waffle maker. Leftovers can be kept in the fridge and used as a snack if wished.

Grain-Free, Gluten-Free, Dairy-Free, Suitable for Vegetarians

Makes 4 large waffles

Ingredients

1 tbsp melted coconut oil

6 eggs

1 tbsp maple syrup

2 tsp vanilla extract

1 tsp psyllium husks

Pinch of salt

½ tsp bicarbonate of soda

1 tsp baking powder

3 tbsp coconut flour

1–2 tbsp cocoa powder

Coconut yogurt or natural yogurt, to serve

Handful of mixed berries, to serve

Method

▶ In a blender, beat together the coconut oil, eggs, maple syrup and vanilla extract. Add the remaining ingredients and process until smooth and thick. Allow the mixture to sit for 5 minutes to thicken.

▶ Grease a waffle iron.

▶ When hot, pour in the batter and cook according to the manufacturer's instructions.

▶ Serve with coconut yogurt or natural yogurt and berries.

Nutritional information per serving

Calories	Protein	Carbohydrates	Total fat
214kcal	11.6g	11.5g of which sugars 4.4g	12.9g of which saturates 6.3g

CACAO COURGETTE BREAD

This is a simple grain-free bread, great for breakfast or as a snack. You can make up a batch, then slice and freeze it for future use.

Grain-Free, Gluten-Free, Dairy-Free, Suitable for Vegetarians

Makes one 1lb loaf

Ingredients

130g/4½oz almond flour

2–3 tbsp cacao powder

¼ tsp sea salt

½ tsp bicarbonate of soda

2 large eggs

2 tbsp coconut oil, melted

2 tbsp maple syrup

1 tbsp vanilla extract

1 courgette (zucchini), grated

Method

▸ In a food processor combine the almond flour and cacao powder. Pulse in the salt and bicarbonate of soda.

▸ Pulse in the eggs, coconut oil, maple syrup and vanilla, and then the courgette.

▸ Transfer the batter to a greased loaf pan.

▸ Bake at 180°C/350°F, gas mark 4, for 35–40 minutes. Cool in the tin before turning out.

Nutritional information per slice (8 slices)

Calories	Protein	Carbohydrates	Total fat
166kcal	5.9g	6g of which sugars 3.1g	13.1g of which saturates 3.3g

BERRY MUFFINS

For a healthy carb 'fix', try these delicious grain-free muffins. Perfect for a healthy breakfast on-the-go, snack or lunchbox filler. These also freeze well.

Grain-Free, Gluten-Free, Dairy-Free, Suitable for Vegetarians

Makes 6

Ingredients

60g/2½oz coconut flour, sifted
½ tsp sea salt
½ tsp bicarbonate soda
6 eggs

2 tbsp honey
30g/1oz coconut oil
1 tbsp vanilla extract
60g/2½oz blueberries

Method

▸ In a small bowl, combine the coconut flour, salt and bicarbonate of soda.

▸ In a blender process the eggs, honey, oil and vanilla until smooth. Add the coconut flour, salt and bicarbonate of soda and blend – the mixture will stiffen.

▸ Gently fold in the blueberries.

▸ Place batter into paper-lined muffin tins.

- Bake at 180°C/350°F, gas mark 4, for 20–25 minutes. Allow to cool before removing from the tin.

Nutritional information per muffin

Calories	Protein	Carbohydrates	Total fat
189kcal	7.7g	12g of which sugars 6.5g	12g of which saturates 7.3g

SUPER GREENS FRITTATA

This is ideal for breakfast – cold or hot – and could be prepared the day before. For a lighter version, you can whisk up the egg whites separately and then fold into half of the egg yolks only.

Grain-Free, Gluten-Free, Dairy-Free, No Added Sugar, Suitable for Vegetarians

Serves 4

Ingredients

2 tbsp olive oil

Large handful of spring greens or spinach, chopped

½ red onion, chopped

1 courgette (zucchini), sliced thinly

Sea salt and freshly ground black pepper

2 garlic cloves, crushed

1 tomato, deseeded and chopped

8 eggs, whisked

1 tsp onion powder

½ tsp paprika, or to taste

Handful of coriander (cilantro) leaves, chopped

Method

- Heat the oil in an oven-proof frying pan over a medium heat. When hot, add the greens, onion, courgette, salt, pepper and garlic.
- Cover and cook until vegetables are tender (about 5–7 minutes), stirring occasionally.
- Stir in the tomato. Cook, uncovered, for 5 minutes more or until the liquid evaporates.
- Combine the eggs with the spices and coriander and whisk until frothy.
- Pour the eggs over the vegetable mixture and stir gently. Cover, reduce the heat and cook for 15 minutes.

- ▸ Meanwhile, preheat the grill. Place the frittata under the grill for 2–3 minutes until lightly golden and set.
- ▸ Invert onto a plate, slice and serve warm or cold.

Nutritional information per serving

Calories	Protein	Carbohydrates	Total fat
167kcal	13.7g	1.9g of which sugars 1.5g	11.5g of which saturates 3.2g

QUICK MEXICAN BAKED EGGS

Eggs are a nutritious option for breakfast and they're a good source of high-quality protein and energizing B vitamins, particularly choline (see Chapter 7). They are also a useful source of iodine and selenium, both important for healthy thyroid function. This easy recipe is also delicious as a lunch option served with salad.

Grain-Free, Gluten-Free, Dairy-Free, No Added Sugar, Suitable for Vegetarians

Serves 2–4

Ingredients

1 tbsp olive oil

1 red pepper, finely chopped

½ red onion, diced

1 garlic clove, crushed

400g/14oz can chopped tomatoes

1 tsp honey (optional)

Sea salt and freshly ground black pepper

400g/14oz can black-eyed beans, drained and rinsed

4 large eggs

Small handful of fresh coriander (cilantro), chopped

½ red onion, sliced

Lime wedges

Method

- ▸ Put the olive oil in a large frying pan over a high heat and fry the red pepper and half the onion for 2 minutes. Mix through the garlic and cook for a further minute.
- ▸ Add the tomatoes and honey, season with sea salt and freshly ground black pepper and allow to simmer away gently for 8 minutes until the sauce has thickened slightly. Stir through the beans until combined.

- Make four wells in the tomato sauce with the back of a spoon and crack in the eggs. Grind a little freshly ground black pepper over the top. Cover the pan with a lid and cook for 6–8 minutes or until the egg whites are no longer translucent.
- When cooked, garnish with fresh coriander leaves, the remaining thinly sliced red onion and lime wedges. Serve straight away with some toasted sourdough bread.

Nutritional information per 2 servings

Calories	Protein	Carbohydrates	Total fat
344kcal	23.6g	34g of which sugars 18.1g	12.5g of which saturates 3.3g

SWEET POTATO FRITTERS WITH POACHED EGGS

Crispy sweet fritters – rich in antioxidants, carotenoids, vitamins A and C – make a wonderful alternative to standard hash browns. Top these with a poached egg for an energizing breakfast.

Grain-Free, Gluten-Free, Dairy-Free, No Added Sugar, Suitable for Vegetarians

Serves 4

....

Ingredients

2 medium carrots, grated

1 sweet potato, peeled and grated

1 shallot, diced

3 eggs, whisked

½ tsp sea salt

1 tbsp coconut flour

Coconut oil for frying

4 poached eggs, to serve

....

Method

- In a large bowl combine the carrots, sweet potato, shallot and eggs. Stir the salt and coconut flour into the carrot mixture.
- Heat a frying pan and add some coconut oil. Place large spoonfuls of the batter into the pan and fry on each side until brown and crisp. Place on kitchen paper to drain and repeat with the remaining batter.
- Serve with a poached egg.

Calories	Protein	Carbohydrates	Total fat
228kcal	12.4g	15.9g of which sugars 6.4g	12.7g of which saturates 3.7g

TOFU VEGETABLE SCRAMBLE

This is a quick and simple recipe that's ideal if you're allergic to eggs or if you want a vegan option. The nutritional yeast flakes provide B vitamins and a lovely cheesy flavour to the tofu. The turmeric has anti-inflammatory properties (see Chapter 8) and also imparts a vibrant colour to the dish.

Grain-Free, Gluten-Free, Dairy-Free, No Added Sugar, Suitable for Vegetarians

Serves 4

. . . .

Ingredients

1 tbsp olive oil

1 onion, diced

450g/1lb firm tofu, crumbled

6 sundried tomatoes, drained and chopped

Large handful of spinach

3 tbsp nutritional yeast flakes

2 tbsp tamari

½ tsp turmeric

Sea salt and freshly ground black pepper

. . . .

Method

▶ Heat the oil in a frying pan. Add the onion and sauté for 3 minutes until soft. Add the tofu and tomatoes, and cook for 2 minutes.

▶ Add the remaining ingredients and cook for a further 5 minutes. Season to taste.

Nutritional information per serving

Calories	Protein	Carbohydrates	Total fat
168kcal	15.6g	5.9g of which sugars 1.2g	9.1g of which saturates 1.1g

LUNCHES
RICH GREENS SOUP

A cleansing, refreshing soup packed with alkalizing greens. The addition of avocado provides a creaminess, as well as some healthy monounsaturated fat.

Grain-Free, Gluten-Free, Dairy-Free, No Added Sugar, Suitable for Vegetarians

Serves 4

....

Ingredients

1 tbsp olive oil	400g/14oz spinach leaves
4 spring onions (scallions), chopped	500ml/1 pint vegetable stock
1 leek, chopped	Juice of ½ lime
2 celery sticks, chopped	½ tsp Himalayan salt
1 garlic clove, crushed	1 ripe avocado
1 green chilli, deseeded and diced	1 tsp flaxseed oil

....

Method

▸ Heat the olive oil in a large pan and sauté the spring onion, leek, celery, garlic and chilli. Cook for 5 minutes until the vegetables are soft. Add the spinach and stir until wilted. Pour in the vegetable stock. Simmer for 5 minutes.

▸ Combine with the remaining ingredients in a high-speed blender and blend until smooth.

▸ Pour into bowls to serve.

Nutritional information per serving

Calories	Protein	Carbohydrates	Total fat
133kcal	4.3g	3.8g of which sugars 3g	11g of which saturates 1.8g

CREAMY RED PEPPER SOUP

This is a speedy, antioxidant-packed soup. It's an excellent source of vitamins C and E and carotenoids, including lycopene, studied for its potential anti-cancer properties. The cashew nuts provide protein and a creamy texture to the soup.

Grain-Free, Gluten-Free, Dairy-Free, No Added Sugar, Suitable for Vegetarians

Serves 4

....

Ingredients

250g/9oz ripe vine tomatoes, halved

1 onion, quartered

2 garlic cloves, crushed

1 tbsp olive oil

4 roasted red peppers, drained

75g/3oz cashews, soaked for 1–2 hours and then drained

400ml/14fl oz hot vegetable or chicken stock

Himalayan salt and freshly ground black pepper to taste

Juice of ½ lemon

1 tbsp nutritional yeast flakes

2 pinches cayenne pepper

Pinch of smoked paprika

Dairy-Free Macadamia Pesto (see recipe), to serve (optional)

....

Method

▸ Preheat the oven to 190°C/375°F, gas mark 5. Place the tomatoes, onion and garlic on a baking tray. Drizzle over the oil and toss to coat. Bake in the oven for 20 minutes.

▸ Place the remaining ingredients in a blender or food processor and process until smooth. Warm in a pan to serve.

▸ Spoon into bowls and top with a little pesto if you wish.

Nutritional information per serving (without pesto)

Calories	Protein	Carbohydrates	Total fat
215kcal	13.7g	18g of which sugars 13.7g	12.6g of which saturates 2.3g

DAIRY-FREE MACADAMIA PESTO

Make up this pesto in advance and keep in the fridge for 3–4 days. It's delicious as a topping for soup but can also be stirred through cooked vegetables or rice, or use as a salad dressing.

Grain-Free, Gluten-Free, Dairy-Free, No Added Sugar, Suitable for Vegetarians

....

Ingredients

50g/2oz basil leaves

2 tbsp nutritional yeast flakes

60g/2½ oz macadamia nuts

5 tbsp olive oil or flaxseed oil

Pinch of Himalayan salt

2 tsp lemon juice

Method

▸ Pulse all the ingredients in a food processor until broken down to your desired consistency. (You can leave a little texture to the finished pesto.)

Nutritional information per tbsp

Calories	Protein	Carbohydrates	Total fat
87kcal	1.2g	0.9g of which sugars 0.2g	8.8g of which saturates 1.2g

PINEAPPLE GAZPACHO

A light, refreshing chilled soup. The pineapple core contains the anti-inflammatory enzyme bromelain (see Chapter 8).

Grain-Free, Gluten-Free, Dairy-Free, No Added Sugar, Suitable for Vegetarians

Serves 4

Ingredients

1 small pineapple, peeled and chopped, including the core

1 cucumber peeled, seeded and coarsely chopped

1 green chilli, deseeded and chopped

1 tbsp lime juice

150ml/5fl oz pineapple juice or coconut water

1 tbsp olive oil

75g/3oz flaked almonds, toasted

Handful of mint leaves, chopped

Handful of basil leaves, chopped

Sea salt and freshly ground black pepper

Method

▸ Finely chop ¼ of the pineapple and reserve. Coarsely chop the remaining pineapple. Place in a blender with the cucumber, chilli, lime juice, pineapple juice, oil, half of the almonds and half of the mint and basil leaves. Purée until smooth. Taste and season. Stir in the chopped pineapple.

▸ Spoon into shallow soup bowls. Top with the remaining almonds and herbs.

Calories	Protein	Carbohydrates	Total fat
198kcal	4.9g	15.1g of which sugars 14.9g	13g of which saturates 1.2g

BROCCOLI PEAR SOUP

A lovely light, creamy soup rich in detoxifying glucosinolates from the broccoli (see Chapter 6).

Grain-Free, Gluten-Free, Dairy-Free, Nut-Free, No Added Sugar, Suitable for Vegetarians

Serves 4

Ingredients

600ml/1 pint vegetable stock

1 onion, finely chopped

1 celery stick, chopped

1 garlic clove, crushed

1 small potato, chopped

Juice of ½ lemon

1 tbsp tamari

400g/14oz fresh broccoli, cut into small pieces

2 ripe pears, cored, peeled and chopped

Sea salt and freshly ground black pepper to taste

Method

- Put the stock, onion, celery, garlic, potato, lemon juice and tamari in a large saucepan and bring to the boil.
- Add the broccoli and simmer for 3–4 minutes until the broccoli is just tender.
- Process the soup with the pears in a blender to create a thick, smooth soup. Season to taste.
- Spoon into bowls and drizzle with a little tamari or olive oil to taste.

Nutritional information per serving

Calories	Protein	Carbohydrates	Total fat
92kcal	5.6g	14.2g of which sugars 10.2g	1.3g of which saturates 0.2g

ASIAN CHICKEN NOODLE SOUP

Home-made chicken soup has a long history of traditional use for immune system health. This Asian version includes additional immune-supporting ingredients, such as garlic, ginger and chillies. Mirin is a Japanese condiment based on rice wine.

Gluten-Free, Dairy-Free

Serves 4

....

Ingredients

800ml/1½ pints chicken stock

3 tbsp tamari

1 tbsp white miso paste

1 tsp maple syrup or honey

2 star anise

2 cinnamon sticks

1 red chilli, deseeded and chopped

2cm piece of fresh root ginger, grated

2 tbsp mirin

200g/7oz buckwheat noodles, rice noodles or kelp noodles

200g/7oz bean sprouts or sprouted mung beans

1 pak choi, shredded

Bunch of spring onions (scallions), finely chopped (optional)

6 shitake mushrooms, sliced

350g cooked chicken, shredded

Bunch of coriander (cilantro) leaves

Freshly ground black pepper

2 tsp sesame oil

....

Method

▸ Place the stock, tamari, miso, maple syrup, spices and mirin in a large saucepan and bring to the boil.

▸ If using the buckwheat or rice noodles, cook in a pan of boiling water according to the instructions. Drain and refresh under cold running water. For kelp noodles, soak in water and then drain.

▸ Add the bean sprouts, pak choi, spring onions and mushrooms, and simmer for a couple of minutes. Divide the noodles and chicken between four bowls. Pour over the hot soup and finish with coriander, freshly ground black pepper and a drizzle of sesame oil.

Nutritional information per serving (with plain rice noodles)

Calories	Protein	Carbohydrates	Total fat
387kcal	37.5g	41.6g of which sugars 5.5g	7.5g of which saturates 0.8g

NORI AVOCADO MAKI ROLLS

Using minced parsnip as 'rice' makes this a nutritious low-carb option. Pack your sushi with plenty of colourful vegetables. You could also add some strips of tofu or smoked salmon.

Grain-Free, Gluten-Free, Dairy-Free, No Added Sugar, Suitable for Vegetarians

Serves 4

....

Ingredients

4 shiitake mushrooms, finely sliced

1 tbsp tamari

1 large parsnip

30g/1oz pine nuts

1 tsp tahini

Pinch of sea salt

Freshly ground black pepper

1 tsp apple cider vinegar

4 nori sheets, cut in half along the central line

1 ripe avocado, sliced

1 carrot, cut into julienne strips strips

Handful of alfalfa sprouts

....

Method

▸ Place the mushrooms in a bowl and pour over the tamari. Coat thoroughly and leave to marinate for 15–30 minutes.

▸ Process the parsnip and pine nuts in a food processor until very fine. Add the tahini, salt, pepper and vinegar, and pulse to combine.

▸ Place a sheet of nori, shiny side down, on top of a sushi-rolling mat. Spoon a little parsnip rice on the top half of the nori and press down.

▸ Place the avocado slices over the rice in a horizontal line. Arrange the shitake mushrooms and carrot strips on top, and finally place on top the alfalfa sprouts.

▸ Using the rolling mat, roll the nori tightly. Wet the edge of the nori sheet to help it seal. Using a sharp knife, cut the sushi into 6 pieces. Repeat with the remaining nori sheets.

Nutritional information per serving

Calories	Protein	Carbohydrates	Total fat
148kcal	4.4g	6.8g of which sugars 4g	11.5g of which saturates 1.6g

KALE SALAD WITH SWEET TAHINI DRESSING

Grain-Free, Gluten-Free, Dairy-Free, Nut-Free, Suitable for Vegetarians

Serves 4

....

Ingredients

70g/2½oz white miso

75g/3oz tahini

2 tbsp tamari

2 tbsp maple syrup

3–4 tbsp water

1 tbsp nutritional yeast flakes (optional)

Himalayan salt or herbal salt

250g/9oz bag of kale, chopped

200g/7oz cherry tomatoes, halved

1 red pepper, diced

Large handful of sprouted seeds (e.g. alfalfa)

....

Method

▶ Place the miso, tahini, tamari, maple syrup, water and nutritional yeast flakes in a blender and process to form a thick dressing. Season.

▶ Place the kale in a large bowl. Pour over the dressing and massage the dressing into the kale with your hands to 'wilt' the kale. Add the cherry tomatoes, pepper and alfalfa, and toss lightly.

Nutritional information per serving

Calories	Protein	Carbohydrates	Total fat
227kcal	10.7g	14.8g of which sugars 9.3g	13.6g of which saturates 1.8g

MEXICAN LETTUCE WRAP

This vegan dish uses omega-rich walnuts to create a chunky pâté.

Grain-Free, Gluten-Free, Dairy-Free, Suitable for Vegetarians

Serves 4

....

Ingredients

Little gem lettuce, leaves separated

Lime Guacamole (see recipe), to serve

Roasted Pepper Mayonnaise (see recipe; optional)

Walnut pâté

115g/4oz walnuts
60g/2½oz sundried tomatoes
2 fresh tomatoes
2 tsp onion powder

2 tsp cumin powder
2 tsp garlic salt
1 red chilli, deseeded and diced

Method

▸ Place all the pâté ingredients in a food processor and blend until chunky. Season to taste. To serve, place a spoonful of the mixture into a lettuce leaf. Top with guacamole and mayonnaise and serve.

Nutritional information per serving (lettuce with walnut pâté only)

Calories	Protein	Carbohydrates	Total fat
284kcal	5.6g	3.2g of which sugars 2.7g	27.9g of which saturates 3.2g

WATERCRESS, APPLE AND WALNUT SALAD WITH CREAMY MUSTARD DRESSING

A light, nutrient-rich salad. Watercress is packed with antioxidant phytochemicals, vitamin C and beta-carotene. It also provides folate and calcium for bone support.

Grain-Free, Gluten-Free, Dairy-Free, No Added Sugar, Suitable for Vegetarians

Serves 4

Ingredients

1 large romaine lettuce, torn into 2cm pieces
1 bunch of watercress, stems removed
60g/2½oz seedless grapes, cut in half

1 apple, diced
2 sticks celery, finely diced
Small handful of fresh flat-leaf parsley, chopped

100g/3½oz walnuts, roughly broken up and lightly toasted, to serve

Dressing

½ tsp Dijon mustard
2 tbsp apple cider vinegar
2 tbsp flaxseed oil
2 tbsp olive oil

2–3 tbsp water
1 tbsp cashew nut butter
Sea salt and freshly ground black pepper to taste

Method

▸ Tear the lettuce and watercress by hand and transfer to a bowl with the grapes, apple and celery. Scatter over the chopped parsley.

▸ Put all the dressing ingredients in a blender and process until smooth – add a little water if the dressing is too thick.

▸ Toss the salad with the dressing just before serving. Scatter over the walnuts to serve.

Nutritional information per serving

Calories	Protein	Carbohydrates	Total fat
403kcal	8.2g	5.9g of which sugars 5.7g	37.8g of which saturates 4.5g

SEEDED FATTOUSH SALAD

This Middle Eastern-style salad is normally served with croutons. Instead, we've used crumbled seeded crackers for a lovely crunchy flavour and to keep the meal gluten-free. The sumac spice adds a tart flavour. Serve the salad with some protein (e.g. chickpeas, roast chicken).

Grain-Free, Gluten-Free, Dairy-Free, Nut-Free, Suitable for Vegetarians

Serves 4

Ingredients

1 cos lettuce, shredded

225g/8oz cherry tomatoes, halved

4 spring onions (scallions), chopped

1 cucumber, deseeded and sliced

8 radishes, thinly sliced

1 red pepper, diced

Handful of parsley, chopped

Handful of mint, chopped

4 *Tomato Seeded Crackers* (see recipe)

1 tsp sumac

Dressing

Juice and zest of 1 lemon

3 tbsp olive oil

2 tbsp flaxseed oil

2 tsp honey

1 tbsp pomegranate molasses

Sea salt and freshly ground black pepper

Method

▸ Combine the lettuce, tomatoes, spring onions, cucumber, radishes, pepper and herbs in a large bowl. Break up the crackers and sprinkle over the salad. Sprinkle over the sumac and toss lightly.

▸ Make up the dressing by whisking all the ingredients together. Season to taste. Pour over the salad just before serving.

Nutritional information per serving

Calories	Protein	Carbohydrates	Total fat
295kcal	6.9g	15.2g of which sugars 10.9g	23.5g of which saturates 3.1g

QUINOA TABBOULEH WITH POMEGRANATE

Quinoa is a delicious nutrient-packed seed that is used as a grain, in a similar way to couscous. This colourful, herb-rich salad is perfect for packed lunches.

Grain-Free, Gluten-Free, Dairy-Free, Nut-Free, No Added Sugar, Suitable for Vegetarians

Serves 4

Ingredients

180g/6oz quinoa

500ml/1 pint vegetable stock

Juice of 2 lemons

5 tbsp olive oil

1 red onion, finely diced

1 tsp ground cumin

1 tsp sea salt

1 cucumber, deseeded, and chopped

4 plum tomatoes, deseeded and finely diced

Handful of parsley, chopped

Handful of mint chopped

Seeds from 1 pomegranate

1 preserved lemon, rind only, finely chopped

Method

▸ Place the quinoa in a pan and pour over the vegetable stock. Bring to the boil. Cover and reduce the heat to a simmer. Simmer for 15 minutes. Turn off the heat and allow to stand for 5 minutes. Fluff up with a fork. Add the remaining ingredients and toss well. Season to taste.

Nutritional information per serving

Calories	Protein	Carbohydrates	Total fat
280kcal	7.9g	30.1g of which sugars 8.6g	14.1g of which saturates 1.9g

ROASTED BABY BEETS WITH TEMPEH AND WALNUT DRESSING

Beetroots are used traditionally for supporting bile flow, which is important for eliminating toxins. Tempeh is a type of fermented soy. It's an excellent source of protein and calcium. It is rich in isoflavones, which may help to support hormonal balance (see Chapter 9).

Grain-Free, Gluten-Free, Dairy-Free, Suitable for Vegetarians

Serves 4

Ingredients

8 baby beetroot, peeled and whole, or 4 medium beetroot, peeled and halved

4 tbsp extra virgin olive oil

350g/12oz tempeh cut into chunks

Juice and zest of 1 lemon

1 tsp sea salt

2 garlic cloves, crushed

Freshly ground black pepper

Bag of mixed green salad leaves, to serve

Dressing

3 tbsp sherry vinegar

4 tbsp walnut or hazelnut oil

½ tsp Dijon mustard

1 tsp honey

Handful of parsley, chopped

Sea salt and freshly ground black pepper

Method

▶ Heat the oven to 200°C/400°F, gas mark 6. Place the beetroot on a large piece of foil-backed baking paper. Drizzle with 1 tbsp of the olive oil and season. Wrap to form a parcel.

▶ Place the tempeh on a baking tray. Mix together the remaining oil, lemon juice, salt and garlic. Pour over the tempeh. Cover with foil. Roast for 30 minutes. Remove the foil from the tempeh and roast for a further 10 minutes until the tempeh is golden and the beetroots are tender.

▶ Slice the beetroot thickly. Whisk together the dressing ingredients.

- Place the beetroot and tempeh on a platter and drizzle over the dressing ingredients while the beetroots are still warm. Serve with a mixed green salad.

Nutritional information per serving

Calories	Protein	Carbohydrates	Total fat
448kcal	19.4g	11.5g of which sugars 6.7g	35.7g of which saturates 3.5g

BITTER GREENS WITH GRAPEFRUIT AND AVOCADO

A simple, clean-tasting salad. Bitter greens can help stimulate digestive juices. They are also rich in folate, antioxidant carotenoids and minerals including calcium, magnesium and iron.

Grain-Free, Gluten-Free, Dairy-Free, Nut-Free, No Added Sugar, Suitable for Vegetarians

Serves 4

....

Ingredients

Large handful of rocket (arugula)

Large handful of watercress

Large handful of baby spinach

2 red grapefruits, peeled

2 avocados, peeled and sliced

1 red onion, diced

Handful of basil leaves, chopped

Dressing

30g/1oz black olives, finely chopped

2 tbsp apple cider vinegar

4 tbsp olive oil

1 tbsp walnut oil

1 tbsp lemon juice

Sea salt and freshly ground black pepper

....

Method

- Place the rocket, watercress and spinach leaves in a large bowl. Cut the grapefruit into segments and add to the salad with the avocado and red onion. Sprinkle over the basil leaves.
- Mix all the ingredients together for the dressing. Season to taste. Drizzle over the salad to serve.

Nutritional information per serving

Calories	Protein	Carbohydrates	Total fat
273kcal	4.8g	8.4g of which sugars 7.5g	24.3g of which saturates 4g

VIETNAMESE CHICKEN SALAD WITH CHILLI LIME DRESSING

A fresh, protein-packed salad. The dressing is tangy, lightly spiced and bursting with fresh flavours. A wonderfully energizing dish.

Grain-Free, Gluten-Free, Dairy-Free, Nut-Free, No Added Sugar

Serves 4

Ingredients

500ml/1 pint chicken stock

3 skinless chicken breasts

2 carrots, cut into julienne strips

1 red pepper, cut into julienne strips

1 cucumber, deseeded and thinly sliced

1 red onion, finely diced

Handful of fresh mint leaves, chopped

Handful of fresh coriander (cilantro) leaves, chopped

Dressing

125ml/4fl oz lime juice

1 tbsp honey

1 garlic clove, crushed

½ red chilli, deseeded and diced

2 tbsp fish sauce

1 tbsp fresh coriander (cilantro) leaves

Freshly ground black pepper

Method

▸ Bring the stock to the boil in a medium pan. Add the chicken and simmer for 10 minutes. Turn off the heat and allow to stand for 15 minutes. Remove the chicken and shred.

▸ Combine all the vegetables in a large bowl with the chicken. Make up the dressing by whisking all the ingredients together. Toss in the dressing and sprinkle over the herbs to serve. Season with a little freshly ground black pepper to taste.

Nutritional information per serving

Calories	Protein	Carbohydrates	Total fat
186kcal	27.5g	11.6g of which sugars 11.2g	3.1g of which saturates 0.9g

GREEK CHICKEN SALAD WITH ROASTED OLIVES

This summery Mediterranean salad makes a substantial meal and any leftovers will keep for the next day. The addition of anchovies in the dressing increases the omega 3 content of the dish.

Grain-Free, Gluten-Free, Nut-Free, No Added Sugar

Serves 4

. . . .

Ingredients

Marinade

Juice and zest of 2 lemons

3 tbsp olive oil

2 tsp chopped fresh oregano

Sea salt and freshly ground black pepper

2 skinless chicken breasts

Vinaigrette

1 anchovy, rinsed and chopped

10 capers, finely chopped

5 tbsp red wine vinegar

1 garlic clove, crushed

4 tbsp extra virgin olive oil

2 tbsp flaxseed oil

Salad

250g/9oz cherry tomatoes, halved

1 red onion, chopped

1 cucumber, seeded, peeled and sliced into thick slices

150g/5oz *Roasted Herb and Lemon-Scented Olives* (see recipe)

1 Romaine lettuce, shredded

150g/5oz feta cheese, crumbled (optional)

. . . .

Method

▸ Combine the marinade ingredients and marinate the chicken for 1 hour.

▸ Place all the vinaigrette ingredients in a jar and shake well.

▸ Preheat a frying pan and pan fry the chicken for 6–7 minutes on each side until cooked through. Rest, then slice.

▸ Combine all the salad ingredients together. Add the feta if using and the chicken. Toss with a little of the dressing to serve.

Nutritional information per serving

Calories	Protein	Carbohydrates	Total fat
458kcal	28.2g	7g of which sugars 6.2g	34.2g of which saturates 8.8g

PRAWN AND SEA VEGETABLE SALAD WITH UMEBOSHI DRESSING

Sea vegetables are rich in many minerals including calcium, copper, iodine, iron, magnesium, manganese, molybdenum, phosphorus, potassium, selenium, vanadium and zinc. They also contain sulphated polysaccharides called fucoidans which are known for their anti-inflammatory properties. This Japanese-style salad contains umeboshi, pickled sour plum used for its digestive benefits.

Grain-Free, Gluten-Free, Dairy-Free, Nut-Free

Serves 4

Ingredients

20 large cooked prawns

2 carrots, cut into julienne strips

1 red pepper, cut into thin strips

1 cucumber, deseeded and thinly sliced into rounds

Handful of mint leaves, chopped

Handful of coriander (cilantro) leaves, chopped

25g/1oz mixed sea vegetables, soaked for 15 minutes, then drained thoroughly

Dressing

1 tsp umeboshi paste

Juice of ½ lemon

2 tsp tahini

2 tsp sesame oil

2 tsp tamari

1 tsp rice vinegar or apple cider vinegar

2 tsp honey, yacon syrup or maple syrup

Method

▸ Place the dressing ingredients in a blender and process to combine.

▸ Combine the prawns, carrots, red pepper, cucumber, herbs and sea vegetables in a bowl. Just before serving pour over the dressing and mix well.

Nutritional information per serving

Calories	Protein	Carbohydrates	Total fat
98kcal	7.3g	5.9g of which sugars 5.6g	4.8g of which saturates 0.7g

SEARED BEEF SALAD WITH CORIANDER PESTO

Choose grass-fed beef, as this is richer in omega 3 fats. It is also a good source of CLA, a healthy fat that promotes energy production and a lean body composition. Using pumpkin seeds and seed oil in the pesto is a great way to increase the omega 3 content of this dish.

Grain-Free, Gluten-Free, Dairy-Free

Serves 4

Ingredients

400g/14oz beef fillet or sirloin steak

1 tbsp olive oil

Large bag of mixed greens (e.g. rocket/arugula, watercress, baby spinach)

1 red onion, thinly sliced

250g/9oz cherry tomatoes, halved

Juice of 2 limes

Pesto

60g/2½oz fresh coriander (cilantro) leaves

30g/1oz pumpkin seeds

20g/¾oz cashew nuts

2 cloves garlic, chopped

Juice and zest of 1 lime

125ml/4fl oz extra-virgin olive oil

30ml/1fl oz pumpkin seed oil or walnut oil

1 red chilli, deseeded and finely chopped

Marinade

1 red chilli, deseeded and chopped

1 garlic clove, crushed

1 tbsp honey

3 tbsp olive oil

Method

▸ Make the pesto. Place the ingredients in a food processor and blend until smooth. Check for seasoning.

▸ Mix the marinade ingredients together. Pour over the fillet and leave to marinate for 1–2 hours or overnight.

▸ Remove the meat from the marinade. Heat the oil in a frying pan and sear the beef on each side. Place in a roasting dish and roast at

190°C/375°F, gas mark 5, for 20 minutes until cooked. Allow to rest for 10 minutes, then slice thinly.

▸ Place the green leaves, onions and tomatoes in a bowl and toss together. Top with the beef and drizzle over the pesto to serve.

Nutritional information per serving (with 1 tbsp pesto)

Calories	Protein	Carbohydrates	Total fat
403kcal	26.5g	8.3g of which sugars 7.5g	29.2g of which saturates 5.6g

WARM SALAD OF BUTTERNUT SQUASH WITH SWEET AND SOUR DRESSING

Warm salads provide comforting nourishment in the cooler months, without having to resort to high-carb dishes. Roasting butternut squash brings out its wonderful sweet, caramel flavour. The beans provide protein to help keep blood sugar levels stable.

Grain-Free, Gluten-Free, Dairy-Free, Suitable for Vegetarians

Serves 4

Ingredients

1kg/2lb butternut squash, peeled and cut into chunks

5 tbsp olive oil or coconut oil, melted

1 tsp sea salt

Pinch of freshly ground black pepper

2 garlic cloves, crushed

3 tbsp red wine vinegar

1–2 tbsp honey or maple syrup

1 red onion, sliced

Pinch of red chilli powder or flakes, or cayenne pepper

Handful of rocket (arugula) or spinach leaves

1 x 400g/14oz can soy beans or mixed beans

4 tbsp toasted pine nuts

2 tbsp chopped fresh mint

Method

▸ Preheat the oven to 200°C/400°F, gas mark 6. Toss the butternut squash in 2 tbsp oil and place on a large baking sheet. Season with salt and pepper. Bake for 20 minutes.

▸ Heat the remaining oil in a frying pan and add the garlic and cook for 2 minutes, then pour in the vinegar, honey, onion and chilli, and simmer for about 3 minutes until syrupy.

▸ Place the rocket, beans and butternut squash in a bowl. Drizzle over the dressing with the pine nuts and mint to serve.

Nutritional information per serving

Calories	Protein	Carbohydrates	Total fat
387kcal	9.6g	36.6g of which sugars 19.8g	22.3g of which saturates 2.3g

PAN-FRIED SALMON WITH SWEET SOY KELP NOODLES SALAD

Kelp noodles are low in carbs, yet rich in micronutrients, including iodine, important for metabolism and thyroid function. If you prefer, you could use buckwheat or rice noodles instead.

Grain-Free, Gluten-Free, Dairy-Free, Nut-Free

Serves 4

....

Ingredients

4 salmon fillets, boneless

1 tbsp coconut oil

250g/9oz kelp noodles

350g/12oz sprouting broccoli, cut into 2–3cm pieces

1 garlic clove, crushed

Handful of sprouted seeds/beans, to serve

1 tbsp sesame seeds, to serve

Dressing

5 tbsp tamari mixed with 1 tbsp coconut sugar or xylitol

2 red chillies, deseeded and chopped

3 garlic cloves, crushed

2 tsp grated ginger

Juice of 2 limes

1 tbsp rice vinegar

1 tbsp raw honey

2 tsp omega oil blend or flaxseed oil

....

Method

▸ Mix all the dressing ingredients together. Pour a little of the dressing over the salmon and marinate for 30 minutes. Heat the oil in a frying pan and pan fry the salmon for 3–5 minutes on each side until cooked. Alternatively, you could steam the salmon for 5–7 minutes. Cool and flake into large pieces.

▸ Soak the kelp noodles according to packet instructions and drain thoroughly.

- Blanch the broccoli in boiling water for a couple of minutes. Place in cold water to stop the cooking. Drain well and dry in a tea towel.
- Place the noodles in a large bowl. Pour over the dressing and mix well.
- Heat the oil in a pan and stir the garlic and broccoli to coat in the oil – about 1–2 minutes. Toss into the noodles with the salmon. Add a handful of sprouted seeds and sprinkle over the sesame seeds to serve.

Nutritional information per serving

Calories	Protein	Carbohydrates	Total fat
319kcal	26.4g	11.6g of which sugars 10.9g	18.6g of which saturates 4.6g

SNACKS
LIME GUACAMOLE
Guacamole is a nutrient-rich spread. This one has a wonderful tangy flavour with the addition of lime and a dash of cumin. It works well as a snack with vegetable sticks, crackers or oat cakes.

Grain-Free, Gluten-Free, Dairy-Free, Nut-Free, No Added Sugar, Suitable for Vegetarians

Serves 4

Ingredients

2 ripe avocados

Juice and zest of 1 lime

½ tsp Himalayan salt

2 tomatoes, diced

1 tsp cumin

1 garlic clove, crushed

Small handful of coriander (cilantro) leaves, chopped

Method
- Mash up the avocado, then mix in the remaining ingredients.

Nutritional information per serving

Calories	Protein	Carbohydrates	Total fat
102kcal	1.5g	2.1g of which sugars 1.3g	10.1g of which saturates 2.1g

COURGETTE HUMMUS

A bean-free dip with a creamy and rich texture, packed with calcium and magnesium.

Grain-Free, Gluten-Free, Dairy-Free, Nut-Free, No Added Sugar, Suitable for Vegetarians

Serves 8

....

Ingredients

2 large courgettes (zucchini), chopped

Juice and zest of 1 lemon

1 tsp sea salt

1–2 tsp cumin to taste

120g/4½oz tahini (sesame seed paste)

2 garlic cloves, crushed

4 tbsp olive oil or omega 3 oil blend

....

Method

▶ Simply place all the ingredients in a food processor and process until smooth.

Nutritional information per serving

Calories	Protein	Carbohydrates	Total fat
166kcal	3.6g	1g of which sugars 0.8g	16.6g of which saturates 2.4g

TOMATO NUT CHEESE

A protein-packed dairy-free alternative to cheese. Use this as a dip or a spread for crackers, bread or pizza bases. You can eat this straightaway, but if you leave it to ferment it develops a tasty sour flavour.

Grain-Free, Gluten-Free, Dairy-Free, No Added Sugar, Suitable for Vegetarians

Serves 6

....

Ingredients

60g/2½oz cashew nuts

60g/2½oz macadamia nuts

2 tsp lemon juice

¼ tsp salt

4 sundried tomatoes in oil, drained

1 tbsp nutritional yeast

60ml/2fl oz water

1 tsp probiotic powder or empty the contents of 1–2 capsules (*Lactobacillus*)

Method

▸ Grind all the ingredients in a food processor. This can be eaten straight away. Alternatively, cover and leave at room temperature for 12 hours to 'ferment' if wished. This will keep in the fridge for 3–4 days.

Nutritional information per serving

Calories	Protein	Carbohydrates	Total fat
163kcal	3.6g	3g of which sugars 1g	15.2 of which saturates 2.4g

BEET MINT DIP

A refreshing, clean-tasting dip. Beetroots are useful for promoting detoxification and helping to maintain healthy blood pressure. Beetroot also contains an energizing mix of iron and folate, important for red blood cell formation.

Grain-Free, Gluten-Free, Dairy-Free, Suitable for Vegetarians

Serves 6

Ingredients

200g/7oz cooked beetroot

Handful of fresh mint leaves

125g/4½oz cashew nuts

1 tbsp apple cider vinegar

1 tsp maple syrup

2 tsp tamari

1 tbsp flaxseed or olive oil

Pinch of sea salt

Method

▸ Place all the ingredients in a food processor and process until smooth. Add a little more oil if needed to achieve a smooth consistency.

Nutritional information per serving

Calories	Protein	Carbohydrates	Total fat
152kcal	4.5g	4.3g of which sugars 0.1g	11.6g of which saturates 2.2g

BALSAMIC FIG SPREAD

A sweet spread that's a perfect complement to cooked fish, cheese or meats, but equally delicious spread on raw crackers for a healthy snack.

Grain-Free, Gluten-Free, Dairy-Free, Suitable for Vegetarians

Serves 8

....

Ingredients

150g/5oz macadamia nuts, soaked overnight

175ml/6fl oz water

1 tsp probiotic powder or the contents of 1–2 capsules (*Lactobacillus*)

Juice of ½ lemon

2 tbsp honey, coconut nectar or maple syrup

2 tbsp balsamic vinegar

4 dried figs, finely chopped

2 tbsp finely chopped shallot

1 tsp fresh rosemary, finely chopped

2 tbsp nutritional yeast

Himalayan salt and freshly ground black pepper to taste

....

Method

▸ Place the soaked macadamia nuts and water in a high-speed blender and blend until smooth. Stir in the probiotic powder and lemon juice.

▸ Line a sieve with cheesecloth. Pour in the nut mixture, fold the cheesecloth over the top and set on a plate. Leave out to culture for 24 hours.

▸ Place the honey and vinegar in a bowl and add the figs. Allow to soak for 1 hour.

▸ Place the 'cheese' and remaining ingredients in a blender and pulse to combine – do not over-process. Keep some texture. This will keep in the fridge for 3–4 days.

Nutritional information per serving

Calories	Protein	Carbohydrates	Total fat
180kcal	3g	8.6g of which sugars 7.7g	14.7g of which saturates 2.1g

OLIVE TAPENADE

Olives are a rich source of monounsaturated fats as well as heart-healthy phytochemicals. This tapenade is delicious spread on crackers or oat cakes.

Grain-Free, Gluten-Free, Dairy-Free, Nut-Free, No Added Sugar, Suitable for Vegetarians

Serves 6

....

Ingredients

100g/4oz pitted olives	2 tbsp basil leaves
1 garlic clove, crushed	1 tbsp lemon juice
1 tbsp capers	Olive oil for blending

....

Method

▸ Whizz all the ingredients together with enough oil to make a paste.

Nutritional information per serving

Calories	Protein	Carbohydrates	Total fat
19kcal	0.3g	0.2g of which sugars 0.1g	1.9g of which saturates 0.3g

BASIC MAYONNAISE

This mayonnaise is surprisingly easy to make. The trick is to use a really fresh egg and to make sure that all the ingredients are at room temperature before you start. The mayo can be stored in the fridge for a couple of days.

Grain-Free, Gluten-Free, Dairy-Free, No Added Sugar, Suitable for Vegetarians

Serves 6

....

Ingredients

1 large egg yolk, at room temperature	1 tsp white vinegar
1½ tsp lemon juice	150ml/5fl oz light olive oil or a light nut oil (e.g. macadamia nut oil)
¼ tsp Dijon mustard	
¼ tsp salt	

Method

▶ Place the egg and lemon juice in a blender or food processor. Add the mustard, salt, vinegar and 2–3 tbsp of the oil. Process for a few seconds.

▶ With the processor running very slowly, drizzle in the remaining oil. This should take a couple of minutes to form a thick emulsion.

Nutritional information per tbsp (15g)

Calories	Protein	Carbohydrates	Total fat
118kcal	0.3g	0g	13g of which saturates 1.9g

ROASTED PEPPER MAYONNAISE

An egg-free mayonnaise – perfect as a dip or spread or used as a dressing for salads and coleslaw.

Grain-Free, Gluten-Free, Dairy-Free, No Added Sugar, Suitable for Vegetarians

Serves 6

Ingredients

125g/4½oz cashew nuts
1 pickled chilli, drained and chopped
1 roasted red pepper
½ tsp cider vinegar

1 tbsp lemon juice
Pinch of garlic salt
Water to blend

Method

▶ Simply combine all the ingredients in a blender with a little water until smooth. Season to taste.

Nutritional information per tbsp (15g)

Calories	Protein	Carbohydrates	Total fat
72kcal	2.2g	2.2g of which sugars 0.6g	6g of which saturates 1.2g

KALE-ONAISE

A sneaky way to get more greens in your diet. Delicious used as a dip or spread on oat cakes.

Grain-Free, Gluten-Free, Dairy-Free, Nut-Free, No Added Sugar, Suitable for Vegetarians

Ingredients

Large handful of chopped kale, large stems removed

½ tsp sea salt

2 garlic cloves, chopped

125g/4½oz *Basic Mayonnaise* (see recipe)

Zest and juice of 1 lemon to taste

Method

▶ In a food processor, combine the kale leaves, salt and garlic. Process until finely chopped. Add in the mayonnaise, lemon zest and lemon juice, and process until smooth.

Nutritional information per tbsp (15g)

Calories	Protein	Carbohydrates	Total fat
66kcal	0.3g	0.2g of which sugars 0.1g	7.1g of which saturates 1.1g

ROASTED HERB AND LEMON-SCENTED OLIVES

The roasting helps draw out some of the moisture in the olives, making them slightly more dense and even more delicious. As the olives roast, they also soak in the flavours from the aromatics, giving them a bright, tangy, garlicky flavour.

Grain-Free, Gluten-Free, Dairy-Free, Nut-Free, No Added Sugar, Suitable for Vegetarians

Serves 8

Ingredients

150g/5oz black pitted olives, drained

150g/5oz Greek Kalamata pitted olives, drained

6 garlic cloves, crushed

4 fresh thyme sprigs

4 rosemary sprigs

Zest of ½ lemon, finely shredded

60ml/2½fl oz olive oil

Juice of ½ lemon

Pinch of sea salt

Method

▸ Preheat the oven to 200°C/400°F, gas mark 6.

▸ In a medium bowl, combine all the ingredients and mix well. Transfer the olive mixture to a shallow baking dish.

▸ Bake for 20 minutes. Cool in the baking dish before using.

Nutritional information per serving

Calories	Protein	Carbohydrates	Total fat
108kcal	0.5g	0.3g of which sugars 0.1g	11.6g of which saturates 1.7g

CAULIFLOWER MUNCHIES

These are a great snack option – you can eat them raw, bake them in the oven or dehydrate them.

Grain-Free, Gluten-Free, Dairy-Free, Suitable for Vegetarians, No Added Sugar

Serves 8

Ingredients

1 cauliflower, cut into small pieces	1 tsp olive oil
2–3 tbsp nutritional yeast	2 tsp tamari or coconut aminos liquid
Garlic salt or sea salt to taste	Pinch of ground cumin powder
Freshly ground black pepper to taste	Pinch of cayenne pepper or paprika

Method

▸ Place all the ingredients in a large bag or bowl. Mix thoroughly and leave to stand for 5 minutes.

▸ Dehydrate if wished overnight or bake in an oven at 180°C/350°F, gas mark 4 for 15–20 minutes until crisp.

Nutritional information per serving

Calories	Protein	Carbohydrates	Total fat
30kcal	3.2g	2.5g of which sugars 0.8g	0.9g of which saturates 0.1g

SALTED VINEGAR AND ONION KALE CHIPS

Crunchy kale crisps make a tremendously healthy snack and are an ideal alternative to conventional high-fat processed crisps. These will keep well in an airtight container for 3–4 days.

Grain-Free, Gluten-Free, Dairy-Free, Suitable for Vegetarians, No Added Sugar

Serves 8

Ingredients

75g/3oz cashew nuts, ideally soaked for 2 hours and then drained

1 shallot, chopped

2 tbsp nutritional yeast flakes

½ tsp garlic salt

4 soft large dates, chopped

2 tbsp lemon juice

2 tbsp water

2 tbsp apple cider vinegar

250g/9oz bag of chopped kale

Method

▶ Blend all the ingredients except the kale until thick. Add a little more water if needed. Place the kale in a bowl and pour over the sauce. Massage thoroughly with your hands. Place on a teflex sheet and dehydrate for 4–6 hours. Then flip over the kale and place on the mesh sheet and dehydrate for a further 6–8 hours until crisp.

▶ For an oven-baked version: Preheat the oven to 150°C/300°F, gas mark 2. Place the kale on a lined baking tray and bake for 15–20 minutes. Carefully turn the kale over and cook for a further 5 minutes.

Nutritional information per serving

Calories	Protein	Carbohydrates	Total fat
82kcal	4.2g	4.7g of which sugars 2.6g	5.1 of which saturates 1g

SPICED GLAZED NUTS

This combination of spices, maple syrup and salt is a great way to liven up nuts. You can bake these in the oven or use a dehydrator.

Grain-Free, Gluten-Free, Dairy-Free, Suitable for Vegetarians

Serves 10

Ingredients

250g/9oz mixed nuts (cashews, almonds, macadamia nuts)

½ tsp sea salt

1 tsp lemon juice

1 tsp curry powder

½ tsp cumin powder

2 tbsp maple syrup

Method

▸ Soak the nuts in water for 1 hour and then drain. Mix together the remaining ingredients and toss with the nuts.

▸ Preheat the oven to 150°C/300°F, gas mark 2. Spread the nuts on a greased, lined baking sheet and bake for 10–15 minutes, stirring occasionally during cooking until lightly golden. Cool before using. These nuts can also be dehydrated. Spread on to a teflex-lined dehydrator tray and dehydrate for 12–16 hours until dry.

Nutritional information per heaped tbsp (30g)

Calories	Protein	Carbohydrates	Total fat
157kcal	5g	4.5g of which sugars 2.8g	13.3g of which saturates 1.6g

COCONUT CINNAMON BREAD

A simple gluten- and grain-free bread. The addition of coconut buttercream or 'manna' creates a delicious creamy texture. Add plenty of cinnamon, which can help with stabilizing blood sugar.

Grain-Free, Gluten-Free, Dairy-Free, Suitable for Vegetarians, No Added Sugar

Serves 10

Ingredients

6 eggs

2 tbsp coconut manna or use coconut oil, softened

1 tsp vanilla extract

2 tsp ground cinnamon

40g/1½oz coconut flour

1 tbsp ground flaxseed

½ tsp bicarbonate of soda

1 tsp baking powder

30g/1oz desiccated coconut, plus a little for sprinkling

Method

- Preheat the oven to 180°C/350°F, gas mark 4.
- Whisk the eggs, coconut manna, vanilla and cinnamon in a blender.
- Add the coconut flour, flaxseed, bicarbonate and baking powder, and blend until smooth. Stir in the desiccated coconut.
- Pour into a 1lb loaf tin and sprinkle over a little more desiccated coconut. Bake for 30–40 minutes until light brown and cooked through. Allow to cool, then slice.

Nutritional information per slice

Calories	Protein	Carbohydrates	Total fat
116kcal	4.9g	3.2g of which sugars 0.4g	9.3g of which saturates 5.6g

TOMATO SEEDED CRACKERS

A high-protein cracker, grain-free and gluten-free. Perfect for snacks or as an accompaniment to soups and salads. These will keep well in an airtight container.

Grain-Free, Gluten-Free, Dairy-Free, Suitable for Vegetarians, No Added Sugar

Makes 20–24 crackers

Ingredients

225g/8oz cashew nuts

115g/4oz flaxseeds

50g/2oz shelled hemp seeds

50g/2oz sunflower seeds

30g/1oz natural protein powder (e.g. pea, hemp)

3 tbsp nutritional yeast flakes

1 tsp onion powder

1 tsp garlic salt

4 sundried tomatoes

3 tomatoes, chopped

Juice of ½ lemon

Method

- Soak the nuts in water for 1 hour and then drain. Place the nuts and seeds in a food processor and process until fine. Add the remaining ingredients and process to form a thick paste, adding water if necessary.

- Spread the batter onto 2–3 teflex-lined dehydrator sheets to form 3 squares. Score the batter into small cracker shapes. Dehydrate for 6 hours until dry. Flip the crackers onto mesh sheets and dehydrate until crispy for another 6 hours.
- Alternatively, to bake these crackers, preheat the oven to 150°C/300°F, gas mark 2. Spread the batter as above on separate trays and bake for 25–30 minutes until crisp.

Nutritional information per cracker

Calories	Protein	Carbohydrates	Total fat
119kcal	5.1g	4.5g of which sugars 0.9g	9.1g of which saturates 1.3g

MAIN MEALS
MEAT
SLOW COOKED ZA'ATAR LAMB SHOULDER

Za'atar is a Middle Eastern herb-and-spice mix consisting mainly of dried oregano, salt and sesame seeds. It's great as a marinade for lamb. This slow-cooked, melt-in-the-mouth meat needs 5 hours in the oven but very little preparation.

Grain-Free, Gluten-Free, Dairy-Free, Nut-Free, No Added Sugar

Serves 8

Ingredients

3 tbsp za'atar

1 tbsp sumac

4 tbsp olive oil

2kg/4½lb shoulder of lamb

Sea salt and freshly ground black pepper

2 onions, sliced

6 garlic cloves, peeled but left whole

300ml/10fl oz chicken stock

Handful of mint, chopped

1 tbsp red wine vinegar

Method

- Combine the za'atar, sumac and oil, and mix to a paste. Rub all over the lamb and marinate overnight in the fridge if possible.
- Preheat the oven to 150°C/300°F, gas mark 2. Lay the onions and garlic in a roasting tray. Season with salt and pepper. Cook until you can pull the meat apart easily with two forks.

- ▶ Remove the lamb from the oven and place it on a chopping board. Cover it with foil and leave it to rest.
- ▶ Pour away most of the fat from the roasting tray. Add the stock, stirring gently Simmer for a few minutes to reduce the liquid and then add the mint and vinegar. Serve with the lamb.

Nutritional information per serving

Calories	Protein	Carbohydrates	Total fat
532kcal	36.1g	1.6g of which sugars 0.8g	42.4g of which saturates 17.9g

MOROCCAN BEEF TAGINE

A comforting, warming dish, the beef steak is cooked gently and slowly with a range of antioxidant-rich vegetables, nuts and dried fruit to create a complete meal in a bowl.

Grain-Free, Gluten-Free, Dairy-Free, No Added Sugar

Serves 4

....

Ingredients

500g/1lb braising steak cut into thick slices

1 tbsp ras el hanout spice mix

1 tbsp ground cumin

1 tsp ground coriander (cilantro)

1 tsp ground cinnamon

Sea salt and freshly ground black pepper

2 tbsp olive oil

1 onion, finely sliced

1 garlic clove, crushed

2cm piece ginger, grated

1 x 400g/14oz can chickpeas drained

1 x 400g/14oz can chopped tomatoes

500ml/1 pint vegetable stock

1 small butternut squash, cut into cubes

150g/5oz ready-to-eat prunes

1 tbsp pomegranate molasses

2 tbsp flaked almonds

Handful of coriander (cilantro), chopped

....

Method

- ▶ Place the beef in a bowl. Add the spices, seasoning and olive oil and massage into the meat. Leave for several hours to marinate.
- ▶ Heat a little more oil in a large casserole and fry the beef. (For an even healthier option, you can skip this 'browning' stage.) Add the onion,

garlic and ginger, and sauté for 5 minutes. Tip in the chickpeas and tomatoes, then pour in the stock and stir. Bring to the boil, then put the lid on the pan and reduce to a simmer for 1 hour.

▶ Add the butternut squash and prunes, and simmer on a very low heat for another hour. Stir in the pomegranate molasses and scatter over the almonds and coriander.

Nutritional information per serving

Calories	Protein	Carbohydrates	Total fat
417kcal	38.5g	2.4g of which sugars 21g	16.8g of which saturates 3g

KOREAN SPICED VENISON

Venison is a good source of B vitamins, including B12, and the minerals iron, selenium, zinc and copper. Wild venison is particularly high in protein and low in fat, making it especially energizing. This lightly spiced dish full of Korean flavours is delicious served with pickled vegetables and a large leafy green salad. Beef could be used if venison is not available.

Grain-Free, Gluten-Free, Dairy-Free, Nut-Free

Serves 4

....

Ingredients

400g/14oz loin venison cut into thick slices

Vegetable pickles and a leafy green salad, to serve

Marinade

75ml/3fl oz mirin

3 tbsp tamari

1 tsp coconut sugar or xylitol

2 garlic cloves, crushed

Pinch of chilli flakes

1 tbsp sesame salt

2cm piece of grated root ginger

4 spring onions (scallions), chopped

....

Method

▶ Mix all the marinade ingredients together. Pour over the venison and refrigerate for 2 hours or overnight.

▶ Preheat the oven to 200°C/400°F, gas mark 6.

- Heat a large, heavy-based frying pan. Add the venison and sear on each side for a couple of minutes. Put the venison in a roasting tin and place in the preheated oven for about 10–12 minutes for rare meat, a bit longer for medium-rare or medium. Remove from the oven and allow to rest for ten minutes. This will ensure moist meat before slicing.
- Serve with raw cauliflower pickles and a leafy green salad.

Nutritional information per serving

Calories	Protein	Carbohydrates	Total fat
125kcal	22.7g	2.5g of which sugars 2.2g	1.7g of which saturates 0.8g

SAFFRON CHICKEN SKEWERS WITH CHIMMICHURI SAUCE

This punchy, smoky-flavoured sauce makes a wonderful marinade for chicken and turkey. Prepare ahead and keep the sauce chilled for up to 2–3 days.

Grain-Free, Gluten-Free, Dairy-Free, Nut-Free, No Added Sugar

Serves 4

....

Ingredients

Pinch of saffron, infused in 1 tbsp boiling water

Pinch of ground cumin

1 garlic clove, crushed

1 tbsp red wine vinegar

2 tbsp olive oil

3 skinless chicken breasts, cut into cubes

1 red pepper, cut into chunks

Chimmichuri sauce

1 green chilli, deseeded and chopped

2 garlic cloves, crushed

Bunch of coriander (cilantro), chopped

Bunch of parsley, chopped

½ tsp smoked paprika

100ml/4fl oz olive oil

3 tbsp red wine vinegar

Sea salt and freshly ground black pepper

....

Method

- Combine the saffron, cumin, garlic, vinegar and 1 tbsp of the olive oil in a bowl. Add the chicken and coat all over. Leave to marinate in the fridge for 1 hour. Thread the chicken and pepper onto skewers.

- ▸ To make the sauce, place all the ingredients in a food processor and pulse to combine. This can be kept in the fridge for 1 day.
- ▸ Preheat the grill. Place the chicken and pepper skewers on a baking sheet and grill for 5–8 minutes until golden and cooked through. Serve with the chimmichuri sauce.

Nutritional information per serving (with 2 tbsp sauce)

Calories	Protein	Carbohydrates	Total fat
335kcal	24.7g	3g of which sugars 2.5g	24.6g of which saturates 3.7g

MISO GINGER BAKED CHICKEN

A Japanese-inspired dish. Miso is deliciously savoury and comforting, and has an intensely rich flavour that makes an ideal marinade for chicken. Miso is a form of fermented soy, packed with antioxidants and a useful source of vitamin K for bone and cardiovascular health.

Grain-Free, Gluten-Free, Dairy-Free

Serves 4

....

Ingredients

8 small chicken thighs, boned and with skin left on

75g/3oz white miso paste

2 tbsp root ginger, finely grated

4 tbsp mirin

6 tbsp apple cider vinegar

8 shallots, peeled and halved

1 tbsp olive oil

200ml/7fl oz chicken stock

100g/3½oz walnuts, broken

1½ tbsp maple syrup

1 tbsp chopped tarragon

....

Method

- ▸ Place the chicken in a large bowl. Stir together the miso, ginger, mirin and vinegar, and pour the mixture over the chicken. Coat thoroughly. Cover and leave in the fridge to marinate, ideally overnight.
- ▸ Preheat the oven to 200°C/400°F, gas mark 6.
- ▸ Place the shallots in a baking dish and drizzle with oil. Place the chicken on top of the shallots with the marinade. Pour over the stock.

- Bake in the oven for 30 minutes until cooked. Remove the chicken and shallots from the pan. Pour the cooking juices into a pan with the walnuts and maple syrup and simmer for a couple of minutes.
- Serve the chicken with the sauce spooned on top and the tarragon scattered over.

Nutritional information per serving

Calories	Protein	Carbohydrates	Total fat
450kcal	32.7g	9.6g of which sugars 5g	29.4g of which saturates 4.6g

LEMON HARISSA TURKEY LEAF WRAPS

Lettuce leaves are ideal for making low-carb wraps. These are delicious with the dipping sauce.

Grain-Free, Gluten-Free, Dairy-Free, Nut-Free

Serves 4

Ingredients

400g/14oz turkey mince

1 egg yolk

1 preserved lemon, chopped

2 tsp harissa paste

1 tsp ground cumin

Handful of coriander (cilantro) leaves

Sea salt and freshly ground black pepper

Little gem lettuce leaves, to serve

Easy dipping sauce

2 tbsp Chinese rice vinegar

2 tsp maple syrup or honey

Splash of fish sauce

Squeeze of lime juice

Grated ginger

Method

- Preheat the oven to 180°C/350°F, gas mark 4. Place the mince, egg, preserved lemon, harissa paste, cumin, coriander and seasoning in a food processor and blend to a chunky paste. Shape into patties or little balls.
- Place on a non-stick baking tray, brush with oil and cook for 20 minutes until golden and cooked through.

- ▸ Mix together the ingredients for the dipping sauce.
- ▸ Serve the patties in the lettuce leaves with the dipping sauce.

Nutritional information per serving

Calories	Protein	Carbohydrates	Total fat
208kcal	29.5g	3.3g of which sugars 3.2g	8.3g of which saturates 2.4g

GRAIN-FREE PIZZA

A good all-round low-carb pizza, grain- and gluten-free. Choose a range of toppings according to taste.

Grain-Free, Gluten-Free, Suitable for Vegetarians, No Added Sugar
Serves 6

....

Ingredients

1 aubergine (eggplant), skin removed

1 egg

40g/1½oz ground flaxseed

40g/1½oz almond flour

1 tbsp olive oil

Sea salt and pepper

1 tbsp nutritional yeast flakes

½ tsp onion powder

Olive oil for greasing

Selection of toppings to taste (e.g. passata, olives, artichoke hearts, mushrooms, cooked chicken or beef, mozzarella cheese)

....

Method

- ▸ Preheat the oven to 190°C/375°F, gas mark 5.
- ▸ Grate the aubergine. Place in a bowl with the egg, flaxseed, almond flour and oil. Season well and add the nutritional yeast flakes and onion powder. Mix thoroughly, adding a little more oil if needed to create a soft dough.
- ▸ Grease a baking sheet and line with baking parchment. Spread the dough into a thin circle.
- ▸ Bake in the oven for 20–25 minutes until crisp.
- ▸ Flip over and brush with a little olive oil, then cook for a further 10 minutes.
- ▸ Spoon over the toppings and return to the oven for 10–15 minutes.

Nutritional information per serving (with cheese, mushrooms, artichokes, tomatoes and olives)

Calories	Protein	Carbohydrates	Total fat
172kcal	8g	4.8g of which sugars 1.7g	13.7g of which saturates 3.5g

MACADAMIA DUKKAH-CRUSTED SEA BASS WITH GREEN BEANS AND ROCKET

Dukkah is a traditional Egyptian condiment. Here it is used to coat salmon fillets to create a dinner dish rich in protein and anti-inflammatory omega 3 fats. The pomegranate molasses create a tangy sweet-and-sour dressing that is equally delicious drizzled over meats.

Grain-Free, Gluten-Free, Dairy-Free

Serves 4

Ingredients

4 sea bass fillets, boneless, skin on

1 tsp coconut oil

Dukkah

50g/2oz hazelnuts, blanched

50g/2oz Macadamia nuts

1 tbsp cumin seeds

2 tbsp coriander (cilantro) seeds

250g/9oz green beans

200g/7oz bag of rocket (arugula) leaves

2 tbsp onion seeds

2 tbsp sesame seeds

2 tbsp desiccated coconut

Sea salt and freshly ground black pepper

Dressing

3 tbsp pomegranate molasses

1 tbsp lemon juice

1 garlic clove, crushed

Pinch of ground cumin

5 tbsp extra virgin olive oil

Method

▸ For the dukkah, heat a frying pan over a medium heat until hot. Add the nuts and toast for 1–2 minutes, or until pale golden-brown. Add the remaining dukkah ingredients and continue to toast, stirring constantly, for 1–2 minutes.

▸ Blend the mixture in a food processor to a coarse powder. Season, to taste, with salt and freshly ground black pepper and set aside.

- Mix together the dressing ingredients and set aside.
- Coat each fish fillet with dukkah on the skinless side and place on a plate. Heat the oil in a frying pan. Cook the fish, skin-side down for 3 minutes or until golden. Reduce the heat to medium, turn the fish over and cook for 5 minutes or until just cooked through. Keep warm.
- Blanch the green beans in boiling water for 2 minutes. Drain and toss with the rocket. Divide between four plates.
- Place the fish on each plate with a little of the dressing. Sprinkle over a little additional dukkah to serve.

Nutritional information per serving (with 1 tbsp dressing)

Calories	Protein	Carbohydrates	Total fat
462kcal	27.7g	9.6g of which sugars 7.4g	38.5g of which saturates 8.9g

BAKED HALIBUT WITH SPICED TOMATO RELISH

Halibut is a firm white fish with a delicate, sweet flavour. It is surprisingly rich in omega 3 fats and an excellent source of selenium, an important antioxidant mineral that is also required for thyroid function. The tomato relish is also delicious with egg dishes.

Grain-Free, Gluten-Free, Dairy-Free

Serves 4

....

Ingredients

4 halibut steaks
½ tsp ground coriander (cilantro)

Sea salt and freshly ground black pepper
Olive oil

Spiced Tomato Relish

1 tbsp olive oil
1 garlic clove, crushed
2 tsp fresh root ginger, grated
1 shallot, finely chopped
4 tbsp apple cider vinegar

1 x 400g/14oz can chopped tomatoes
Pinch of cinnamon
Pinch of ground cloves
2–3 tbsp xylitol

Method

- To make the relish, heat the oil in a pan and sauté the garlic and ginger for 1 minute. Add the remaining ingredients and bring the mixture to the boil. Simmer for 30 minutes until the mixture is thick and sticky. Stir it occasionally to prevent it burning. Allow to cool.

- Preheat oven to 220°C/425°F, gas mark 7. Lightly coat a baking sheet with olive oil. Season the halibut steaks all over with coriander, salt and freshly ground black pepper.

- Rub the halibut with plenty of olive oil and place skin-side down in a hot ovenproof pan over a medium heat. Cook the halibut for 3 minutes and then transfer to the oven to roast for 5 minutes. Remove from the oven, turn the halibut steaks over and return to the oven to roast for another 5 minutes, or until cooked through.

- Remove from the oven and place on warmed plates. Spoon over the relish to serve.

Nutritional information per serving

Calories	Protein	Carbohydrates	Total fat
170kcal	22.8g	11.5g of which sugars 10.6g	5.2g of which saturates 0.7g

TURMERIC GLAZED FISH WITH CUCUMBER PICKLE

Turmeric is widely used for its anti-inflammatory properties, and its active constituent curcumin shows great promise in the management of many age-related health problems (see Chapter 8). This is a simple Asian-style dish, great for when time is short. The pickle can be prepared in advance and kept in the fridge for a couple of days.

Grain-Free, Gluten-Free, Dairy-Free

Serves 4

Ingredients

2 tbsp olive oil

1 tsp turmeric

Pinch of coconut sugar or xylitol

Sea salt and freshly ground black pepper

4 firm white fish fillets

Cucumber Pickle

1 tbsp mirin

1 tbsp rice vinegar

1 tsp sesame oil

1 cucumber

Fresh coriander (cilantro) leaves, chopped

....

Method

▸ Mix together the oil, turmeric, sugar and seasoning in a bowl. Add the fish fillets and toss to coat. Marinate for 30 minutes.

▸ Whisk together the mirin, vinegar and oil. Use a potato peeler and peel long ribbons from the cucumber. Toss in the dressing along with the chopped coriander and set aside.

▸ Heat a little oil in a frying pan and add the fish. Cook on each side for 5–6 minutes until cooked through. Serve with the cucumber pickle.

Nutritional information per serving

Calories	Protein	Carbohydrates	Total fat
137kcal	18.8g	1.2g of which sugars 1.2g	6.1g of which saturates 0.9g

THAI SALMON FISHCAKES

A great prepare-ahead recipe, these fishcakes can also be frozen. Sweet potato is rich in antioxidant carotenoids and vitamin C. Salmon is a great source of anti-inflammatory omega 3 fats.

Gluten-Free, Dairy-Free, No Added Sugar

Makes 8 fishcakes

....

Ingredients

2 tbsp olive oil

2 shallots, finely chopped

1 red chilli, chopped

150g/5oz cooked salmon

175g/6oz mashed sweet potato

Pinch of cayenne pepper

Grated zest and juice of 1 lime

Sea salt and freshly ground black pepper

2 eggs, beaten

125g/4½oz breadcrumbs, gluten-free if needed, or oatmeal or polenta

Method

▶ Preheat the oven to 200°C/400°F, gas mark 6.

▶ Heat the oil in a pan and add the shallots, chilli, salmon and sweet potato, and stir for a couple of minutes. Mash the ingredients together with a wooden spoon, then add the cayenne pepper, the lime zest and juice, and season. Form into balls.

▶ Beat the eggs and pour onto a large plate. Place the breadcrumbs on another plate. Roll the balls in the egg, flatten slightly and then dip in the breadcrumbs.

▶ Place on a lined or greased baking tray and bake for 20–25 minutes until golden.

Nutritional information per fishcake

Calories	Protein	Carbohydrates	Total fat
151kcal	7.5g	17.1g of which sugars 3.6g	5.8g of which saturates 1g

PARCHMENT-BAKED FISH WITH TAMARIND AND LIME

Tamarind is rich in polysaccharides (a type of dietary fibre), shown to promote a healthy balance of bugs in the gut and help stabilize blood sugar levels. Easy to find now as a purée, it is a great addition to marinades for fish and meat.

Grain-Free, Gluten-Free, No Added Sugar, Nut-Free

Serves 4

Ingredients

1 tbsp butter	A few red onion slices
Grated zest of 1 lime	4 slices of fresh ginger root
2 tbsp lime juice	2 garlic cloves, sliced
4 sea bass fillets	8 dried curry leaves
2 tsp tamarind paste	2 tsp coriander (cilantro) seeds
Lime slices	Lime wedges and salad to serve

Method

▶ Preheat the oven to 180°C/350°F, gas mark 4.

▶ Mix together the butter and lime zest and juice.

- Place each fish fillet in the centre of a square piece of baking parchment. Smear the top of each fillet with the tamarind paste. Place the lime slices on the top and scatter over the onion, ginger, garlic, curry leaves and coriander seeds. Dot with the lime butter.
- Close up the parcels and scrunch up the edges to seal. Place on a baking tray and bake for 15 minutes until cooked through.
- Serve with lime wedges and salad.

Nutritional information per serving

Calories	Protein	Carbohydrates	Total fat
140kcal	19.7g	2.5g of which sugars 0.7g	5.7g of which saturates 2.4g

GRILLED MACKEREL WITH SWEET AND SOUR MUSHROOMS

The oily flesh of mackerel combines beautifully with the tangy balsamic-infused mushrooms. Mackerel's good levels of B vitamins and magnesium make it an energizing food. It is also an excellent source of omega 3 fats. Any leftover mushrooms can be served with salad or cold meats.

Grain-Free, Gluten-Free, Dairy-Free, Nut-Free

Serves 4

Ingredients

30g/1oz dried mushrooms

2 tbsp olive oil

1 onion, finely diced

1 tbsp rosemary, chopped

250ml/8fl oz balsamic vinegar

200ml/7fl oz chicken stock

1 tbsp redcurrant jelly

150g/5oz button mushrooms, sliced

4 mackerel fillets, skin on

Juice and zest of 1 lemon

Sea salt and freshly ground black pepper

Method

- Soak the dried mushrooms in boiling water and leave for 20 minutes. Strain and reserve the liquid. Roughly chop the mushrooms.

- Heat 1 tbsp of the oil in a frying pan and sauté the onion until soft. Add the rosemary, vinegar and stock, and bring to the boil. Simmer for 10 minutes until the liquid has reduced by half. Add the redcurrant jelly, the soaked mushrooms and the fresh button mushrooms. Simmer for 2–3 minutes until the mushrooms are soft. If the sauce becomes dry add a little of the reserved mushroom liquid.
- Score the skin on the mackerel fillets. Place on a baking sheet skin-side up. Season the mackerel well, squeeze a few drops of lemon juice and a sprinkling of zest over each fillet, and drizzle with the remaining olive oil. Place under the grill for 5–7 minutes until cooked through.
- Serve the mackerel fillets with the mushroom sauce.

Nutritional information per serving

Calories	Protein	Carbohydrates	Total fat
280kcal	20.8g	8.7g of which sugars 3.8g	16.6g of which saturates 3.4g

ASIAN CAULIFLOWER 'RICE' STIR FRY

A great alternative to rice: minced cauliflower! This makes a delicious low-carb stir fry – perfect for a speedy meal.

Grain-Free, Gluten-Free, Dairy-Free

Serves 4

. . . .

Ingredients

1 small head of cauliflower, separated into florets

20 large raw prawns

1 tbsp coconut oil

2 large eggs, beaten

1 small onion, finely chopped

1 garlic clove

1 piece of fresh root ginger, grated

100g/3½oz sliced shitake mushrooms

Handful of coriander (cilantro) leaves, chopped

1–2 tbsp of Braggs Aminos or tamari

2 tsp fish sauce to taste

2 tsp rice vinegar to taste

Handful of basil, chopped

Handful of mint, chopped

Marinade

1 tbsp chilli sauce   Juice of 1 lime

1 tsp honey or maple syrup

....

Method

▶ Place the cauliflower in a food processor and pulse until finely chopped.

▶ Place the prawns in a bowl. Mix together the marinade ingredients and pour over the prawns – leave for 1 hour.

▶ Heat a little oil in a frying pan and pour in the beaten egg to form an omelette. Remove from the pan and slice thinly.

▶ Add a little more coconut oil to the pan, then sauté the onion, garlic and ginger. Add the mushrooms and cauliflower and season. Place the lid on the pan and steam fry for 5 minutes. Once softened, add the Aminos or tamari, fish sauce, vinegar and herbs. Just before serving, add the prawns and egg.

Nutritional information per serving

Calories	Protein	Carbohydrates	Total fat
129kcal	10.6g	8.3g of which sugars 7.7g	5.9g of which saturates 2.9g

SEARED SCALLOPS WITH GREMOLATA

Gremolata is a wonderful mixture of finely chopped garlic, lemon zest and parsley – a great antioxidant and anti-inflammatory combination, which adds a fabulous flavour to the scallops.

Grain-Free, Gluten-Free, Dairy-Free, Nut-Free

Serves 4

....

Ingredients

Large handful of parsley, chopped

1 garlic clove, crushed

Zest of 1 lemon

16 scallops, cleaned and trimmed

Olive oil for cooking

200g/7oz cherry tomatoes, halved

Rocket (arugula) leaves or watercress, to serve

Dressing

Juice of 1 lemon

5 tbsp olive oil

1 tbsp honey or xylitol

Sea salt and freshly ground black pepper

....

Method

▸ Whisk together the lemon juice, olive oil and honey in a bowl and season.

▸ Mix the parsley, garlic and lemon zest in a separate bowl.

▸ Drizzle the scallops with a little olive oil and season with salt and pepper. Heat a griddle or frying pan and sear the scallops 1 minute on each side. Place the scallops in a bowl with the tomatoes. Pour over the dressing and toss. Spoon onto plates, then sprinkle over the parsley mixture.

▸ Serve with rocket leaves or watercress.

Nutritional information per serving

Calories	Protein	Carbohydrates	Total fat
153kcal	6.6g	6.4g of which sugars 5.3g	11.9g of which saturates 1.8g

CHILLI AND LIME SPICED SARDINES

A speedy recipe packed with protein and healthy omega 3 fats. Sardines are also a great source of B12, essential for energy and healthy nerve function.

Grain-Free, Gluten-Free, Dairy-Free, Nut-Free

Serves 4

....

Ingredients

8 x 60g/2½oz sardines, gills removed, scaled and gutted

1 tbsp harissa paste

1 clove garlic, finely chopped

1 tbsp olive oil

Juice of 2 limes

Sea salt and freshly ground black pepper

Bag of leafy green lettuce leaves, to serve

1 ripe avocado, sliced, to serve

Method

- Butterfly the sardines by removing the heads, trimming the fins and cutting open the fish from the belly to the tail. Open out the fish and place flesh-side down on a chopping board, pressing down firmly along the backbone with your fingers until the fish is flattened.
- Turn the fish over and carefully and slowly pull out the backbone, cutting it off at the tail end. Remove any small bones left behind.
- Mix together the harissa paste, garlic, olive oil and lime juice and season. Pour the mixture over the sardines and marinate for 15 minutes.
- Preheat the grill to high. Cook the sardines for about 3 minutes on each side until the flesh is opaque.
- Serve with the lettuce leaves and avocado.

Nutritional information per serving

Calories	Protein	Carbohydrates	Total fat
242kcal	21.5	1.5g of which sugars 1g	16.6g of which saturates 4.1g

VEGETARIAN
TEMPEH COCONUT CURRY

A deliciously creamy curry, lightly spiced and packed with an array of antioxidant vegetables. Tempeh is bland-tasting on its own but by marinating in the curry paste it takes on the delicious flavours of the spices.

Grain-Free, Gluten-Free, Dairy-Free, Suitable for Vegetarians

Serves 4

Ingredients

350g/12oz tempeh, cubed

4 tbsp tamari

Juice of 3 limes

2 tbsp coconut oil

400ml/14fl oz can coconut milk

2 courgettes (zucchini), chopped into chunks

1 small sweet potato, peeled and chopped into chunks

1 red pepper, deseeded and chopped into chunks

150g/5oz mangetout

1 tsp coconut sugar

Handful of coriander (cilantro) leaves, chopped

Paste

2 red chillies, deseeded and chopped	2cm piece of root ginger, grated
1 lemongrass, roughly chopped	2 garlic cloves
1 small onion, roughly chopped	A little water to blend
½ red pepper, deseeded and roughly chopped	Sea salt and freshly ground black pepper
Handful of coriander (cilantro) leaves	

Method

▶ Place all the paste ingredients in a food processor and process to form a thick paste.

▶ Place the tempeh in a bowl and pour over the tamari and lime juice. Marinate for 1 hour.

▶ Heat the oil in a large frying pan. Add the tempeh, reserving the marinade, and pan-fry until golden. Remove and set aside. Add 4 tbsp of the paste and fry for a couple of minutes. Stir in the coconut milk, courgette, sweet potato and pepper, and cook for 10 minutes until just tender. Add the mangetout, tempeh, coconut sugar and remaining marinade, and simmer for a couple of minutes. Garnish with coriander leaves and serve.

Nutritional information per serving

Calories	Protein	Carbohydrates	Total fat
299kcal	22.6g	27.1g of which sugars 16.3g	11.1g of which saturates 4.2g

QUINOA NUT BURGERS

These delicious vegan patties contain protein and healthy fats, thanks to the combination of quinoa and almonds. The nutritional yeast flakes provide B vitamins and they impart a wonderful nutty, cheesy flavour to the burgers.

Gluten-Free, Dairy-Free, Suitable for Vegetarians, No Added Sugar
Makes 8, serves 4

Ingredients

100g/3½oz dry quinoa

1 tsp bouillon powder

250ml/8fl oz water

250g/9oz almonds

1 clove garlic, chopped

1 tbsp balsamic vinegar

1 tbsp tamari

1 tbsp tomato paste

2 tbsp nutritional yeast flakes

Pinch of sea salt

1 onion, finely chopped

60g/2½oz sundried tomatoes, drained and chopped

1 tbsp coconut oil

Basic Mayonnaise or *Roasted Pepper Mayonnaise* (see recipes), to serve

Method

▶ Place the quinoa in a pan with the bouillon power and water. Bring to the boil. Put the lid on and turn the heat to a gentle simmer. Cook for 15 minutes. Turn off the heat and allow the quinoa to cool.

▶ In a food processor, process the almonds, garlic, vinegar, tamari, tomato paste, nutritional yeast flakes and salt. Purée until the nuts are very finely ground and becoming a little sticky. Add the onion and sundried tomatoes, and pulse together until the mixture starts to stick together. Add the quinoa and pulse again until incorporated.

▶ Shape the mixture into patties and chill for 30 minutes.

▶ Heat a little coconut oil in a frying pan and cook the patties in batches for about 5–6 minutes before turning over and cooking for a further 2–3 minutes until golden brown.

▶ Serve with salad and mayonnaise.

Nutritional information per burger

Calories	Protein	Carbohydrates	Total fat
284kcal	10.2g	10.9g of which sugars 3g	22.1g of which saturates 1.9g

ASPARAGUS AND COURGETTE SPAGHETTI WITH RED PEPPER MARINARA SAUCE

A light low-carbohydrate dish using strips of asparagus and courgette (zucchini) as 'pasta' and served with a rich, creamy pepper sauce.

Grain-Free, Gluten-Free, Dairy-Free, Suitable for Vegetarians, No Added Sugar

Serves 4

Ingredients

3 courgettes (zucchini)

1 bunch of asparagus

2 tbsp extra virgin olive oil

2 tbsp freshly squeezed lemon juice

Sea salt

1 tbsp tamari

4 dates

4 sundried tomatoes, drained

Handful of basil leaves, chopped, to serve

Marinara Sauce

60g/2½oz pine nuts

1 red pepper

1 tomato

2 tsp lemon juice

Method

▶ Using a swivel potato peeler, peel long thin strips from the courgettes and asparagus. Place in a bowl with the olive oil, lemon juice and salt. Cover and refrigerate for at least half an hour and up to 2 hours. The lemon juice will tenderize the asparagus.

▶ To make the sauce, simply place all the ingredients in a food processor and blend until smooth. Season to taste.

▶ Toss the sauce and vegetables together. Scatter over the basil leaves to serve.

Nutritional information per serving

Calories	Protein	Carbohydrates	Total fat
215kcal	5.5g	7.4g of which sugars 7.1g	18.1g of which saturates 1.8g

TOFU SKEWERS WITH ROMESCO SAUCE

Romesco sauce normally contains bread. This grain-free option is packed with protein and makes an ideal accompaniment to skewers of golden tofu.

Grain-Free, Gluten-Free, Dairy-Free, Suitable for Vegetarians, No Added Sugar

Serves 4

Ingredients

1 tsp ground cumin

2 tbsp extra virgin olive oil

Juice of 1 lemon

1 garlic clove, crushed

Romesco Sauce

2 roasted red peppers from a jar, drained

4 ripe vine tomatoes, chopped

3 tbsp extra virgin olive oil

30g/1oz hazelnuts

30g/1oz almonds

1 tsp onion powder

400g/14oz firm tofu, cut into cubes

Pinch of sea salt

Freshly ground black pepper

1 red pepper, cut into chunks

1 garlic clove

1 tsp smoked paprika

Pinch of cayenne pepper

1–2 tbsp red wine vinegar

Sea salt and freshly ground black pepper

Method

▸ Mix together the cumin, oil, lemon juice and garlic. Place the tofu in a bowl and pour over the marinade. Season. Cover and leave for 1 hour.

▸ Place all the ingredients for the sauce in a food processor and process until smooth.

▸ Thread the tofu and red pepper pieces onto skewers. Brush with the remaining marinade. Place on a baking tray and grill for about 6 minutes, turning during cooking until golden. Serve with the Romesco sauce.

Nutritional information per serving

Calories	Protein	Carbohydrates	Total fat
325kcal	12.9g	11.6g of which sugars 10.4g	25.3g of which saturates 3g

CARROT RIBBON NOODLES WITH ALMOND SATAY SAUCE

This recipe uses almond nut butter to make a creamy sauce, which is gently tossed into strips of carrots. You can use a potato peeler or spiralizer to create carrot noodles. Alternatively, kelp noodles could be used.

Grain-Free, Gluten-Free, Dairy-Free, Suitable for Vegetarians, No Added Sugar

Serves 4

Ingredients

4–5 carrots, spiralized

1 red pepper, cut into thin strips

Large handful of baby spinach

Handful of coriander (cilantro), chopped

Handful of mint, chopped

Handful of parsley, chopped

2 spring onions (scallions), finely chopped (optional)

2 tbsp sesame seeds

Almond Satay Sauce

60g/2½oz almond nut butter

1 tbsp maple syrup

1 tbsp rice vinegar

1 garlic clove, crushed

½ tsp ground cumin

3 tbsp tamari

1 tsp grated ginger

2 tbsp coconut cream

2–3 tbsp water

Sea salt to taste

Method

▶ Blend all the sauce ingredients together and add enough water to make a thick sauce.

▶ In a large bowl, combine the rest of the ingredients, except the onion and seeds. Add the almond sauce and toss to coat. Garnish with spring onion and sesame seeds just before serving.

Nutritional information per serving

Calories	Protein	Carbohydrates	Total fat
245kcal	6.2g	17.8g of which sugars 15.5g	17.5g of which saturates 4.1g

MEDITERRANEAN TARTS WITH GOAT'S CHEESE

A simple Mediterranean-style tart using almond flour for the pastry base. Warm or cold, these are delicious with a colourful leafy salad.

Grain-Free, Gluten-Free, Suitable for Vegetarians

Serves 4

Ingredients

180g/6oz almond flour

1 tbsp ground chia seeds

Pinch of sea salt

1 tbsp finely chopped fresh rosemary

2–3 tbsp butter or coconut oil melted

Water to bind as needed

Colourful salad leaves, to serve

Filling

1 tbsp olive oil	1 tsp thyme, chopped
1 garlic clove, crushed	2 tsp balsamic vinegar
½ small red onion, finely chopped	1 tbsp xylitol
12 cherry tomatoes, halved	4 slices of goat's cheese

Method

▸ Preheat the oven to 180°C/350°F, gas mark 4.

▸ In a food processor combine the almond flour, chia seeds, salt and rosemary. Pulse in the butter or oil and add a little water if needed to combine. Line four mini tartlet tins with circles of baking parchment. Press in the dough to form the tart shells.

▸ Bake for 15–20 minutes, until lightly brown.

▸ To make the filling, heat the oil in a frying pan and sauté the garlic and onion gently for 5 minutes to soften. Add the tomatoes, thyme, vinegar and xylitol, and cook for a further 5 minutes to caramelize the tomatoes.

▸ Spoon the tomatoes into the centre of the tarts. Top with a slice of cheese.

▸ Turn the oven up to 200°C/400°F, gas mark 6. Bake for 10 minutes until the cheese is soft. Serve with a colourful salad.

Nutritional information per tart

Calories	Protein	Carbohydrates	Total fat
368kcal	12g	9.2g of which sugars 6.1g	32.2g of which saturates 8.4g

SWISS CHARD SAUTÉ

Swiss chard and kale are 'super greens', packed with plenty of vitamins, minerals and antioxidants. Serve this dish with some protein, such as scrambled egg, tofu or crumbled feta cheese.

Grain-Free, Gluten-Free, Dairy-Free, Suitable for Vegetarians

Serves 4

Ingredients

2 tbsp olive oil

1 red onion, cut in half and then sliced

Pinch of sea salt

1 garlic clove, crushed

60g/2½oz raisins

A little water for cooking

400g/14oz Swiss chard or kale, stems removed and cut into small pieces

2 tsp maple syrup

1 tsp lemon juice

Freshly ground black pepper

60g/2½oz toasted pine nuts

Method

▸ In a large sauté pan heat the oil and add the onion and salt. Sauté for 10 minutes to caramelize the onion.

▸ Add the garlic and raisins and stir well. Add a splash of water and the Swiss chard and a little more salt. Stir well until the greens wilt, about 2–3 minutes.

▸ Add the maple syrup and lemon juice and season to taste. Toss in the pine nuts to serve.

Nutritional information per serving

Calories	Protein	Carbohydrates	Total fat
230kcal	6.1g	14.3g of which sugars 14g	16.5g of which saturates 1.5g

DESSERTS AND SWEET TREATS
FRUIT PARFAIT

An easy-to-assemble fruity treat which is also delicious for breakfast. Vary the fruit according to the season. You can prepare this in advance and keep chilled in the fridge until needed.

Grain-Free, Gluten-Free, Dairy-Free, Suitable for Vegetarians

Serves 6

Ingredients

60g/2½oz walnuts

1 tbsp flaxseed

1 tbsp chia seeds

60g/2½oz almonds

100g/3½oz dates, chopped

1 tsp cinnamon

100g/3½oz strawberries, sliced

100g/3½oz raspberries

100g/3½oz blueberries

Nut Yogurt (see recipe)

Method

▸ Place the nuts and seeds in a food processor and process to form chunky crumbs. Add the dates and cinnamon and process to combine.

▸ Mix all the berries together. Spoon the berries into 6 glasses, top with a little yogurt and then a spoonful of the nut mixture. Repeat the layers, finishing with the nuts. Chill until required.

Nutritional information per serving

Calories	Protein	Carbohydrates	Total fat
340kcal	9.2g	21.1g of which sugars 16.7g	24.5g of which saturates 3.4g

CHOCOLATE LIME MOUSSE

This rich and creamy chocolate mousse is packed with healthy monounsaturated fats, potassium and B vitamins, thanks to the addition of avocado. Rich in antioxidants too, this is a delicious heart-healthy dessert

Grain-Free, Gluten-Free, Dairy-Free, Suitable for Vegetarians

Serves 4

Ingredients

Juice of 2 limes

40g/1½oz raw cacao powder

2 ripe avocados, pitted and peeled

100g/3½oz soft pitted dried dates

2–3 tbsp honey

2 tbsp melted coconut butter

Method

▸ Place all the ingredients in a food processor and blend until smooth. Sweeten with a little more honey if needed. This will firm up slightly if it is chilled for 1 hour before serving.

Nutritional information per serving

Calories	Protein	Carbohydrates	Total fat
279kcal	3.5g	31.8g of which sugars 25.4g	15.1g of which saturates 6.5g

LEMON AND PASSIONFRUIT KEFIR PANNA COTTA

Kefir has a wonderful tangy, sour taste, which complements the sweetness of the passionfruit. A great way to increase your intake of beneficial bacteria.

Serves 4

Grain-Free, Gluten-Free, Suitable for Vegetarians

....

Ingredients

8 passionfruit

2 tbsp agar agar flakes

Juice and zest of 2 lemons

500ml/1 pint *Kefir* (see recipe); milk or coconut

1 tbsp vanilla extract

2 tbsp honey or maple syrup

....

Method

▸ Scoop out the flesh from the passionfruit and pass through a sieve into a bowl. Reserve 1 tbsp of the seeds from the sieve.

▸ Place the agar agar flakes in the lemon juice and heat to dissolve completely. Place the kefir, vanilla, honey, lemon zest, half of the passionfruit juice and agar mixture in a blender and blend for 3–5 minutes. Pour into moulds and refrigerate until set, about 2–3 hours.

▸ Mix the reserved passionfruit seeds into the remaining juice.

▸ Dip each mould into a bowl of hot water, loosen the edges and turn each panna cotta out onto a plate. Spoon over the passionfruit seeds and juice to serve.

Nutritional information per serving

Calories	Protein	Carbohydrates	Total fat
131kcal	5g	17.4g of which sugars 17.4g	5g of which saturates 3g

CARAMEL PEAR TART WITH CHOCOLATE DRIZZLE

A sensational grain-free tart filled with soft pears and a sweet nutty caramel sauce. This is also delicious served as a frozen dessert.

Grain-Free, Gluten-Free, Dairy-Free, Suitable for Vegetarians

Serves 8

Ingredients

2 ripe pears, peeled and thinly sliced

Crust

250g/9oz almonds, ground until fine

100g/3½oz soft dates

Caramel Filling

60g/2½oz Macadamia nuts, soaked for 1 hour

75g/3oz dates, pitted, soaked for 30 minutes

4–6 tbsp *Classic Almond Milk* (see recipe) or coconut milk

150g/5oz melted chocolate for drizzling

1 tsp vanilla extract

Pinch of sea salt

2 tbsp maple syrup

1 tbsp vanilla extract

½ tsp ground cinnamon

½ tsp sea salt

Method

▸ To make the crust, combine the almond, dates, vanilla and salt in a food processor and pulse until well combined.

▸ Press the mixture into a 20cm/8-inch springform cake tin or loose-bottom tart tin, pressing down firmly. Place the crust in the refrigerator while you make the filling.

▸ For the filling, drain and rinse the nuts and dates. In a food processor or high-powered blender, combine all the ingredients, adding enough almond or coconut milk to create a smooth, thick sauce.

▸ Spoon the caramel sauce into the tin. Place the pears in a shallow bowl. Arrange the pears over the caramel and drizzle over the chocolate.

Nutritional information per serving

Calories	Protein	Carbohydrates	Total fat
429kcal	9g	33.4g of which sugars 33g	28.6g of which saturates 5.4g

TROPICAL GOJI SORBET

An antioxidant-packed sorbet making use of superfood powders and fruits. The water kefir provides plenty of probiotics, but if you don't have this, use coconut water instead. Baobab is an African fruit, rich in antioxidants.

Grain-Free, Gluten-Free, Dairy-Free, Suitable for Vegetarians

Serves 6

....

Ingredients

60g/2½oz goji berries

Juice of 4 passionfruits

2 ripe mangos, cut into chunks

2 peaches, chopped

2 tsp superfood berry powder or acai berry powder

2 tsp baobab powder

¼ tsp guar gum or xanthum gum

100ml/4fl oz *Water Kefir* (see recipe) or coconut water

....

Method

▶ Soak the goji berries in the passion fruit juice to soften for 30 minutes. Put in a blender with the rest of the ingredients and blend until smooth.

▶ Pour into an ice cream maker and churn according to the manufacturer's instructions. Alternatively, pour into a shallow container and freeze for 2 hours. Then process again in a food processor or blender to prevent ice crystals forming. Return to the freezer and freeze until firm. Take out of the freezer 20 minutes before serving.

Nutritional information per serving

Calories	Protein	Carbohydrates	Total fat
104kcal	1.3g	19g of which sugars 16.3g	2.4g of which saturates 0.1g

ROASTED BANANA, CARAMEL KEFIR ICE CREAM

A delicious, rich and creamy ice cream. Roasting the bananas in their skins intensifies their sweet flavour. For an extra special treat, drizzle over a little melted dark chocolate to serve.

Grain-Free, Gluten-Free, Suitable for Vegetarians

Serves 8

Ingredients

3 bananas	1 tbsp vanilla extract
250ml/8fl oz coconut milk	2 tbsp coconut oil
125g/4½oz dates	Sea salt to taste
4 tbsp almond nut butter	500ml/1 pint *Kefir* (see recipe)
4 tbsp honey or maple syrup	1 tbsp coconut sugar or xylitol
2 tbsp lucuma powder	60g/2½oz toasted almonds, roughly chopped

Method

▸ Roast the bananas in the oven at 180°C/350°F, gas mark 4 with their skins on for 20 minutes until blackened. Allow to cool, then peel.

▸ To make the caramel, place the coconut milk, dates, nut butter, honey, lucuma, vanilla, coconut oil and salt in a food processor and blend until smooth and creamy. Set aside.

▸ Place the kefir, coconut sugar and bananas in a blender and purée. Churn in an ice cream maker. As it begins to harden, stir in the caramel and chopped toasted nuts. Freeze until required. Allow to soften in the fridge for 20 minute before serving.

Nutritional information per serving

Calories	Protein	Carbohydrates	Total fat
288kcal	6.1g	35.7g of which sugars 33.1g	14g of which saturates 4.3g

DANDELION ROOT 'MOCHA' ICE CREAM

Dandelion root is a great liver and digestive support. Dandelion coffee provides a caffeine-free alternative and adds a richness to this ice cream. Maca helps nourish and strengthen the adrenal glands, while the glutamine and probiotics support digestive health.

Grain-Free, Gluten-Free, Dairy-Free, Suitable for Vegetarians

Serves 8

Ingredients

125g/4½oz almonds

750ml/1½ pints water

180g/6oz cashews

45g/1½oz unsweetened shredded/ desiccated coconut

60g/2½oz dates

75g/3oz maple syrup, honey or coconut nectar

1 tbsp vanilla extract

1 tbsp maca root powder

2 tbsp dandelion root coffee granules

2 tbsp lemon juice

60g/2½oz coconut oil, melted

3 tbsp raw cacao powder

1 tsp probiotic powder (such as *Lactobacillus*)

1 tbsp glutamine powder

1 tbsp lecithin granules

Pinch of salt

Method

▶ Blend all the ingredients in a high-speed blender until smooth.

▶ Pour into an ice cream maker and freeze according to the manufacturer's instructions. Alternatively, place in a shallow freezer-proof container and freeze until firm. For a smoother texture, place back in the food processor and blend to remove any crystals, and then refreeze.

▶ Remove from the freezer 20 minutes before serving to allow it to soften slightly.

Nutritional information per serving

Calories	Protein	Carbohydrates	Total fat
402kcal	10.7g	22.7g of which sugars 13.5g	29.6g of which saturates 11.4g

SUPER GREENS MINT CHOCOLATE CHIP ICE CREAM

An easy way to cram in some extra greens into your diet. Use chocolate chips or grated chocolate to provide some texture to the ice cream.

Grain-Free, Gluten-Free, Dairy-Free, Suitable for Vegetarians

Serves 6

Ingredients

125g/4½oz cashew nuts, soaked in water for 2 hours and then drained

250ml/8fl oz coconut water

2 tsp super green food powder

1 tsp probiotics

1 tsp colostrum powder or glutamine powder

1 tbsp vanilla extract

60g/2½oz unsweetened coconut flakes

60g/2½oz maple syrup or honey

60g/2½oz coconut butter

Dash peppermint extract

Pinch of sea salt

30g/1oz dark chocolate chips, dairy-free if needed

Method

▶ Put the nuts and coconut water in the blender and process until smooth. Add all the other ingredients, except the chocolate chips, and blend.

▶ Pour the mixture into an ice cream maker and churn, adding in the chocolate chips. Then freeze to harden. Allow to stand at room temperature for 10–15 minutes before serving.

Nutritional information per serving

Calories	Protein	Carbohydrates	Total fat
337kcal	5.8g	15.9g of which sugars 11.8g	27.8g of which saturates 16.8g

RICH CHOCOLATE CAKE

A rich, grain-free chocolate cake that is ideal for birthdays or as a special treat. Serve plain or top with the creamy dairy-free icing.

Grain-Free, Gluten-Free, Dairy-Free, Suitable for Vegetarians

Serves 10

Ingredients

60g/2½oz coconut flour

25g/1oz cocoa powder

½ tsp sea salt

tsp bicarbonate of soda

Zest of 1 orange (optional)

5 eggs

125ml/4fl oz light olive oil

75g/3oz xylitol

60g/2½oz honey

2 tsp vanilla extract

Chocolate icing (optional)

45g/1½oz raw cacao powder

60g/2½oz coconut butter

75g/3oz maple syrup, honey or coconut nectar

1 tsp vanilla

....

Method

▸ Preheat the oven to 180°C/350°F, gas mark 4.

▸ In a food processor combine the flour, cocoa, salt and bicarbonate of soda and orange zest if using.

▸ Using a hand-held whisk or blender, beat together the eggs, oil, xylitol, honey and vanilla. Gradually add to the dry ingredients and continue to blend in the processor until smooth.

▸ Lightly grease 20cm/8-inch spring-form cake tin.

▸ Pour the batter into the cake tin and bake for 35–40 minutes.

▸ Remove from the oven and allow to cool completely before removing from the tin.

▸ To make the icing, simply blend all the ingredients together. Spread over the top of the cooled cake.

Nutritional information per serving (without icing)

Calories	Protein	Carbohydrates	Total fat
220kcal	4.5g	15.5g of which sugars 11.5g	16.7g of which saturates 3.7g

SUPERFOOD FUDGE

This is a delicious creamy fudge which contains protein and superfoods to energize the body. This can be frozen and cut into bite-size pieces, providing a fabulous sweet treat whenever you fancy one. Tocotrienols powder is a concentrated source of bioavailable vitamin E, an important antioxidant to protect brain function and maintain cell integrity. It has a mild, sweet flavour and is a great addition to smoothies, chocolates and desserts. As it is sensitive to heat, do not cook with it.

Grain-Free, Gluten-Free, Dairy-Free, Suitable for Vegetarians

Makes 20 pieces

Ingredients

60g/2½oz cashew nut butter

150g/5oz cacao butter, melted

½ tsp vanilla

4 tbsp honey or coconut nectar

60g/2½oz xylitol or coconut sugar

3 tbsp lucuma powder

2 tsp baobab powder

1 tbsp collagen powder

1 tbsp tocotrienols powder

1 tsp acai powder

Pinch of sea salt

225g/8oz almonds

100g/3½oz coconut flour

Method

▸ Place the cashew nut butter, cacao butter, vanilla, honey and xylitol in a blender and process until smooth.

▸ Place the remaining ingredients in a food processor and process until fine. Then add the wet ingredients and process to combine. Transfer the batter into a lined, greased 20cm/8-inch square tin. Freeze for 30 minutes, then transfer to the fridge. Cut into squares to serve.

Nutritional information per serving

Calories	Protein	Carbohydrates	Total fat
177kcal	4.5g	12.4g of which sugars 7.2g	12.8g of which saturates 3.5g

ALMOND CHOCOLATE CHIP COOKIES

A simple, delicious grain-free cookie which includes protein and healthy fats to help stabilize blood sugar levels. Almonds are a great source of calcium, phosphorous and magnesium for bone health.

Grain-Free, Gluten-Free, Soy-Free, Dairy-Free

Makes 12

Ingredients

60g/2½oz almond nut butter

60g/2½oz xylitol

125ml/4fl oz *Classic Almond Milk* (see recipe) or coconut milk

1 tbsp vanilla extract

2 tbsp honey or yacon syrup

2 tbsp raw cacao powder

60g/2½oz coconut flour

30g/1oz almonds, ground until fine

Pinch of sea salt

60g/2½oz chocolate chips or raw cacao nibs

Method

▶ Preheat the oven to 180°C/350°F, gas mark 4.

▶ Place the nut butter, xylitol, milk, vanilla and honey in a food processor and blend until smooth. Add the cacao powder, coconut flour, almonds and sea salt and process to form a sticky dough. Pulse in the chocolate chips.

▶ Roll the dough into small balls, then press onto a lined baking tray and shape into circles. Bake in the oven for 10 minutes until golden. Allow to cool for 5 minutes before transferring to a cooling rack.

Nutritional information per cookie

Calories	Protein	Carbohydrates	Total fat
131kcal	2.8g	16.5g of which sugars 11.3g	7g of which saturates 2.1g

REFERENCES

CHAPTER 1

1. Carey, N. (2012) *The Epigenetics Revolution*. Australia: Allen and Unwin.
2. Ribarič, S. (2012) 'Diet and aging.' *Oxidative Medicine and Cell Longevity*. Epub, 13 August 2012.
   Martin, S.L., Hardy, T.M. and Tollefsbol, T.O. (2013) 'Medicinal chemistry of the epigenetic diet and caloric restriction.' *Current Medicinal Chemistry 20*, 32, 4050–9.
3. Li, Y., Daniel, M. and Tollefsbol, T.O. (2011) 'Epigenetic regulation of caloric restriction in ageing.' *BMC Medicine 9*, 98. Available at www.biomedcentral.com/1741-7015/9/98, accessed on 14 January 2014.
   Cava, E. and Fontana, L. (2013) 'Will calorie restriction work in humans?' *Aging 5*, 7, 507–14.
4. Ribarič 2012.
   Rochon, J., Bales, C.W., Ravussin, E., Redman, L.M. *et al.* (2011) 'Design and conduct of the CALERIE study: comprehensive assessment of the long-term effects of reducing intake of energy.' *Journal of Gerontology 66*, 1, 97–108.
   Meydani, M., Das, S., Band, M., Epstein, S. and Roberts, S. (2011) 'The effect of caloric restriction and glycemic load on measures of oxidative stress and antioxidants in humans: results from the CALERIE Trial of Human Caloric Restriction.' *Journal of Nutrition, Health and Aging 15*, 6, 456–60.
5. Martin, S.L., Hardy, T.M. and Tollefsbol, T.O. (2013) 'Medicinal chemistry of the epigenetic diet and caloric restriction.' *Current Medicinal Chemistry 20*, 32, 4050–9.
   Ribaric 2012.
6. Teiten, M.H., Dicato, M. and Diederich, M. (2013) 'Curcumin as a regulator of epigenetic events.' *Molecular Nutrition and Food Research 57*, 9, 1619–29.
7. Schramm, L. (2013) 'Going green: The role of the green tea component EGCG in chemoprevention.' *Journal of Carciogenesis and Mutagenesis 4*, 142, 1000142.
8. Gerhauser, C. (2013) 'Epigenetic impact of dietary isothiocyanates in cancer chemoprevention.' *Current Opinion in Clinical Nutrition and Metabolic Care 16*, 4, 405–10.
9. Ribarič 2012.
   Gerhauser. C. (2013) 'Cancer chemoprevention and nutri-epigenetics: state of the art and future challenges.' *Topics in Current Chemistry 329*, 73–132.
   Kelly, G. (2010) 'A review of the sirtuin system, its clinical implication and the potential role of dietary activators like resveratrol. Part 1.' *Alternative Medicine Review 15*, 3, 245–63.
   Kelly, G. (2010) 'A review of the sirtuin system, its clinical implication and the potential role of dietary activators like resveratrol. Part 2.' *Alternative Medicine Review 15*, 4, 313–28.
10. Carey 2012; Ribarič 2012.
11. Egger, G. (2012) 'In search of a germ theory equivalent for chronic disease.' *Preventing Chronic Disease*, Epub 10 May 2012.
12. Zhang, X., Lin, S., Funk, W.E. and Hou, L. (2013) 'Environmental and occupational exposure to chemicals and telomere length in human studies.' *Occupational and Environmental Medicine 70*, 1, 743–9.
13. Heaney, R.P. (2003) 'Long-latency deficiency disease: insights from calcium and vitamin D.' *American Journal of Clinical Nutrition 78*, 5, 912–9.
    Ames, B. (2010) 'Prevention of mutation, cancer and other age-associated disease by optimizing micronutrient intake.' *Journal of Nucleic Acids*, Epub 22 September 2010. Available at www.ncbi.nlm.nih.gov/pubmed/20936173, accessed on 14 January 2014.

14. Ornish, D., Lin, J., Chan, J.M., Epel, E. *et al.* (2013) 'Effect of comprehensive lifestyle changes on telomerase activity and telomere length in men with biopsy-proven low-risk prostate cancer: 5-year follow-up of a descriptive pilot study.' *Lancet Oncology 14*, 11, 1112–20.
15. Buettner, C. (2012) *The Blue Zones* (2nd edition). Washington, DC: National Geographic.

CHAPTER 2

1. Butt, M.S., Shahzadi, N., Sharif, M.K. and Nasir, M. (2007) 'Guar gum: a miracle therapy for hypercholesterolemia, hyperglycemia and obesity.' *Critical Reviews in Food Science and Nutrition 47*, 4, 389–96.
   Gunness, P. and Gidley, M.J. (2010) 'Mechanisms underlying the cholesterol-lowering properties of soluble dietary fibre polysaccharides.' *Food and Function 1*, 2, 149–55.
2. Foster-Powell, K., Holt, S.H. and Brand-Miller, J.C. (2002) 'International table of glycemic index and glycemic load values: 2002.' *American Journal of Clinical Nutrition 76*, 1, 5–56.
3. Hooper, L., Summerbell, C.D., Higgins, J.P., Thompson, R.L. *et al.* (2012) 'Reduced or modified dietary fat for preventing cardiovascular disease.' *Cochrane Database of Systematic Reviews*, 3.
4. Derbyshire, E. (2012) 'Trans fats: implications for health.' *Nursing Standard 27*, 3, 51–6.
5. Kossoff, E.H., Zupec-Kania, B.A. and Rho, J.M. (2009) 'Ketogenic diets: an update for child neurologists.' *Journal of Child Neurology 24*, 8, 979–88.
6. Cao, G., Alessio, H.M.J. and Cutler, R.G. (1993) 'Oxygen-radical absorbance capacity assay for antioxidants.' *Free Radical Biology and Medicine 14*, 3, 303–11.
7. Sapone, A., Bai, J., Ciacci, C., Dolinsek, J. *et al.* (2012) 'Spectrum of gluten-related disorders: consensus on new nomenclature and classification.' *BMC Medicine 10*, 13.
8. Buettner, D. (2008) *Blue Zones: Lessons for Living Longer from the People Who've Lived the Longest*. Washington, DC: National Geographic.
9. World Cancer Research Fund (2007) *Food, Nutrition, Physical Activity and the Prevention of Cancer: A Global Perspective*. Chapter 12. Available at www.dietandcancerreport.org/cancer_resource_center/downloads/Second_Expert_Report_full.pdf, accessed on 15 October 2013.
10. Cava, E. and Fontana, L. (2013) 'Will calorie restriction work in humans?' *Aging 5*, 7, 507–14.
11. Walford, R.L., Mock, D., Verdery, R. and MacCallum, T. (2002) 'Calorie restriction in biosphere 2: alterations in physiologic, hematologic, hormonal, and biochemical parameters in humans restricted for a 2-year period.' *Journals of Gerontology 57*, 6, B211–24.
12. Meydani, M., Das, S., Band, M., Epstein, S. and Roberts, S. (2011) 'The effect of caloric restriction and glycemic load on measures of oxidative stress and antioxidants in humans: results from the CALERIE Trial of Human Caloric Restriction.' *Journal of Nutrition, Health and Aging 15*, 6, 456–60.
13. Wilcox, B.J., Wilcox, D.C., Todoriki, H., Fujiyoshi, A. *et al.* (2007) 'Caloric restriction, the traditional Okinawan diet, and healthy aging: the diet of the world's longest-lived people and its potential impact on morbidity and life span.' *Annals of the New York Academy of Sciences 1115*, 434–55.
14. Masoro, E.J. (2005) 'Overview of calorie restriction and ageing.' *Mechanisms of Ageing and Development 126*, 9, 913–22.
15. Bloomer, R.J., Kabir, M.M., Canale R.E., Trepanowski, J.F. *et al.* (2010) 'Effect of a 21 day Daniel Fast on metabolic and cardiovascular disease risk factors in men and women.' *Lipids in Health and Disease 9*, 94.
    Meydani *et al.* 2011.
16. Masoro 2005; Bloomer *et al.* 2010.
17. Masoro, E.J. (2007) 'Role of hormesis in life extension by caloric restriction.' *Dose-Response 5*, 2, 163–73.
18. Li, Y., Daniel, M. and Tollefsbol, T.O. (2011) 'Epigenetic regulation of caloric restriction in ageing.' *BMC Medicine 9*, 98. Available at www.biomedcentral.com/1741-7015/9/98, accessed on 14 January 2014.
19. Aksungar, F.B., Topkaya, A.E. and Akyildiz, M. (2007) 'Interleukin-6, C-reactive protein and biochemical parameters during prolonged intermittent fasting.' *Annals of Nutrition and Metabolism 51*, 1, 88–95.

20. Trepanowski, J.F., Canale, R.E., Marshall, K.E., Kabir, M.M. and Bloomer, R.J. (2011) 'Impact of caloric and dietary restriction on markers of health and longevity in humans and animals: a summary of available findings.' *Nutrition Journal 10*, 107.

21. Varady, K.A. and Hellerstein, M.K. (2007) 'Alternate-day fasting and chronic disease prevention: a review of human and animal trials.' *American Journal of Clinical Nutrition 86*, 1, 7–13.

CHAPTER 3

1. Institute for Functional Medicine (2013) *Gastrointestinal Inflammation and Dysbiosis: Addressing Both Local and Systemic Manifestations*. Chapter 1. Institute for Functional Medicine. (Private distribution to conference attendees.)

2. van Heel, D.A. and West, J. (2006) 'Recent advances in coeliac disease.' *Gut 55*, 7, 1037–46.

3. Qin. J., Li, R., Raes, J., Arumugam, M. *et al.* (2010) 'A human gut microbial gene catalogue established by metagenomic sequencing.' *Nature 464*, 7285, 59–65.

4. Diamant, M., Blaak, E.E. and de Vos, W.M. (2011) 'Do nutrient-gut-microbiota interactions play a role in human obesity, insulin resistance and type 2 diabetes?' *Obesity Reviews 12*, 4, 272–81.

5. Aitken, J.D., and Gewirtz, A.T. (2013) 'Gut microbiota in 2012: Toward understanding and manipulating the gut microbiota.' *Nature Reviews Gastroenterology and Hepatology 10*, 2, 72–4.

6. Fasano, A. and Shea-Donohue, T. (2005) 'Mechanisms of disease: the role of intestinal barrier function in the pathogenesis of GI autoimmune diseases.' *Nature Clinical Practice, Gastroenterology and Hepatology 2*, 9, 416–22.

7. Ash, M. (2010) 'Vitamin A: The key to a tolerant immune system?' *Focus: Allergy Research News*, August. Available at www.allergyresearchgroup.com/August-2010-Focus-Vitamin-A-sp-107.html, accessed on 13 May 2014.

8. Egger, G. (2012) 'In search of a germ theory equivalent for chronic disease.' *Preventing Chronic Disease*, Epub 10 May 2012.

9. Institute for Functional Medicine 2013.

10. Rashid, T. and Ebringer, A. (2007) 'Ankylosing spondylitis is linked to Klebsiella: the evidence.' *Clinical Rheumatology 26*, 6, 858–64.

11. Franceschi. F. and Gasbarrini, A. (2007) 'Helicobacter pylori and extragastric diseases.' *Best Practice and Research: Clinical Gastroenterology 21*, 2, 325–34.

12. Danese, S., Semeraro, S., Papa, A., Roberto, I. *et al.* (2005) 'Extraintestinal manifestations in inflammatory bowel disease.' *World Journal of Gastroenterology 11*, 46, 7227–36.

13. Hauge, T., Persson, J. and Danielsson, D. (1997) 'Mucosal bacterial growth in the upper gastrointestinal tracts in alcoholics (heavy drinkers).' *Digestion 58*, 6, 591–5.

14. Maes, M., Kubera, M. and Leunis, J.-C. (2008) 'The gut–brain barrier in major depression: intestinal mucosal dysfunction with an increased translocation of LPS from gram negative enterobacterial (leaky gut) plays a role in the inflammatory pathophysiology of depression.' *Neuroendocrinology Letters 29*, 1, 117–24.

15. de Roest, R.H., Dobbs, B.R., Chapman, B.A., Batman, B. *et al.* (2013) 'The low FODMAP diet improves gastrointestinal symptoms in patients with IBS: a prospective study.' *International Journal of Clinical Practice 67*, 9, 895–903.
    Halmos, E.P., Power, V.A., Shepherd, S.J., Gibson, P.R. and Muir, J.G. (2013) 'A diet low in FODMAPs reduces symptoms of IBS.' *Gastroenterology 146*, 1, 67–75.

16. Force, M., Sparks, W.S. and Ronzio, R.A. (2000) 'Inhibition of enteric parasites by emulsified oil of oregano in vivo.' *Phytotherapy Research 14*, 3 213–4.

17. Castell, D.O. (1975) 'Diet and the lower esophageal sphincter.' *American Journal of Clinical Nutrition 28*, 11, 1296–8.)

18. Fasano, A. (2011) 'Zonulin and its regulation of intestinal barrier function: the biological door to inflammation, autoimmunity and cancer.' *Physiological Reviews 91*, 1, 151–75.
    Zhao, Y., Qin, G., Sun, Z., Che, D., Bao, N. and Zhang, X. (2011) 'Effects of soybean agglutinin on intestinal barrier permeability and tight junction protein expression in weaned piglets.' *International Journal of Molecular Sciences 12*, 12, 8502–12.

Dalla Pellegrina, C., Perbellini, O., Scupoli, M.T., Tomelleri, C. *et al.* (2009) 'Effects of wheat germ agglutinin on human gastrointestinal epithelium: insights from an experimental model of immune/epithelial cell interaction.' *Toxicology and Applied Pharmacology* 237, 2, 146–53.

Katsuya, M., Tanada, T. and McNeil, P. (2007) 'Lectin-based food poisoning: a new mechanism of protein toxicity.' *PLoS One* 2, 8, e687.

19. Söderholm, J.D. (2007) 'Stress-related changes in oesophageal permeability: filling the gaps of GORD?.' *Gut* 56, 9, 1177–80.

20. Hamer, H.M., Jonkers, D., Venema, K., Vanhoutvin, S., Troost, F.J. and Brummer, R.J. (2008) 'Review article: the role of butyrate on colonic function.' *Alimentary Pharmacology and Therapeutics* 27, 2, 104–19.

21. Davidson, G., Kritas, S. and Butler, R. (2007) 'Stressed mucosa.' *Nestle Nutrition Workshop Series Paediatric Programme* 59, 133–42.

22. Valassi, M. (2012) 'Functional foods with digestion-enhancing properties.' *International Journal of Food Sciences and Nutrition* 63, Suppl 1, 82–9.

23. Yoon, S., Grundmann, O, Koepp, L. and Farrell, L. (2011) 'Management of irritable bowel syndrome (IBS) in adults: conventional and complementary/alternative approaches.' *Alternative Medicine Review* 16, 2, 134–51.

24. Fasano and Shea-Donohue 2005.

25. Rapin, J.R. and Wiernsperger, N. (2010) 'Possible links between intestinal permeability and food processing: a potential therapeutic niche for glutamine.' *Clinics (Sao Paulo)* 65, 6, 635–43.

26. Gillie, O. (2006) 'A new government policy is needed for sunlight and vitamin D.' *British Journal of Dermatology* 154, 1052–61.

Gillie, O. (2011) 'Sunlight robbery: the failure of UK policy on vitamin D. In search of evidence-based public health policy.' Paper presented at the Vitamin D Experts' Forum, London, April 2011.

27. Leung, W.C., Hessel, S., Méplan, C., Flint, J. *et al.* (2009) 'Two common single nucleotide polymorphisms in the gene encoding beta-carotene 15,15'-monoxygenase alter beta-carotene metabolism in female volunteers.' *FASEB Journal* 23, 4, 1041–53.

28. Swidsinski, A., Loening-Baucke, V., Theissing, F., Engelhardt, H. *et al.* (2006) 'Comparative study of intestinal mucus barrier in normal and inflamed colon.' *Gut* 56, 3, 343–50.

29. Willcox, D.C., Willcox, B.J., Todoriki, H. and Suzuki, M. (2009) 'The Okinawan diet: health implications of a low-calorie, nutrient-dense, antioxidant-rich dietary pattern low in glycaemic load.' *Journal of the American College of Nutrition* 28, Suppl, 500–16S.

CHAPTER 4

1. Stevens, G.A., Singh, G.M., Lu, Y., Danaei, G. *et al.* (2012) 'National, regional, and global trends in adult overweight and obesity prevalences.' *Population Health Metrics* 10, 1, 22.

2. The Health and Social Care Information Centre (2013) 'Statistics on obesity, physical activity and diet –England 2013.' Available at www.hscic.gov.uk/catalogue/PUB10364, accessed on 11 September 2013.

3. University of Oxford (2009) 'Moderate obesity takes years off life expectancy.' *Science Daily*. Available at www.sciencedaily.com/releases/2009/03/090319224823.htm, accessed on 12 September 2013.

Sassi, F. and Devaux, M. (2012) *The Organisation for Economic Co-operation and Development (OECD) Obesity Update 2012.* Available at www.oecd.org/health/healthpoliciesanddata/49716427.pdf, accessed on 24 January 2014.

4. The Health and Social Care Information Centre (2013) 'Statistics on obesity, physical activity and diet – England 2013.' Available at www.hscic.gov.uk/catalogue/PUB10364, accessed on 11 September 2013.

5. Lukaczer, D. (2005) 'The Epidemic of Insulin Insensitivity.' In D.S. Jones (ed.) *The Textbook of Functional Medicine.* Gig Harbor, WA: Institute for Functional Medicine.

6. Luevano-Contreras, C. and Chapman-Novakofski, K. (2010) 'Dietary advanced glycation end products and aging.' *Nutrients* 2, 12, 1247–65.

7.   Smith, B.W. and Adams, L.A. (2011) 'Non-alcoholic fatty liver disease.' *Critical Reviews in Clinical Laboratory Sciences 48*, 3, 97–113.
     Cho, L.W. (2011) 'Metabolic syndrome.' *Singapore Medical Journal 52*, 11, 779–85.
8.   Cho 2011.
9.   Doyle, S.L., Donohoe, C.L, Lysaght, J. and Reynolds, J.V. (2012) 'Visceral obesity, metabolic syndrome, insulin resistance and cancer.' *Proceedings of the Nutrition Society 71*, 1, 181–9.
10. Panza, F., Frisardi, V., Capurso, C., Imbimbo, B.P. *et al.* (2010) 'Metabolic syndrome and cognitive impairment: current epidemiology and possible underlying mechanisms.' *Journal of Alzheimer's Disease 21*, 3, 691–724.
     Kroner. Z. (2009) 'The relationship between AD and diabetes: type 3 diabetes?' *Alternative Medicine Review 14*, 4, 373–9.
11. Kozumplik, O. and Uzan, S. (2011) 'Metabolic syndrome in patients with depressive disorder: features of comorbidity.' *Psychiatria Danubina 23*, 1, 84–8.
12. Kershaw, E.E. and Flier J.S. (2004) 'Adipose tissue as an endocrine organ.' *Journal of Clinical Endocrinology and Metabolism 89*, 6, 2548–56.
     Fain, J.N. (2006) 'Release of interleukins and other inflammatory cytokines by human adipose tissue is enhanced in obesity and primarily due to the nonfat cells.' *Vitamins and Hormones 74*, 443–77.
13. Diamond, F. (2002) 'The endocrine function of adipose tissue.' *Growth, Genetics and Hormones 18*, 2, 17–22.
14. Diabetes UK (2010) '"Active Fat" campaign launched.' Available at www.diabetes.org.uk/About_us/News_Landing_Page/Active-Fat-campaign-launched, accessed on 24 January 2014.
15. Jiang, L., Tian, W., Wang, Y., Rong, J. *et al.* (2012) 'Body mass index and susceptibility to knee osteoarthritis: a systematic review and meta-analysis.' *Joint, Bone, Spine 79*, 3, 291–7.
16. Hampel, H., Abraham, N.S. and El-Serag, H.B. (2005) 'Meta-analysis: obesity and the risk for gastroesophageal reflux disease and its complications.' *Annals of Internal Medicine 43*, 3, 199–211.
17. Knutson, K.L., Spiegel, K., Penev, P. and Van Cauter, E. (2007) 'The metabolic consequences of sleep deprivation.' *Sleep Medicine Reviews 11*, 3, 163–78.
18. Fain, J.N. (2006) 'Release of interleukins and other inflammatory cytokines by human adipose tissue is enhanced in obesity and primarily due to the nonfat cells.' *Vitamins and Hormones 74*, 443–77.
19. Carter, S., Caron, A., Richard, D. and Picard, F. (2013) 'Role of leptin resistance in the development of obesity in older patients.' *Clinical Interventions in Aging 8*, 829–44.
20. Kershaw, E.E. and Flier, J.S. (2004) 'Adipose tissue as an endocrine organ.' *Journal of Clinical Endocrinology and Metabolism 89*, 6, 2548–56.
21. Diamond 2002.
22. Diamond 2002.
23. Durukulasuriya, L.R., Stas, S. Lastra, G., Manrique, C. and Sowers, J.R. (2011) 'Hypertension in obesity.' *Medical Clinics of North America 95*, 5, 903–17.
24. Quistorff, B. and Grummett, N. (2003) 'Transformation of sugar and other carbohydrates into fat in humans.' *Ugeskrift for Laeger 165*, 15, 1551–2.
25. Miller, M. and Cappuccio, E. (2007) 'Inflammation, sleep, obesity and cardiovascular disease.' *Current Vascular Pharmacology 5*, 93–102.
26. Yamamoto, T. (2003) 'Brain mechanisms of sweetness and palatability of sugars. *Nutrition Reviews 61*, Suppl 5, S5–S9.
     Pelchat, M.L. (2002) 'Of human bondage: food craving, obsession, compulsion and addiction.' *Physiology and Behaviour 76*, 3, 347–52.
27. Anderson, I.M, Parry-Billings, M., Newsholme, E.A., Fairburn, C.G. and Cowen, P.J. (1990) 'Dieting reduces plasma tryptophan and alters brain 5HTP function in women.' *Psychological Medicine 20*, 785–91.
28. Wurtman, R.J. and Wurtman, J.J. (1996) 'Brain serotonin, carbohydrate-craving, obesity and depression.' *Advances in Experimental Medicine and Biology 398*, 35–41.
29. Cangiano, C., Ceci, F. and Cascino, A. (1992) 'Eating behaviour and adherence to dietary prescriptions in obese adult subjects treated with 5-hydroxytryptophan.' *American Journal of Clinical Nutrition 56*, 863–7.

Cangiano, C., Lavano, A. and Del Ben, M. (1998) 'Effects of oral 5-hydroxytryptophan on energy intake and macronutrient selection in non-insulin dependent diabetic patients.' *International Journal of Obesity Related Metabolism Disorders 22*, 648–54.

Rondanelli, M., Klersy C., Iadarola, P., Monteferrario, F. and Opizzi, A. (2009) 'Satiety and amino-acid profile in overweight women after a new treatment using a natural plant extract sublingual spray formulation.' *International Journal of Obesity (London) 33*, 10, 1174–82.

Rondanelli, M., Opizzi, A., Falilva, M., Bucci, M. and Perna, S. (2012) 'Relationship between the absorption of 5HTP from an integrated diet, by means of Griffonia simplicifolia extract, and the effect on satiety in overweight females after oral spray administration.' *Eating and Weight Disorders 17*, 1, e22–8.

30. Redmond, G.P. (2004) 'Thyroid dysfunction and women's reproductive health.' *Thyroid 14*, Suppl 1, S5–15.

31. Million, M., Lagier, J.C., Yahav, D. and Paul, M. (2013) 'Gut bacterial microbiota and obesity.' *Clinical Microbiology and Infection 19*, 4, 305–13.

32. Baillie-Hamilton, P. (2002) 'Chemical toxins: a hypothesis to explain the global obesity epidemic.' *Journal of Alternative and Complementary Medicine 8*, 2, 185–92.

33. Hyman, M. (2007) 'Systems biology, toxins, obesity and functional medicine.' *Thirteenth International Symposium of the IFM*, 134–9.

34. Quistorff and Grummett 2003.

35. Hooper, L., Summerbell, C.D., Higgins, J.P., Thompson, R.L. *et al.* (2001) 'Reduced or modified dietary fat for prevention of cardiovascular disease.' *Cochrane Database of Systematic Reviews 3*, CD002137.

36. Nicolle, L. and Hallam, A. (2010) 'PUFA Imbalances.' In L. Nicolle and A. Woodriff Beirne (eds) *Biochemical Imbalances in Disease*. London: Singing Dragon.

37. Tishinsky, J.M., Dyck, D.J. and Robinson, L.E. (2012) 'Lifestyle factors increasing adiponectin synthesis and secretion.' *Vitamins and Hormones 90*, 1–30.

38. Clegg, M.E. (2010) 'Medium-chain triglycerides are advantageous in promoting weight loss although not beneficial to exercise performance.' *International Journal of Food Sciences and Nutrition 61*, 7, 653–79.

St-Onge, M.P. (2005) 'Dietary fats, teas, dairy, and nuts: potential functional foods for weight control?' *American Journal of Clinical Nutrition 81*, 1, 7–15.

39. Willett, W.C. (2006) 'Ask the doctor. I have heard that coconut is bad for the heart and that it is good for the heart. Which is right?' *Harvard Heart Letter 17*, 1, 8.

Feranil, A.B., Duazo, P.L., Kuzawa, C.W. and Adair, L.S. (2011) 'Coconut oil is associated with a beneficial lipid profile in pre-menopausal women in the Philippines.' *Asia Pacific Journal of Clinical Nutrition 20*, 2, 190–5.

40. Derbyshire, E. (2012) 'Trans fats: implications for health.' *Nursing Standard 27*, 3, 51–6.

41. Hua Y., Clark, S., Ren, J. and Sreejayan, N. (2012) 'Molecular mechanisms of chromium in alleviating insulin resistance.' *Journal of Nutritional Biochemistry 23*, 4, 313–9.

42. Wang, Z.Q. and Cefalu, W.T. (2010) 'Current concepts about chromium supplementation in type 2 diabetes and insulin resistance.' *Current Diabetes Reports 10*, 2, 145–51.

43. Rumawas, M.E., McKeown, N.M., Rogers, G., Meigs, J.B., Wilson, P.W. and Jacques, P.F. (2006) 'Magnesium intake is related to improved insulin homeostasis in the Framingham offspring cohort.' *Journal of the American College of Nutrition 25*, 6, 486–92.

Ma, B., Lawson, A.B., Liese, A.D., Bell, R.A. and Mayer-Davis, E.J. (2006) 'Dairy, magnesium and calcium intake in relation to insulin sensitivity: approaches to modeling a dose-dependent association.' *American Journal of Epidemiology 164*, 5, 449–58.

Song, Y., Manson, J.E. and Liu, S. (2004) 'Dietary magnesium intake in relation to plasma insulin levels and risk of type 2 diabetes in women.' *Diabetes Care 27*, 1, 59–65.

44. Song *et al.* 2004.

Larsson, S.C. and Wolk, A. (2007) 'Magnesium intake and risk of type 2 diabetes: a meta-analysis.' *Journal of Internal Medicine 262*, 208.

45. He, K., Liu, K., Daviglus, M.L., Morris, S.J *et al.* (2006) 'Magnesium intake and incidence of metabolic syndrome among young adults.' *Circulation 113*, 13, 1675–82.

46. Lopez-Ridaura, R., Willett, W.C., Rimm, E.B., Liu, S. *et al.* (2004) 'Magnesium intake and risk of type 2 diabetes in men and women.' *Diabetes Care 27*, 1, 134–40.

47. Pham, P.C., Pham, P.M., Pham, S.V., Miller, J.M. and Pham, P.T. (2007) 'Hypomagnesemia in patients with type 2 diabetes.' *Clinical Journal of the American Society of Nephrology 2*, 2, 366–73.

48. Mooren, F.C., Krüger, K., Völker, K., Golf, S.W., Wadepuhl, M. and Kraus, A. (2011) 'Oral magnesium supplementation reduces insulin resistance in non-diabetic subjects – a double-blind, placebo-controlled, randomized trial.' *Diabetes, Obesity and Metabolism 13*, 3, 281–4.

49. Rodriguez-Moran, M. and Guerro-Romero, F. (2003) 'Oral magnesium supplementation improves insulin sensitivity and metabolic control in type 2 diabetic subjects: a randomized double-blind controlled trial.' *Diabetes Care 26*, 4, 1147–52.

Yokota, K., Kato, M., Lister, F., Ii, H. *et al.* (2004) 'Clinical efficacy of magnesium supplementation in patients with type 2 diabetes.' *Journal of the American College of Nutrition 23*, 5, 506S–509S.

Barbagallo, M. and Dominquez, L.J. (2007) 'Magnesium metabolism in type 2 diabetes mellitus, metabolic syndrome and insulin resistance.' *Archives of Biochemistry and Biophysics 458*, 1, 40–7.

50. Jeukendrup, A.E. and Randell, R. (2011) 'Fat burners: nutrition supplements that increase fat metabolism.' *Obesity Reviews 12*, 10, 841–51.

Suzuki, Y., Miyoshi, N. and Isemura, M. (2012) 'Health-promoting effects of green tea.' *Proceedings of the Japan Academy – Series B: Physical and Biological Sciences 88*, 3, 88–101.

51. Kim, A., Chiu, A., Barone, M.K., Avino, D. *et al.* (2011) 'Green tea catechins decrease total and LDL cholesterol: a systematic review and meta-analysis.' *Journal of the American Dietetic Association 111*, 1, 1720–9.

52. Suzuki *et al.* 2012.

53. Wolfram, S. (2007) 'Effects of green tea and EGCG on CV and metabolic health.' *Journal of the American College of Nutrition 26*, 4, 373S–88S.

54. Suzuki *et al.* 2012; Wolfram 2007.

55. Khan, A., Safdar, M., Ali Khan, M.M., Khattak, K.N. and Anderson, R.A. (2003) 'Cinnamon improves glucose and lipids of people with type 2 diabetes.' *Diabetes Care 26*, 12, 3215–8.

56. Akilen, R., Tsiami, A., Devendra, D. and Robinson, N. (2010) 'Glycated haemoglobin and blood pressure-lowering effects of cinnamon in multi-ethnic type 2 diabetic patients in the UK: a randomized, placebo-controlled, double-blind clinical trial.' *Diabetic Medicine 27*, 10, 1159–67.

Davis, P.A. and Yokoyama, W. (2011) 'Cinnamon intake lowers fasting blood glucose: meta-analysis.' *Journal of Medicinal Food 14*, 9, 884–9.

57. Davis and Yokoyama 2011.

58. Cao, H., Polansky, M.M. and Anderson, R.A. (2007) 'Cinnamon extract and polyphenols affect the expression of tristetraprolin, insulin receptor and GLUT-4 in mouse 3T3-L1 adipocytes.' *Archives of Biochemistry and Biophysics 459*, 2, 214–22.

59. Cheng, D.M., Kuhn, P., Poulev, A., Rojo, L.E., Lila, M.A. and Raskin, I. (2012) 'In vivo and in vitro antidiabetic effects of aqueous cinnamon extract and cinnamon polyphenol-enhanced food matrix.' *Food Chemistry 135*, 4, 2994–3002.

60. Vinson, J.A., Burnham, B.R. and Nagendran, M.V. (2012) 'Randomized, double-blind, placebo-controlled, linear dose, crossover study to evaluate the efficacy and safety of a green coffee bean extract in overweight subjects.' *Diabetes, Metabolic Syndrome and Obesity 5*, 21–7.

61. Bhatti, S.K., O'Keefe, J.H. and Lavie, C.J. (2013) 'Coffee and tea: perks for health and longevity?' *Current Opinion in Clinical Nutrition and Metabolic Care 16*, 6, 688–97.

62. Gray, N. (2013) 'Green coffee bean compound may help to control blood sugar.' Available at www.nutraingredients.com/Research/Green-coffee-bean-compound-may-help-control-blood-sugar-Study/?utm_source=newsletter_weekly&utm_medium=email&utm_campaign=Newsletter%2BWeekly&c=l9sQcvaQXiXwpFfOjJYVXmzfPSt2WE5y, accessed on 20 April 2013.

63. Wedick, N.M., Brennan, A.M., Sun, Q., Hu, F.B., Mantzoros, C.S. and van Dam, R.M. (2011) 'Effects of caffeinated and decaffeinated coffee on biological risk factors for type 2 diabetes: a randomized controlled trial.' *Nutrition Journal 10*, 93.

64. Hemmerle, H., Burger, H.J., Below, P. Schubert, G. *et al.* (1997) 'Chlorogenic acid and synthetic chlorogenic acid derivatives: novel inhibitors of hepatic glucose-6-phosphate translocase.' *Journal of Medicinal Chemistry 40*, 2, 137–45.

65. Thom, E. (2007) 'The effect of chlorogenic acid enriched coffee on glucose absorption in healthy volunteers and its effect on body mass when used long-term in overweight and obese people.' *Journal of International Medical Research* 35, 6, 900–8.

66. Couet, C., Delarue, J., Ritz, P., Antoine, J.M. and Lamisse, F. (1997) 'Effect of dietary fish oil on body fat mass and basal fat oxidation in healthy adults.' *International Journal of Obesity and Related Metabolic Disorders* 21, 8, 637–43.
    Golub, N., Geba, D., Mousa, S.A., Williams, G. and Block, R.C. (2011) 'Greasing the wheels of managing overweight and obesity with omega 3 fatty acids.' *Medical Hypotheses* 77, 6, 1114–20.

67. Sugiura, T. (2009) 'Physiological roles of 2-arachidonoylglycerol, an endogenous cannabinoid receptor ligand.' *Biofactors* 25, 1, 88–97.

68. Lee, J.H., O'Keefe, J.H., Lavie, C.J., Marchioli, R. and Harris, W.S. (2008) 'Omega 3 fatty acids for cardioprotection.' *Mayo Clinic Proceedings* 83, 3, 324–9.
    Tziomalos, K., Athyros, V.G. and Mikhailidis, D.P. (2007) 'Fish oils and vascular disease prevention: an update.' *Current Medicinal Chemistry* 14, 24, 2622–8.
    Milte, C.M., Coates, A.M., Buckley, J.D., Hill, A.M. and Howe, P.R. (2008) 'Dose-dependent effects of DHA-rich fish oil on erythrocyte DHA and blood lipid levels.' *British Journal of Nutrition* 99, 5, 1083–8.

69. Abeywardena, M.Y. and Patten, G.S. (2011) 'Role of omega-3 long-chain PUFAs in reducing cardio-metabolic risk factors.' *Endocrine, Metabolic and Immune Disorders – Drug Targets* 11, 3, 232.
    Mozaffairan, D. and Wu, J.H. (2012) 'Omega-3 fatty acids and cardiovascular health: are effects of EPA and DHA shared or complementary? *Journal of Nutrition* 142, 3, 614S–625S.

70. Abeywardena and Pattan 2011.
    Hall, W.L. (2009) 'Dietary saturated and unsaturated fats as determinants of blood pressure and vascular function.' *Nutrition Research Reviews* 22, 1, 18–38.

71. Lopez-Huertas, E. (2012) 'The effect of EPA and DHA on MetS patients: a systematic review of RCTs.' *British Journal of Nutrition* 107, Suppl 2, S185–94.

72. Lee *et al.* 2008.

73. Rondanelli *et al.* 2009; Rondanelli *et al.* 2012.

74. Chen, D., Liu, Y., He, W., Wang, H. and Wang, Z. (2012) 'Neurotransmitter-precursor-supplement intervention for detoxified heroic addicts.' *Journal of Huazhong University of Science and Technology Medical Sciences* 32, 3, 422–7.

75. D'Orazio, N., Gemello, E., Gammone, M.A., de Girolamo, M., Ficoneri, C., and Riccioni, G. (2012) 'Fucoxantin: a treasure from the sea.' *Marine Drugs* 10, 3, 604–16.

76. Abidov, M., Ramazanov, Z., Seifulla, R. and Grachev, S. (2010) 'The effects of Xanthigen in the weight management of obese premenopausal women with non-alcoholic fatty liver disease and normal liver fat.' *Diabetes, Obesity and Metabolism* 12, 1, 72–81.

77. Lau, F.C., Golakoti, T., Krishnaraju, A.V. and Sengupta, K. (2011) 'Efficacy and tolerability of Merastin™: a randomized, double-blind, placebo-controlled study.' *FASEB Journal* 25, 601.

78. Ngondi, J.L., Oben, J.E. and Minka, S.R. (2005) 'The effect of Irvingia gabonensis seeds on body weight and blood lipids of obese subjects in Cameroon.' *Lipids in Health and Disease* 4, 12.
    Oben, J.E., Ngondi, J.L., Momo, C.N., Agbor, G.A. and Sobgui, C.S.M. (2008) 'The use of a Cissus quadrangularis/Irvingia gabonensis combination in the management of weight loss: a double-blind placebo-controlled study.' *Lipids in Health and Disease* 7, 12.

79. Gout, B., Bourges, C. and Paineau-Dubreuil, S. (2010) 'Satiereal, a Crocus sativus L extract, reduces snacking and increases satiety in a randomized placebo-controlled study of mildly overweight, healthy women.' *Nutrition Research* 30, 5, 305–13.

80. Preuss, H.G., Echard, B., Bagchi, D. and Stohs, S. (2007) 'Inhibition by natural dietary substances of gastrointestinal absorption of starch and sucrose in rats 2. Subchronic studies.' *International Journal of Medical Sciences* 4, 4, 209–15.

81. Sood, N., Baker, W.L. and Coleman, C.I. (2008) 'Effect of glucomannan on plasma lipid and glucose concentrations, body weight, and blood pressure: systematic review and meta-analysis.' *American Journal of Clinical Nutrition* 88, 4, 1167–75.

82. Barrett, M.L. and Udani, J.K. (2011) 'A proprietary alpha-amylase inhibitor from white bean (Phaseolus vulgaris): a review of clinical studies on weight loss and glycemic control.' *Nutrition Journal* 10, 24.

83. Ostman, E., Granfeldt, Y., Persson, L. and Björk, I. (2005) 'Vinegar supplementation lowers glucose and insulin responses and increases satiety after a bread meal in healthy subjects.' *European Journal of Clinical Nutrition 59*, 9, 983–8.

84. Amorim Adegboye, A.R. and Linne, Y.M. (2013) 'Diet or exercise, or both, for weight reduction in women after childbirth.' *Cochrane Database of Systematic Reviews*, CD005627.

85. Umpierre, D., Ribeiro, P.A., Schaan, B.D. and Ribeiro, J.P. (2013) 'Volume of supervised exercise training impacts glycaemic control in patients with type 2 diabetes: a systematic review with meta-regression analysis.' *Diabetologia 56*, 2, 242–51.

86. Oliveira, C., Simões, M., Carvalho, J. and Ribeiro, J. (2012) 'Combined exercise for people with type 2 diabetes mellitus: a systematic review.' *Diabetes Research and Clinical Practice 98*, 2, 187–98.

87. Tamashiro, K.L., Sadai, R.R., Shively, C.A., Karatsoreos, I.N. and Reagan, L.P. (2011) 'Chronic stress, metabolism and metabolic syndrome.' *Stress 14*, 5, 468–74.

88. Martins, R.C., Andersen, M.L. and Tufik, S. (2008) 'The reciprocal interaction between sleep and type 2 diabetes mellitus: facts and perspectives.' *Brazilian Journal of Medical and Biological Research 41*, 3, 180–7.

Miller and Cappuccio 2007.

CHAPTER 5

1. Denny, A. and Butriss, J. (2007) *Plant Foods and Health*. London: British Nutrition Foundation.

Davi, G., Falco, A. and Patrono, C. (2005) 'Lipid peroxidation in diabetes mellitus.' *Antioxidants and Redux Signaling 7*, 1–2, 256–68.

Nunomura, A., Castellani, R.J., Zhu, X., Moreira, P.I., Perry, G. and Smith, M.A. (2006) 'Involvement of oxidative stress in Alzheimer Disease.' *Journal of Neuropathology and Experimental Neurology 65*, 7, 631–41.

Wood-Kaczmar, A., Gandhi, S. and Wood, N.W. (2006) 'Understanding the molecular causes of Parkinson's disease.' *Trends in Molecular Medicine 12*, 11, 521–8.

Hitchon, C.A and El-Gabalawy, H.S. (2004) 'Oxidation in rheumatoid arthritis.' *Arthritis Research and Therapy 6*, 6, 265–78.

Cookson, M.R. and Shaw, P.J. (1999) 'Oxidative stress and motor neurone disease.' *Brain Pathology 9*, 1, 165–86.

2. Morganti, P. (2009) 'The photoprotective activity of nutraceuticals.' *Clinics in Dermatology 27*, 166–74.

3. John, E.M. and Sterm, M.C. (2011) 'Meat consumption, cooking practices, meat mutagens and risk of prostate cancer.' *Nutrition and Cancer 63*, 4, 525–37.

4. Knize, M.G., Salmon, C.P., Pais, P. and Felton, J.S. (1999) 'Food heating and the formation of heterocyclic aromatic amine and polycyclic aromatic hydrocarbon mutagens/carcinogens.' *Advances in Experimental Medicine and Biology 459*, 170–93.

5. Derbyshire, E. (2012) 'Trans fats: implications for health.' *Nursing Standard 27*, 3, 51–6.

6. Latreille, J., Kesse-Guyot, E., Malvy, D. Andreeva, V. *et al.* (2013) 'Association between dietary intake of n-3 polyunsaturated fatty acids and severity of skin photoaging in a middle-aged Caucasian population.' *Journal of Dermatological Science 72*, 3, 233–9.

7. Nicolaou, A. (2013) 'Eicosanaoids in skin inflammation.' *Prostaglandins, Leukotrienes and Essential Fatty Acids 88*, 1, 131–8.

8. Muggli, R. (2005) 'Systemic evening primrose oil improves the biophysical skin parameters of healthy adults.' *International Journal of Cosmetic Science 27*, 4, 243–9.

9. Kawamura, A., Ooyama, K., Kojima, K., Kachi, H. *et al.* (2011) 'Dietary supplementation of gamma-linolenic acid improves skin parameters in subjects with dry skin and mild atopic dermatitis.' *Journal of Oleo Science 60*, 12, 597–607.

10. Foster, R.H., Hardy, G. and Alany, R.G. (2010) 'Borage oil in the treatment of atopic dermatitis.' *Nutrition 26*, 7–8, 708–18.

11. Steele, J. and O'Sullivan, I. (2011) *Executive Summary: Adult Dental Health Survey 2009*. London: Health and Social Care Information Centre.

12. Mealey, B.L (2006) 'Periodontal disease and diabetes. A two-way street.' *Journal of the American Dental Association 137*, Suppl, 26S–31S.

Kim, J. and Amar, S. (2006) 'Periodontal disease and systemic conditions: a biodirectional relationship.' *Odontology 94*, 1, 10–21.

13. Kim and Amar 2006.

Skilton, M.R., Maple-Brown, L.J., Kapellas, K., Celermajer, D.S. *et al.* (2011) 'The effect of a periodontal intervention on cardiovascular risk markers in Indigenous Australians with periodontal disease. The PerioCardio study. *BMC Public Health 11*, 729.

Scannapieco, F.A., Bush, R.B. and Paju, S. (2003) 'Association between periodontal disease and risk for atherosclerosis, cardiovascular disease, and stroke: a systematic review.' *Annals of Periodontology 8*, 1, 38–53.

14. Martinez-Maestre, M.A., González-Cejudo, C., Machuca, G., Torrejón, R. and Castelo-Branco, C. (2010) 'Periodontitis and osteoporosis: a systematic review.' *Climacteric 13*, 6, 523–9.

Kim and Amar 2006.

15. Skilton *et al.* 2011.

16. Van der Velden, U., Kuzmanova, D. and Chapple, I.L. (2011) 'Micronutritional approaches to periodontal therapy.' *Journal of Clinical Periodontology 11*, 142–58.

17. Feghali, K., Feldman, M., La, V.D., Santos, J. and Grenier, D. (2012) 'Cranberry proanthocyanidins: natural weapons against periodontal diseases.' *Journal of Agricultural and Food Chemistry 60*, 23, 5728–25.

Bonifait, L. and Grenier, D. (2010) 'Cranberry polyphenols: potential benefits for dental caries and periodontal disease.' *Journal of Canadian Dental Association 76*, a130.

18. Boelsma, E., Henkdriks, H. and Roza, L. (2001) 'Nutritional skin care: health effects of micronutrients and fatty acids.' *American Journal of Clinical Nutrition 73*, 5, 853–64.

19. Boelsma *et al.* 2001.

Morganti, P. (2009) 'The photoprotective activity of nutraceuticals.' *Clinics in Dermatology 27*, 166–74.

Alves-Rodrigues, A. and Shao, A. (2004) 'The science behind lutein.' *Toxicology Letters 150*, 57-83.

Morganti, P., Bruno, C., Guarneri, F., Cardillo, A., Del Ciotto, P. and Valenzano, F. (2002) 'Role of topical and nutritional supplements to modify the oxidative stress.' *International Journal of Cosmetic Science 24*, 6, 331–9.

20. Cross, C.E., Traber, M., Eiserich, J. and van der Vliet, A. (1999) 'Micronutrient antioxidants and smoking.' *British Medical Bulletin 55*, 3, 691–704.

21. Alternative Medicine Review (2005) 'Lutein and zeaxanthin: a monograph.' *Alternative Medicine Review 10*, 2, 128–35.

22. Denny and Butriss 2007.

23. Boelsma *et al.* 2001.

24. Graf, J. (2010) 'Antioxidants and skin care: the essentials.' *Plastic and Reconstructive Surgery 125*, 1, 378–83.

25. World Cancer Research Fund/American Institute for Cancer Research (2007) *Food, Nutrition, Physical Activity and the Prevention of Cancer: A Global Perspective.* Washington, DC: AICR. Available at www.dietandcancerreport.org/cancer_resource_center/downloads/Second_Expert_Report_full.pdf, accessed on 25 January 2014.

26. Denny and Butriss 2007.

D'Archivio, M., Filesi, C., Di Benedetto, R., Gargiulo, R., Giovannini, C. and Masella, R. (2007) 'Polyphenols, dietary sources and bioavailability.' *Annali dell'Istituto Superiore Sanità. 43*, 4, 348–61.

27. Martin, C., Zhang, Y., Tonelli, C. and Petroni, K. (2013) 'Plants, diet and health.' *Annual Review of Plant Biology 64*, 19–46.

Boeing, H., Bechthold, A., Bub, A., Ellinger, S. *et al.* (2012) 'Critical review: vegetables and fruit in the prevention of chronic diseases.' *European Journal of Nutrition 51*, 6, 637–63.

Denny and Butriss 2007.

D'Archivio *et al.* 2007.

He, F.J., Nowson, C.A., Lucas, M. and MacGregor, G.A. (2007) 'Increased consumption of fruit and vegetables is related to a reduced risk of coronary heart disease: meta-analysis of cohort studies.' *Journal of Human Hypertension 21*, 9, 717–28.

Martinez-González, M.A., del Fuente-Arrillaga, C., López-Del-Burgo, C., Vázquez-Ruiz, Z., Benito, S. and Ruiz-Canela, M. (2011) 'Low consumption of fruit and vegetables and risk of chronic disease: a review of the epidemiological evidence and temporal trends among Spanish graduates.' *Public Health Nutrition 14*, 12A, 2309–15.

Hughes, T.F., Andel, R., Small, B.J., Borenstein, A.R.*et al.* (2010) 'Midlife fruit and vegetable consumption and risk of dementia in later life in Swedish twins.' *American Journal of Geriatric Psychiatry 18*, 5, 413–20.

28. D'Archivio *et al.* 2007.

Aolst, B. and Williamson, G. (2008) 'Nutrients and phytochemicals: from bioavailability to bioefficacy and beyond antioxidants.' *Current Opinion in Biotechnology 19*, 2, 73–82..

Martin *et al.* 2013.

29. Mithen, R. (2006) 'Sulphur-Containing Compounds.' In A. Crozier, M.N. Clifford and H. Ashihara (eds) *Plants' Secondary Metabolites: Occurrence, Structure and Role in the Human Diet.* Oxford: Blackwell Publishing.

30. Morganti 2009.

31. Lamberts Healthcare (2011) 'A Study in healthy volunteers to determine the UV protection, the anti-wrinkle properties and the effects on skin elasticity of anthocyanins compared to an inactive placebo after 12 weeks of use.' Unpublished.

32. Alternative Medicine Review (2003) 'Oligomeric proanthocyanidins: monograph.' *Alternative Medicine Review 8*, 4, 442–50.

33. Proksch, E., Segger, D., Degwert, J., Schunck, M., Zaque, V. and Oesser, S. (2014) 'Oral supplementation of specific collagen peptides has beneficial effects on human skin physiology: a double-blind, placebo-controlled study.' *Skin Pharmacology and Physiology 27*, 1, 47–55.

34. Hartog, A., Cozijnsen, M., de Vrij, G. and Garssen, J. (2013) 'Collagen hydrolysate inhibits zymosan-induced inflammation.' *Experimental Biology and Medicine (Maywood) 238*, 7, 798–802.

35. Oba, C., Ohara, H., Morifuji, M., Ito, K., Ichikawa, S., Kawahata, K. and Koga, J. (2013) 'Collagen hydrolysate intake improves the loss of epidermal barrier function and skin elasticity induced by UVB irradiation in hairless mice.' *Photodermatology, Photoimmunology and Photomedicine 29*, 4, 204–11.

36. Alternative Medicine Review (2003) 'Oligomeric proanthocyanidins: monograph.' *Alternative Medicine Review 8*, 4, 442–50.

Christie, S., Walker, A.F., Hicks, S.M. and Abeyaskera, S. (2004) 'Flavonoid supplement improves leg health and reduces fluid retention in pre-menopausal women in a double-blind, placebo-controlled study.' *Phytomedicine 11*, 1, 11–7.

37. Alternative Medicine Review (2009) 'Aesculus hippocastanum.' *Alternative Medicine Review 14*, 3, 278–283.

38. Pittler M.H. and Ernst E. (2004) 'Horse chestnut seed extract for the treatment of chronic venous insufficiency.' *Cochrane Database of Systematic Reviews 2*, CD003230.

39. Rushton D.H. (2002) 'Nutritional factors and hair loss.' *Clinical and Experimental Dermatology 27*, 5, 396–404.

Rushton D.H. (1993) 'Investigating and managing hair loss in apparently healthy women.' *Canadian Journal of Dermatology 5*, 455–61.

40. Bates, B. (1979) *A Guide to Physical Examination* (2nd edition). Philadelphia, PA: J.B. Lippincott.

41. Alternative Medicine Review (2007) 'Biotin.' *Alternative Medicine Review 12*, 1, 73–78.

42. Graf, J. (2010) 'Antioxidants and skin care: the essentials.' *Plastic and Reconstructive Surgery 125*, 1 378–83.

Kerscher, M. and Buntrock, H. (2011) 'Anti-aging creams. What really helps?' *Hautarzt 62*, 8, 607–13.

43. Beitner, H. (2003) 'Randomized, placebo-controlled, double blind study on the clinical efficacy of a cream containing 5% alpha-lipoic acid related to photoageing of facial skin.' *British Journal of Dermatology 149*, 4, 841–9.

44. Jang, M., Cai, L., Udeani, G.O., Slowing, K.V. *et al.* (1997) 'Cancer chemopreventive activity of resveratrol, a natural product derived from grapes.' *Science 275*, 5297, 218–20.

45. Namjoshi, S. and Benson, H.A. (2010) 'Cyclic peptides as potential therapeutic agents for skin disorders.' *Biopolymers 94*, 5, 673–80).
Namjoshi, S., Caccetta, R. and Benson, H.A. (2008) 'Skin peptides: biological activity and therapeutic opportunities.' *Journal of Pharmaceutical Sciences 97*, 7, 2524–42.

CHAPTER 6

1. Silverman, M.N. and Sternberg, E.M. (2012) 'Glucocorticoid regulation of inflammation and its functional correlates: from HPA axis to glucocorticoid receptor dysfunction.' *Annals of the New York Academy of Sciences 1261*, 55–63.
2. Selye, H. (1956) *The Stress of Life*. New York, NY: McGraw Hill.
3. Rosmond, R. (2003) 'Stress induced disturbances of the HPA axis. a pathway to type 2 diabetes?' *Medical Science Monitor 9*, 2, RA35–9.
Pasquali, R., Vicennati, V., Cacciari, M. and Pagotto, U. (2006) 'The hypothalamic-pituitary-adrenal axis activity in obesity and the metabolic syndrome.' *Annals of the New York Academy of Sciences 1083*, 111–28.
4. Bao, A.M. and Swaab, D.F. (2010) 'Corticotropin-releasing hormone and arginine vasopressin in depression focus on the human postmortem hypothalamus.' *Vitamins and Hormones 82*, 339–65.
5. Lupien, S.J., Schwartz, G., Ng, Y.K., Fioccok A. *et al.* (2005) 'The Douglas Hospital Longitudinal Study of Normal and Pathological Aging: a summary of findings.' *Journal of Psychiatry and Neurosciences 30*, 5, 328–34.
6. Kyrou, I. and Tsigos, C. (2008) 'Chronic stress, visceral obesity and gonadal dysfunction.' *Hormones (Athens) 7*, 4, 287–93.
7. Cutolo, M., Foppiani, L. and Minuto, F. (2002) 'Hypothalamic-pituitary-adrenal axis impairment in the pathogenesis of rheumatoid arthritis and polymyalgia rheumatica.' *Journal of Endocrinological Investigation 25*, 10 Suppl, 19–23.
8. Van Houdenhove, B., Van Den Eede, F. and Luyten, P. (2009) 'Does hypothalamic-pituitary-adrenal axis hypofunction in chronic fatigue syndrome reflect a "crash" in the stress system?' *Medical Hypotheses 72*, 6, 701–5.
9. Juruena, M.F. and Cleare, A.J. (2007) 'Overlap between atypical depression, seasonal affective disorder and chronic fatigue syndrome.' *Revista Brasileira de Psiquiatria 29*, Suppl 1, S19–26.
10. Van Houdenhove, B. and Egle, U.T. (2004) 'Fibromyalgia: a stress disorder? Piecing the biopsychosocial puzzle together.' *Psychotherapy and Psychosomatics 73*, 5, 267–75.
11. Wilson, G.R. and Curry, R.W. Jr. (2005) 'Subclinical thyroid disease.' *American Family Physician 72*, 8, 1517–24.
12. Biondi, B. and Cooper, D.S. (2008) 'The clinical significance of subclinical thyroid dysfunction.' *Endocrine Reviews 29*, 1, 76–131.
13. Tagami, T., Tamanaha, T., Shimazu, S., Honda, K. *et al.* (2010) 'Lipid profiles in the untreated patients with Hashimoto thyroiditis and the effects of thyroxine treatment on the subclinical hypothyroidism with Hasimoto thyroiditis.' *Endocrine Journal 57*, 3, 253–8.
14. Roundtree, R. (2011) 'Genetic and Environmental Determinants: Toxins, Toxicity and Biotransformation.' Presentation given at the Applying Functional Medicine in Clinical Practice (AFMCP) symposium, London, October 2011.
15. Kortenkamp, A (2006) 'Breast cancer, oestrogens and environmental pollutants: a re-evaluation from a mixture perspective.' *International Journal of Andrology 29*, 1, 193–8.
16. Felton, J.S. and Malfatti, M.A. (2006) 'What do diet-induced changes in phase I and phase II enzymes tell us about prevention from exposure to heterocyclic amines?' *Journal of Nutrition 136*, 10, Suppl, 2683–4S.
17. Hess, E.V. (2002) 'Environmental chemicals and autoimmune disease: cause and effect.' *Toxicology 181–182*, 65–70.
18. Bártová, J., Procházková, J., Krátká, Z., Benetková, K., Venclíková, Z. and Sterzk, I. (2003) 'Dental amalgam as one of the risk factors in autoimmune diseases.' *Neuro Endocrinology Letters 24*, 1–2, 65–7.

19. McAlindon, T.E., Gulin, J., Chen, T., Klug, T., Lahita, R. and Nuite, M. (2001) 'Indole-3-carbinol in women with SLE: effect on estrogen metabolism and disease activity.' *Lupus 10*, 1, 779–83.

20. Liska, D.J. (1998) 'The detoxification enzyme systems.' *Alternative Medicine Review 3*, 3, 187–98.

21. Williams, A.C., Steventon, G.B., Sturman, S. and Waring, R.H. (1991) 'Hereditary variation of liver enzymes involved with detoxification and neurodegenerative disease.' *Journal of Inherited Metabolic Disease 14*, 4, 431–5.

22. Baillie-Hamilton, P.F. (2002) 'Chemical toxins: a hypothesis to explain the global obesity epidemic.' *Journal of Alternative and Complementary Medicine 8*, 2, 185–92.

23. Kelly, G.S. (2000) 'Peripheral metabolism of thyroid hormones: a review.' *Alternative Medicine Review 5*, 4, 306–33.

24. Kelly 2000; Bártová *et al.* 2003.
    Caride, A., Fernández-Pérez, B., Cabaleiro, T., Tarasco, M. Esquifino, A.I. and Lafuente, A. (2010) 'Cadmium chronotoxicity at pituitary level: effects on plasma ACTH, GH, and TSH daily pattern.' *Journal of Physiology and Biochemistry 66*, 3, 213–20.

25. Nodder, J. (2010) 'Compromised Thyroid and Adrenal Function.' In L. Nicolle and A. Woodriff Beirne (eds) *Biochemical Imbalances in Disease*. London: Singing Dragon.

26. Chek, P. (2011) *Movement as Medicine Webinar, Part 1 and 2*. Vista, CA: CHEK Institute.
    Farhi, D. (1996) *The Breathing Book: Vitality and Good Health through Essential Breath Work*. New York, NY: Henry Holt and Company.
    Yan Lei, S. (2009) *Qi Gong Workout for Longevity*. China: Yan Lei Press.

27. Chek 2011.

28. Kelly 2000.

29. Kelly 2000.

30. Kortenkamp 2006.

31. Coronado, G.D., Beasley, J. and Livaudais, J. (2011) 'Alcohol consumption and the risk of breast cancer.' *Salud Pública de México 53*, 5, 440–7.
    Testino, G. (2011) 'The burden of cancer attributable to alcohol consumption.' *Maedica (Bucharest) 6*, 4, 313–20.

32. World Cancer Research Fund (2011) 'Alcohol and cancer prevention.' Available at www.wcrf-uk.org/cancer_prevention/recommendations/alcohol_and_cancer.php, accessed on 18 January 2012).

33. Li, Y., Hou, M.J., Ma, J., Tang, Z.H., Zhu, H.L. and Ling, W.H. (2005) 'Dietary fatty acids regulate cholesterol induction of liver CYP7alpha1 expression and bile acid production.' *Lipids 40*, 5, 455–62.

34. Nicolle, L. and Bailey, C. (2013) *The Functional Nutrition Cookbook*. London: Singing Dragon.

35. Moon, Y.J., Wang, X. and Morris, M.E. (2006) 'Dietary flavonoids: effects on xenobiotic and carcinogen metabolism.' *Toxicology in Vitro 20*, 2, 187–210.

36. Sartori, S.B., Whittle, N., Hetzenauer, A. and Singewald, N. (2012) 'Magnesium deficiency induces anxiety and HPA axis dysregulation: modulation by therapeutic drug treatment.' *Neuropharmacology 62*, 1, 304–12.

37. Kelly 2000.
    Hess, S.Y. (2010) 'The impact of common micronutrient deficiencies on iodine and thyroid metabolism: the evidence from human studies.' *Best Practice and Research: Clinic Endocrinology and Metabolism 24*, 1, 117–32.
    Zimmerman, M.B. and Köhrle, J. (2002) 'The impact of iron and selenium deficiencies on iodine and thyroid metabolism: biochemistry and relevance to public health.' *Thyroid 12*, 10, 867–78.
    Arthur, J.R. and Beckett, G.J. (1999) 'Thyroid function.' *British Medical Bulletin 55*, 3, 658–68.

38. Enns, C.A. and Zhang, A.S. (2009) 'Iron homeostasis: recently identified proteins provide insight into novel control mechanisms.' *Journal of Biological Chemistry 284*, 2, 711–5.

39. Jaroenporn, S., Yamamoto, T., Itabashi, A., Nakamura, K. *et al.* (2008) 'Effects of pantothenic acid supplementation on adrenal steroid secretion from male rats.' *Biological and Pharmaceutical Bulletin. 31*, 6, 1205–8.

Eisenstein, A.B. (1957) 'Effects of dietary factors on production of adrenal steroid hormones.' *American Journal of Clinical Nutrition* 5, 4, 369–76.

40. Jabbar, A., Yawar, A., Waseem, S., Islam, N. *et al.* (2008) 'Vitamin B12 deficiency common in primary hypothyroidism.' *Journal of the Pakistan Medical Association* 58, 5, 258–61.

Bíčíková, M., Hampl, R., Hill, M., Stanická, S., Tallová, J. and Vondra, K. (2003) 'Steroids, sex hormone-binding globulin, homocysteine, selected hormones and markers of lipid and carbohydrate metabolism in patients with severe hypothyroidism and their changes following thyroid hormone supplementation.' *Clinical Chemistry and Laboratory Medicine* 41, 3, 284–92.

41. Eisenstein 1957.

42. Hess 2010.

43. Goraca, A., Huk-Kolega, H., Piechota, A., Kleniewska, P., Ciejka, E. and Skibska, B. (2011) 'Lipoic acid – biological activity and therapeutic potential.' *Pharmacological Reports* 63, 849–58.

Gardner, A. and Boles, R.G. (2011) 'Beyond the serotonin hypothesis: mitochondria, inflammation and neurodegeneration in major depression and affective spectrum disorders.' *Progress in Neuro-Psychopharmacology and Biological Psychiatry* 35, 3, 730–43.

Ash, M. and Nicolson, G. (2012) 'Mechanisms of membrane repair and the novel role of oral phospholipids (Lipid Replacement Therapy*) and antioxidants to improve membrane function. *Nutri-Link Clinical Education.* Available at www.nleducation.co.uk/resources/ reviews/mechanisms-of-membrane-repair-and-the-novel-role-of-oral-phospholipids-lrt-and-antioxidants/#more-8180, accessed on 10 November 2012.

44. Ames, B.N. (2010) 'Optimal micronutrients delay mitochondrial decay and age-associated diseases.' *Mechanisms of Ageing and Development131*, 7–8, 473–9.

45. Alternative Medicine Review (2007) 'CoQ10: monograph.' *Alternative Medicine Review12*, 2, 159–169.

Alternative Medicine Review (2005) 'Carnitine: a monograph.' *Alternative Medicine Review* 10, 1, 42–50.

Ames 2010.

Goraca, A., Huk-Kolega, H., Piechota, A., Kleniewska, P., Ciejka, E. and Skibska, B. (2011) 'Lipoic acid – biological activity and therapeutic potential.' *Pharmacological Reports* 63, 4, 849–58.

Pekala, J., Patkowska-Sokola, B., Bodkowski, R., Jamroz, D. *et al.* (2011) 'Acetyl-L-carnitine – metabolic functions and meaning in human life.' *Current Drug Metabolism* 12, 7, 667–78.

Storch, A., Jost, W.H., Vieregge, P., Spiegel, J. *et al.* (2007) 'Randomized, double-blind, placebo-controlled trial on symptomatic effects of coenzyme Q(10) in Parkinson's disease.' *Archives of Neurology* 64, 7, 938–44.

Ash and Nicolson 2012.

Nicolson, G., Ellithorpe, R.R., Ayson-Mitchell, C., Jacques, B. and Settineri, R. (2010) 'Lipid replacement therapy with a glycophospholipid-antioxidant-vitamin formulation significantly reduces fatigue within one week.' *Journal of American Nutraceutical Association* 13, 1, 10–14.

46. López-Fando, A., Gómez-Serranillos, M.P., Iglesias, I., Lock, O. and Carratero, M.E. (2004) 'Lepidium peruvianum chacon restores homeostasis impaired by restraint stress.' *Phytotherapy Research 18*, 6, 471–4.

47. Panossian, A., Wikman, G. and Sarris, J. (2010) 'Rosenroot (rhodiola rosea): traditional use, chemical composition, pharmacology and clinical efficacy.' *Phytomedicine 17*, 7, 481-93.

48. Sarris, J., McIntyre, E. and Camfield, D.A. (2013) 'Plant-based medicines for anxiety disorders, part 2: a review of clinical studies with supporting preclinical evidence.' *CNS Drugs 27*, 4, 301–19.

49. Ishaque, S., Shamseer, L., Bukutu, C. and Vohra, S. (2012) 'Rhodiola rosea for physical and mental fatigue: a systematic review.' *BMC Complementary and Alternative Medicine 12*:70.

50. Singh, N., Bhalla, M., de Jager, P. and Gilca, M. (2011) 'An overview on ashwagandha: a Rasayana (rejuvenator) of Ayurveda.' *African Journal of Traditional Complementary and Alternative Medicines 8*, 5 Suppl, 208–13.

51. Chandrasekhar, K., Kapoor, J. and Anishetty, S. (2012) 'A prospective, randomized, double-blind, placebo-controlled study of safety and efficacy of a high-concentration full-spectrum extract of ashwagandha root in reducing stress and anxiety in adults.' *Indian Journal of Psychological Medicine 34*, 3, 255–62.

Sarris and Camfield 2013.

52. Singh *et al.* 2011.
53. Choi, K.T. (2008) 'Botanical characteristics, pharmacological effects and medicinal components of Korean Panax ginseng C A Meyer.' *Acta Pharmacological Sinica 29*, 9, 1109–18.
54. Huang, L., Zhao, H., Huang, B., Zheng, C., Peng, W. and Qin, L. (2011) 'Acanthopanax senticosus: a review of botany, chemistry and pharmacology.' *Die Pharmazie 66*, 2, 83–97.
55. Vuong, Q.V., Bowyer, M.C. and Roach, P.D. (2011) 'L-Theanine: properties, synthesis and isolation from tea.' *Journal of the Science of Food and Agriculture 91*, 11, 1931–9.
56. Yoto, A., Motoki, M., Murao, S. and Yokogoshi, H. (2012) 'Effects of L-theanine or caffeine intake on changes in blood pressure under physical and psychological stresses.' *Journal of Physiological Anthropology 31*, 28.
57. Lyon, M.R, Kapoor, M.P. and Juneja, L.R. (2011. 'The effects of L-theanine (Suntheanine®) on objective sleep quality in boys with attention deficit hyperactivity disorder (ADHD): a randomized, double-blind, placebo-controlled clinical trial.' *Alternative Medicine Review 16*, 4, 348–54.
58. National Institutes of Health (2009) *Dietary Supplement Fact Sheet: Magnesium*. Available at http://dietary-supplements.info.nih.gov/factsheets/magnesium.asp, accessed on 26 June 2012. Volpe, S.L. (2008) 'Magnesium, the metabolic syndrome, insulin resistance and type 2 diabetes mellitus.' *Critical Reviews in Food Science and Nutrition 48*, 3, 293–300.
59. Whitton, C., Nicholson, S.K., Roberts, C., Prynne, C.J. *et al.* (2011) 'National Diet and Nutrition Survey: UK food consumptions and nutrient intakes from the first year of the rolling programme and comparisons with previous surveys. Table.' *British Journal of Nutrition 106*, 12, 1899–914.
60. Chai, W. and Liebman, M. (2005) 'Effect of different cooking methods on vegetable oxalate content.' *Journal of Agricultural and Food Chemistry 53*, 8, 3027–30.
61. Lopez, H.W., Leenhardt, F. and Rémésy, C. (2004) 'New data on the bioavailability of bread magnesium.' *Magnesium Research 17*, 4, 335–40.
    Lopez, H.W., Duclos, V., Coudray, C., Krespine, V. *et al.* (2003) 'Making bread with sourdough improves mineral bioavailability from reconstituted whole wheat flour in rats.' *Nutrition 19*, 6, 524–30.
    Leenhardt, F., Levrat-Verny, M.A., Chanliaud, E. and Rémésy, C. (2005) 'Moderate decrease of pH by sourdough fermentation is sufficient to reduce phytate content of whole wheat flour through endogenous phytase activity.' *Journal of Agricultural and Food Chemistry 53*, 1, 98–102.
62. Coudray, C., Rambeau, M. and Feillet-Coudray, C. (2005) 'Dietary inulin intake and age can significantly affect intestinal absorption of calcium and magnesium in rats: a stable isotope approach.' *Nutrition Journal 4*, 29.
    Coudray, C., Demigné, C. and Rayssiguier, Y. (2003) 'Effects of dietary fibers on magnesium absorption in animals and humans.' *Journal of Nutrition 133*, 1, 1–4.
63. Johnson, S. (2001) 'The multifaceted and widespread pathology of magnesium deficiency.' *Medical Hypotheses 56*, 2, 163–70.
64. Sartori 2012.
65. Johnson 2001.
66. Barbagallo, M. and Dominguez, L.J. (2010) 'Magnesium and aging.' *Current Pharmaceutical Design 16*, 7, 832–9.
    Rosanoff, A., Weaver, C.M. and Rude, R.K. (2012) 'Suboptimal magnesium status in the US: are the health consequences underestimated?' *Nutrition Reviews 70*, 3, 153–64.
67. Barbagallo and Dominguez 2010.
68. Barbagallo and Dominguez 2010.
    Egger, G. (2012) 'In search of a germ theory equivalent for chronic disease.' *Preventing Chronic Disease 9*, E95, Epub.
69. Alraek , T., Lee, M.S., Choi, T.Y., Cao, H. and Liu, J. (2011) 'Complementary and alternative medicine for patients with CFS: a systematic review.' *BMC Complementary and Alternative Medicine 11*, 87.
70. Aydin, H., Deyneli, O., Yavuz, D., Gözü, H. *et al.* (2010) 'Short-term oral magnesium supplementation suppresses bone turnover in postmenopausal osteoporotic women.' *Biological Trace Element Research 133*, 2, 136–43.

Stendig-Lindberg, G., Tepper, R. and Leichter, I. (1993) 'Trabecular bone density in a two year controlled trial of peroral magnesium in osteoporosis.' *Magnes Research 6*, 2, 155–63.

71. Meisel, P., Schwahn, C., Luedemann, J., John, U., Kroemer, H.K. and Kocher, T. (2005) 'Magnesium deficiency is associated with periodontal disease.' *Journal of Dental Research 84*, 10, 937–41.

72. Song *et al.* 2004.
    Larsson, S.C. and Wolk, A. (2007) 'Magnesium intake and risk of type 2 diabetes: a meta-analysis.' *Journal of Internal Medicine 262*, 208.

73. Rumawas, M.E., McKeown, N.M., Rogers, G., Meigs, J.B., Wilson, P.W. and Jacques, P.F. (2006) 'Magnesium intake is related to improved insulin homeostasis in the Framingham Offspring cohort.' *Journal of the American College of Nutrition 25*, 6, 486–92.
    Ma, B., Lawson, A.B., Liese, A.D., Bell, R.A. and Mayer-Davis, E.J. (2006) 'Dairy, magnesium and calcium intake in relation to insulin sensitivity: approaches to modeling a dose-dependent association.' *American Journal of Epidemiology 164*, 5, 449–58.
    Song *et al.* 2004.

74. Pham, P.C., Pham, P.M., Pham, S.V., Miller, J.M. and Pham, P.T. (2007) 'Hypomagnesemia in patients with type 2 diabetes.' *Clinical Journal of the American Society of Nephrology 2*, 2, 366–73.

75. Mooren, F.C., Krüger, K., Völker, K., Golf, S.W., Wadepuhl, M. and Kraus, A. (2011) 'Oral magnesium supplementation reduces insulin resistance in non-diabetic subjects – a double-blind, placebo-controlled, randomized trial.' *Diabetes, Obesity and Metabolism 13*, 3, 281–4.

76. Barbagallo and Dominguez 2007.
    Rodriguez-Moran, M. and Guerro-Romero, F. (2003) 'Oral magnesium supplementation improves insulin sensitivity and metabolic control in type 2 diabetic subjects: a randomized double-blind controlled trial.' *Diabetes Care 26*, 4, 1147–52.
    Yokota, K., Kato, M., Lister, F., Ii, H. *et al.* (2004) 'Clinical efficacy of magnesium supplementation in patients with type 2 diabetes.' *Journal of the American College of Nutrition 23*, 5, 506S–509S.

77. Rosanoff, A. (2005) 'Magnesium and hypertension.' *Clinical Calcium 15*, 2, 255–60.

78. Dickinson, H.O., Nicolson, D.J., Campbell, F., Cook, J.V. *et al.* (2006) 'Magnesium supplementation for the management of essential hypertension in adults.' *Cochrane Database of Systematic Reviews 3*, CD004640.
    Cheriyan, J., O'Shaughnessy, K.M. and Brown, M.J. (2010) 'Primary prevention of CVD: treating hypertension. *Clinical Evidence (Online) 18*, pii: 0214.
    Jee, S.H., Miller, E.R. 3rd, Guallar, E., Singh, V.K., Appel, L.J. and Klag, M.J. (2002) 'The effect of magnesium supplementation on blood pressure: a meta-analysis of randomized clinical trials.' *American Journal of Hypertension 15*, 8, 691–6.

79. Lasserre, B., Spoerri, M., Moullet, V. and Theubet, M.P. (1994) 'Should magnesium therapy be considered for the treatment of coronary heart disease? ii. Epidemiological evidence in outpatients with and without coronary heart disease.' *Magnesium Research 7*, 2, 145–53.

80. Almoznino-Sarafian, D., Berman, S. and Mor, A. (2007) 'Magnesium and C-reactive protein in heart failure: an anti-inflammatory effect of magnesium administration?' *European Journal of Nutrition 46*, 4, 230–7.
    Stepura, O.B. and Martynow, A.I. (2008) 'Magnesium orotate in severe congestive heart failure (MACH).' *International Journal of Cardiology 131*, 2, 293–5.

81. Coudray, C., Rambeau, M., Feillet-Coudray, C., Gueux, E. *et al.* (2005) 'Study of magnesium bioavailability from organic and inorganic Mg salts in Mg-depleted rats using a stable isotope approach.' *Magnesium Research 18*, 4, 215–23.
    Spasov, A.A., Petrov, V.I., Iezhitsa, I.N., Kravchenko, M.S., Kharitonova, M.V. and Ozerov, A.A. (2010) 'Comparative study of magnesium salts bioavailability in rats fed a magnesium-deficient diet.' *Vestnik Rossiĭskoĭ Akademii Meditsinskikh Nauk 2*, 29–37.
    Walker, A.F., Marakis, G., Christie, S. and Byng, M. (2003) 'Mg citrate found more bioavailable than other Mg preparations in a randomised, double-blind study.' *Magnesium Research 16*, 3, 183–91.

82. Firoz, M. and Graber, M. (2001) 'Bioavailability of US commercial magnesium preparations.' *Magnesium Research 14*, 4, 257–62.

CHAPTER 7

1. Dvir, Y. and Smallwood, P. (2008) 'Serotonin syndrome: a complex but easily avoidable condition.' *General Hospital Psychiatry 30*, 3, 284–7.

2. Puri, B. and Lynam, H. (2010) 'Dysregulated Neurotransmitter Function.' In L. Nicolle and A. Woodriff Beirne (eds) *Biochemical Imbalances in Disease.* London: Singing Dragon.

3. Higgins, J.P. and Flicker, L. (2001) 'Lecithin for dementia and cognitive impairment.' *Cochrane Database of Systematic Reviews 3*, CD001015.

4. Allen, P.J. and Feigin, A. (2013) 'Gene-based therapies in Parkinson's Disease.' *Neurotherapeutics 11*, 1, 60–7.

5. Ray, L.A. and Courtney, K.E. (2012) 'Pharmacogenetics of alcoholism: a clinical neuroscience perspective.' *Pharmacogenomics 13*, 2, 129–32.

6. Wise, R.A. (1996) 'Neurobiology of addiction.' *Current Opinion in Neurobiology 6*, 2, 243–51.

7. Avena, N.M. and Bocarsly, M.E. (2011) 'Dysregulation of brain reward systems in eating disorders: Neurochemical information from animal models of binge eating, bulimia nervosa and anorexia nervosa.' *Neuropharmacology 63*, 1, 87–96.

8. Birmingham, C.L. and Gritzner, S. (2006) 'How does zinc supplementation benefit anorexia nervosa?' *Eating and Weight Disorders 11*, 4, e109–11.

9. Gardner, A. and Boles, R.G. (2011) 'Beyond the serotonin hypothesis: mitochondria, inflammation and neurodegeneration in major depression and affective spectrum disorders.' *Progress in Neuro-Psychopharmacology and Biological Psychiatry 35*, 3, 730–43.
   Kidd, P. (2005) 'Neurodegeneration from mitochondrial insufficiency: nutrients, stem cells, growth factors and prospects for brain rebuilding using integrative management.' *Alternative Medicine Review 10*, 4, 268–92.

10. Rao, V.K., Carlson, E.A. and Yan, S.S. (2013) 'Mitochondrial permeability transition pore is a potential drug target for neurodegeneration.' *Biochimica et Biophysica Acta*, Epub ahead of print.

11. Gautier, C.A, Corti, O. and Brice, A. (2013) 'Mitochondrial dysfunctions in Parkinson's disease.' *Revue Neurologique (Paris)*, Epub ahead of print.

12. Hebert, S.L., Lanza, I.R. and Nair, K.S. (2010) 'Mitochondrial DNA alterations and reduced mitochondrial function in aging.' *Mechanisms of Ageing and Development 131*, 7–8, 451–62.

13. Ferrer, I., Martinez, A., Blanco, R., Dalfó, E. and Carmona, M. (2011) 'Neuropathology of sporadic Parkinson disease before the appearance of parkinsonism: preclinical Parkinson disease.' *Journal of Neural Transmission 118*, 5, 821–39.

14. Gorąca, A., Huk-Kolega, H., Piechota, A., Kleniweska, P., Ciejka, E. and Skibska, B. (2011). Lipoic acid – biological activity and therapeutic potential. *Pharmacological Reports 63*, 4, 849–58.
   Gardner, A. and Boles, R.G. (2011) 'Beyond the serotonin hypothesis: mitochondria, inflammation and neurodegeneration in major depression and affective spectrum disorders.' *Progress in Neuro-Psychopharmacology and Biological Psychiatry 35*, 3, 730–43.
   Ash, M. and Nicolson, G. (2012) 'Mechanisms of membrane repair and the novel role of oral phospholipids (Lipid Replacement Therapy®) and antioxidants to improve membrane function. *Nutri-Link Clinical Education.* Available at www.nleducation.co.uk/resources/ reviews/mechanisms-of-membrane-repair-and-the-novel-role-of-oral-phospholipids-lrt-and-antioxidants/#more-8180, accessed on 10 November 2012.
   Kidd 2005 as above).

15. Ames, B.N. (2010) 'Optimal micronutrients delay mitochondrial decay and age-associated diseases.' *Mechanisms of Ageing and Development 131*, 7–8, 473–9.

16. Bentler, S.E., Mart, A.J. and Kuhn, E.M. (2005) 'Prospective observational study of treatments for unexplained chronic fatigue.' *Journal of Clinical Psychiatry 66*, 5, 625–32.
   Alternative Medicine Review (2007) 'CoQ10 monograph.' *Alternative Medicine Review 12*, 2, 159–69.
   Gardner and Boles 2011; Kidd 2005.
   ODS (Office of Dietary Supplements) (2006) *Carnitine dietary supplement fact sheet.* National Institutes of Health. Available at http://ods.od.nih.gov/factsheets/Carnitine-HealthProfessional, accessed on 28 January 2014.

Ash, M. (2012) Mechanisms of membrane repair and the novel role of oral phospholipids (lipid replacement therapy) and AOs to improve membrane function. *NL Education.* Available at www.nleducation.co.uk/resources/reviews/mechanisms-of-membrane-repair-and-the-novel-role-of-oral-phospholipids-lrt-and-antioxidants/#more-8180, accessed on 10 November 2012.

17. Nathan, P.J., Lu, K., Gray, M. and Oliver, C. (2006) 'The neuropharmacology of L-theanine (N-ethyl-L-glutamine): a possible neuroprotective and cognitive enhancing agent.' *Journal of Herbal Pharmacotherapy 6,* 2, 21-30.

    Higashiyama, A., Htay, H.H., Ozeki, M., Juneja, L.R. and Kapoor, M.P. (2011) 'Effects of L-theanine on attention and reaction time response.' *Journal of Functional Foods 3,* 3, 171–8.

    Park, S.K., Jung, I.C., Lee, W.K., Lee, Y.S. *et al.* (2011) 'A combination of green tea extract and L-theanine improves memory and attention in subjects with mild cognitive impairment: a double-blind placebo-controlled study.' *Journal of Medicinal Food 14,* 4, 334–43.

18. Kelly, S.P., Gomez-Ramirez, M., Montesi, J.L. and Foxe, J.J. (2008) 'L-theanine and caffeine in combination affect human cognition as evidenced by oscillatory alpha-band activity and attention task performance.' *Journal of Nutrition 138,* 8, 1572S–1577S.

19. Kirby, S. (2005) 'The positive effects of exercise as a therapy for clinical depression.' *Nursing Times 10,* 13, 28–9.

    Blumenthal, J., Babyak, M.A., Doraiswamy, M., Watkins, L. *et al.* (2007) 'Exercise and pharmacotherapy in the treatment of major depressive disorder.' *Psychosomatic Medicine 69,* 7, 587–96.

20. Martin, B., Mattson, M.P. and Maudsley, S. (2006) 'Caloric restriction and intermittent fasting: two potential diets for successful brain ageing.' *Ageing Research Reviews 5,* 3, 332–53.

21. Gusmão, R., Quintão, S., McDaid, D., Arensman, E. *et al.* (2013) 'Antidepressant utilization and suicide in Europe: an ecological multi-national study.' *PLoS One 8,* 6, e66455.

22. Netdoctor Guide (n.d.) 'Noradrenaline (Norepinephrine).' Available at www.netdoctor.co.uk/heart-and-blood/medicines/noradrenaline.html, accessed on 28 January 2014.

23. Chau, K., Atkinson, S.A. and Taylor, V.H. (2012) 'Are selective serotonin reuptake inhibitors a secondary cause of low bone density?' *Journal of Osteoporosis,* article ID 323061.

    Wu, A., Bencaz, A.F., Hentz, J.G. and Crowell, M.D. (2012) 'Selective serotonin reuptake inhibitors treatment and risk of fractures: a meta-analysis of cohort case-control studies.' *Osteoporosis International 23,* 1, 365–75.

24. Swaab, D.F., Bao, A.M. and Lucassen, P.J. (2005) 'The stress system in the human brain in depression and neurodegeneration.' *Aging Research Reviews 4,* 2, 141–94.

    McEwan, B.S. (2006) 'Protective and damaging effects of stress mediators: central role of the brain.' *Dialogues in Clinical Neuroscience 8,* 4, 367–81).

25. Fetissov, S.O. and Dechelotte, P. (2011) 'The new link between gut-brain axis and neuropsychiatric disorders.' *Current Opinion in Clinical Nutrition and Metabolic Care 14,* 5, 447–82).

    Maes, M., Kubera, M. and Leunis, J.C. (2008) 'The gut–brain barrier in major depression: intestinal mucosal dysfunction with an increased translocation of LPS from gram negative enterobacterial (leaky gut) plays a role in the inflammatory pathophysiology of depression.' *Neuro Endocrinology Letters 29,* 1, 117–24.

26. Harvard Medical School (2006) *Importance of Sleep: Six Reasons Not to Scrimp on Sleep.* Harvard Health Publications. Available at www.health.harvard.edu/press_releases/importance_of_sleep_and_health, accessed on 28 January 2014.

27. Puri and Lynam 2010.

28. Neil, K. (2010) 'Sex Hormone Imbalances.' In L. Nicolle and A. Woodriff Beirne (eds) *Biochemical Imbalances in Disease.* London: Singing Dragon.

29. Buettner, D. (2008) *Blue Zones: Lessons for Living Longer from the People Who've Lived the Longest.* Washington, DC: National Geographic.

30. Neuhoff, C.C. and Schaefer C (2002) 'Effects of laughing, smiling, and howling on mood.' *Psychological Reports 91,* 3 Pt 2, 1079–80.

31. Seasonal Affective Disorder: information, advice and answers from the UK voluntary organisation. Available at www.sad.org.uk, accessed on 21 October 2013.

32. Howland, R.H. (2009) 'An overview of seasonal affective disorder and its treatment options.' *Physician and Sports Medicine 37,* 4, 104–15.

33. Ganji, V., Milone, C., Cody, M.M., McCarty, F. and Wang, Y.T. (2010) 'Serum vitamin D concentrations are related to depression in young adult US population: the Third National Health and Nutrition Examination Survey.' *International Archives of Medicine* 3, 29.

34. Zhang, R. and Naughton, D.P. (2010) 'Vitamin D in health and disease: current perspectives.' *Nutrition Journal 9*, 65.

35. Pogge, E. (2010) 'Vitamin D and Alzheimer's disease: is there a link?' *Consultant Pharmacist 25*, 7, 440–50.

36. Zwart, J.A., Dyb, G., Hagen, K., Ødegård, K.J. *et al.* (2003) 'Depression and anxiety disorders associated with headache frequency. The Nord-Trøndelag Health Study.' *European Journal of Neurology 102*, 2, 147–52.

37. Puri and Lynam 2010.

38. Kokayi, K., Altman, C.H., Callely, R.W. and Harrison, A. (2006) 'Findings of and treatment for high levels of mercury and lead toxicity in Ground Zero rescue and recovery workers and lower Manhattan residents.' *Explore (New York) 2*, 5, 400–7.

39. Shaw, K., Turner, J. and Del Mar, C. (2002) 'Tryptophan and 5-hydroxytryptophan for depression.' *Cochrane Database of Systematic Reviews* 1, CD003198.
     Turner, E.H., Loftis, J.M. and Blackwell, A.D. (2006) 'Serotonin à la carte: supplementation with the serotonin precursor 5-hydroxytryptophan.' *Pharmacology and Therapeutics 109*, 3, 325–38.

40. Karakula, H., Opolska, S., Kowal, A., Domański, M., Plotka, A. and Perzyński, J. (2009) 'Does diet affect our mood? The significance of folic acid and homocysteine.' *Polski Merkuriusz Lekarski 26*, 152, 136–41.

41. Kado, D.M., Karlamangla, A.S., Huang, M.H., Troen, A. *et al.* (2005) 'Homocysteine versus the vitamins folate, B6, and B12 as predictors of cognitive function and decline in older high-functioning adults: MacArthur Studies of Successful Aging.' *American Journal of Medicine 118*, 2, 161–7.

42. Douaud, G., Refsum, H., de Jager, C.A., Jacoby, R. *et al.* (2013) 'Preventing Alzheimer's disease-related gray matter atrophy by B-vitamin treatment.' *Proceedings of the National Academy of Sciences of the USA 110*, 23, 9523–8.

43. Tiemeier, H., van Tuijl, H.R., Hofman, A., Meijer, J., Kiliaan, A.J. and Breteler, M.M.B. (2002) 'Vitamin B12, folate, and homocysteine in depression: the Rotterdam Study.' *American Journal of Psychiatry 159*, 12, 2099–101.
     Ebesunun, M.O., Eruvulobi, H.U., Olangunju, T. and Owoeye, O.A. (2012) 'Elevated plasma homocysteine in association with decreased vitamin B(12), folate, serotonin, lipids and lipoproteins in depressed patients.' *African Journal of Psychiatry (Johannesburg) 15*, 1, 25–9.

44. Abou-Saleh, M.T. and Coppen, A. (2006) 'Folic acid and the treatment of depression.' *Journal of Psychosomatic Research 61*, 3, 285–7.

45. Douaud *et al.* 2013.

46. Coppen, A. and Bolander-Gouaille, C. (2005) 'Treatment of depression: time to consider folic acid and vitamin B12.' *Journal of Psychopharmacology 19*, 1, 59–65.

47. Scaglione, F. and Panzavolta, G.(2014) 'Folate, folic acid and 5-methyltetrahydrofolate are not the same thing.' Xenobiotica, Epub ahead of print.
     Jennings, B.A. and Willis, G. (2014) 'How folate metabolism affects colorectal cancer development and treatment; a story of heterogeneity and pleiotropy.' Cancer Letters pii: S0304-3835(14)00131-1. doi: 10.1016/j.canlet.2014.02.024, Epub ahead of print.

48. Manshadi, D., Ishiguro L., Sohn, K.J., Medline, A. et al (2014). 'Folic Acid supplementation promotes mammary tumor progression in a rat model'. PLoS One 9(1):e84635. doi: 10.1371/journal.pone.0084635. eCollection 2014).

49. Lindzon, G.M., Medline, A., Sohn, K.J., Depeint, F., Croxford, R., Kim Y.I. (2009) 'Effect of folic acid supplementation on the progression of colorectal aberrant crypt foci'. Carcinogenesis (9):1536-43. doi: 10.1093/carcin/bgp152, Epub 18 June, 2009.

50. Jennings and Willis 2014.

51. Vollset, S.E., Clarke, R., Lewington, S., Ebbing, M. et al. (2013) 'Effects of folic acid supplementation on overall and site-specific cancer incidence during the randomised trials: meta-analyses of data on 50,000 individuals'. Lancet 381 (9871):1029-36.

52.   British Dietetic Association (2013) Folic Acid Food Fact Sheet. Available from: www.bda. uk.com/foodfacts/FolicAcid.pdf, accessed 2 April, 2014.

53.   Swardfager, W., Hermann, N., Mazereeuw, G., Goldberger, K., Harimoto, T. and Lanctôt, K.L. (2013) 'Zinc in depression: a meta-analysis.' *Biological Psychiatry 74*, 12 ,872–8.

54.   Swardfager, W., Hermann, N., McIntyre, R.S., Mazereeuw, G. *et al.* (2013) 'Potential roles of zinc in the pathophysiology and treatment of major depressive disorder.' *Neuroscience and Biobehavioral Reviews 37*, 5, 911–29.

      Lai, J., Moxey, A., Nowak, G., Vashum, K., Bailey, K. and McEvoy, M. (2012) 'The efficacy of zinc supplementation in depression: systematic review of randomised controlled trials.' *Journal of Affective Disorders 136*, 1–2, e31–9.

55.   Oma, S., Mawatari, S., Saito, K., Wakana, C. *et al.* (2012) 'Changes in phospholipid composition of erythrocyte membrane in Alzheimer's disease.' *Dementia and Geriatric Cognitive Disorders Extra 2*, 1, 298–303.

56.   Richter, Y., Herzog, Y., Lifshitz, Y., Hayun, R. and Zchut, S. (2013) 'The effect of soybean-derived phosphatidylserine on cognitive performance in elderly with subjective memory complaints: a pilot study.' *Clinical Interventions in Aging 8*, 557–63.

      Vakhapova, V., Cohen, T., Richter, Y., Herzog, Y. and Korczyn, A.D. (2010) 'Phosphatidylserine containing omega-3 fatty acids may improve memory abilities in non-demented elderly with memory complaints: a double-blind placebo-controlled trial.' *Dementia and Geriatric Cognitive Disorders 29*, 5, 467–74.

      Kidd, P.M. (2008) 'Alzheimer's disease, amnestic mild cognitive impairment, and age-associated memory impairment: current understanding and progress toward integrative prevention.' *Alternative Medicine Review 13*, 2, 85–115.

57.   Liu, S.H., Chang, C.D., Chen, P.H., Su, J.R., Chen, C.C. and Chaung, H.C. (2012) 'Docosahexaenoic acid and phosphatidylserine supplementations improve antioxidant activities and cognitive functions of the developing brain on pentylenetetrazol-induced seizure model.' *Brain Research 1451*, 19–26.

58.   Vakhapova *et al.* 2010.

59.   Yurko-Mauro, K. (2010) 'Cognitive and cardiovascular benefits of DHA in aging and cognitive decline.' *Current Alzheimer Research 7*, 3, 190–6.

60.   Hanciles, S. and Pimlott, Z. (2010) 'PUFAs in the Brain.' In L. Nicolle and A. Woodriff Beirne (2010) *Biochemical Imbalances in Disease*. London: Singing Dragon.

61.   Sublette, M.E., Ellis, S.P., Geant, A.L. and Mann, J.J. (2011) Meta-analysis: effects of eicosapentaenoic acid in clinical trials in depression.' *Journal of Clinical Psychiatry 72*, 12, 1577–84.

      Martins, J.G. (2009) 'EPA but not DHA appears to be responsible for the efficacy of omega-3 long chain polyunsaturated fatty acid supplementation in depression: evidence from a meta-analysis of randomized controlled trials.' *Journal of the American College of Nutrition 28*, 5, 25–42.

62.   Savage, V.M. and West, G.B. (2007) 'A quantitative, theoretical framework for understanding mammalian sleep.' *Proceedings of the National Academy of Sciences of the USA 104*, 3, 1051–6.

63.   Machi, M.S., Staum, M., Callaway, C.W., Moore, C. *et al.* (2012) 'The relationship between shift work, sleep and cognition in career emergency physicians.' *Academic Emergency Medicine 19*, 1, 85–91.

      Carskadon, M.A. (2011) 'Sleep's effects on cognition and learning in adolescence.' *Progress in Brain Research 190*, 137–43.

64.   Wang, G., Grone, B., Colas, D., Appelbaum, L. and Mourrain, P. (2011) 'Synaptic plasticity in sleep: learning, homeostasis and disease.' *Trends in Neuroscience 34*, 9, 452–63.

65.   Shaw, C.A. and Tomljenovic, L. (2013) 'Aluminum in the central nervous system (CNS): toxicity in humans and animals, vaccine adjuvants, and autoimmunity.' *Immunologic Research 56*, 2–3, 304–16.

66.   Annweiler, C., Rolland, Y., Schott, A.M., Blain, H. *et al.* (2012) 'Higher vitamin D dietary intake is associated with lower risk of Alzheimer's disease: A 7-year follow-up.' *Journals of Gerontology, Series A, Biological Sciences and Medical Sciences 67*, 11, 1205–11.

67.   Nakano, M., Ubukata, K., Yamamoto, T. and Yamaguchi, H. (2009) 'Effect of pyrroloquinoline quinone (PQQ) on mental status of middle-aged and elderly persons.' *FOOD Style 13*, 7, 50–3.

68. Mahncke, H.W., Bronstone, A. and Merzenich, M.M. (2006) 'Brain plasticity and functional losses in the aged: scientific bases for a novel intervention' *Progress in Brain Research 157*, 81–109.

69. Villaflores, O.B., Chen, Y.J., Chen, C.P., Yeh, J.M. and Wu, T.Y. (2012) 'Curcuminoids and resveratrol as anti-Alzheimer agents.' *Taiwanese Journal of Obstetrics and Gynecology 51*, 4, 515–25.

CHAPTER 8

1. British Pain Society/Galliard Health (2005) 'Pain Survey.' Available at www.britishpainsociety.org/media_surveys.htm, accessed on 31 October 2010.

2. NINDS (National Institute of Neurological Disorders and Stroke) (2001) 'Pain: Hope through Research.' Available at www.ninds.nih.gov/disorders/chronic_pain/detail_chronic_pain.htm, accessed on 28 January 2014.

3. Lloyd, D. and Redmond, N. (2013) 'Does the brain change in response to chronic low back pain?' Pain Relief Foundation. Available at www.painrelieffoundation.org.uk/docs/brain_response_low_back_pain.pdf, accessed on 3 October 2013.

4. Kearney, P.M., Baigent, C., Godwin, J., Halls, H., Emberson, J.R. and Patrono, C. (2006) 'Do selective cyclo-oxygenase-2 inhibitors and traditional non-steroidal anti-inflammatory drugs increase the risk of atherothrombosis? Meta-analysis of randomised trials.' *British Medical Journal 332*, 7553, 1302–8.

5. Katz, N. and Mazer, N.A. (2009) 'The impact of opioids on the endocrine system.' *Clinical Journal of Pain 25*, 2, 170–5.

6. Black, C., Clar, C., Henderson, R., MacEachern, C. *et al.* (2009) 'The clinical effectiveness of glucosamine and chondroitin supplements in slowing or arresting the progression of osteoarthritis of the knee: a systematic review and economic evaluation.' Health and Technology Assessment 13, 52. Available at http://www.hta.ac.uk/fullmono/mon1352.pdf, accessed on 28 January 2014.

   Herrero-Beaumont, G., Ivorra, J.A., Del Carmen Trabado, M., Blanco, F.J. *et al.* (2007) 'Glucosamine sulfate in the treatment of knee osteoarthritis symptoms: a randomized, double-blind, placebo-controlled study using acetaminophen as a side comparator.' *Arthritis and Rheumatism 56*, 2, 555–67.

   Poolsup, N., Suthisisang, C., Channark, P. and Kittikulsuth, W. (2005) 'Glucosamine long-term treatment and the progression of knee osteoarthritis: systematic review of randomized controlled trials.' *Annals of Pharmacotherapy 39*, 6, 1080–7.

7. Wu, D., Huang, Y., Gu, Y. and Fan, W. (2013) 'Efficacies of different preparations of glucosamine for the treatment of osteoarthritis: a meta-analysis of randomised, double-blind, placebo-controlled trials.' *International Journal of Clinical Practice 67*, 6, 585–94.

8. Debbi, E.M., Agar, G., Fichman, G., Ziv, Y.B. *et al.* (2011) 'Efficacy of methylsulfonylmethane supplementation on osteoarthritis of the knee: a randomized controlled study.' *BMC Complementary and Alternative Medicine 11*, 50.

9. Egger, G. (2012) 'In search of a germ theory equivalent for chronic disease.' *Preventing Chronic Disease*, Epub 10 May 2012.

10. Fasano, A. (2011) 'Zonulin and its regulation of intestinal barrier function: the biological door to inflammation, autoimmunity and cancer.' *Physiological Reviews 91*, 1, 151–75.

11. Fasano, A. and Shea-Donohue, T. (2005) 'Mechanisms of disease: the role of intestinal barrier function in the pathogenesis of GI autoimmune diseases.' *Nature Clinical Practice, Gastroenterology and Hepatology 2*, 9, 416–22.

12. Ash, M, (2010) 'Vitamin A: The key to a tolerant immune system?' *Focus: Allergy Research News*, August. Available at www.allergyresearchgroup.com/August-2010-Focus/Vitamin-A-sp-107.html, accessed on 3 April 2014.

13. Fasano (2011)

    Zhao, Y., Qin, G., Sun, Z., Che, D., Bao, N. and Zhang, X. (2011) 'Effects of soybean agglutinin on intestinal barrier permeability and tight junction protein expression in weaned piglets.' *International Journal of Molecular Sciences 12*, 12, 8502–12.

Dalla Pellegrina, C., Perbellini, O., Scupoli, M.T., Tomelleri, C. *et al.* (2009) 'Effects of wheat germ agglutinin on human gastrointestinal epithelium: insights from an experimental model of immune/epithelial cell interaction.' *Toxicology and Applied Pharmacology* 237, 2, 146–53.

Katsuya, M., Tanada, T. and McNeil, P. (2007) 'Lectin-based food poisoning: a new mechanism of protein toxicity.' *PLoS ONE* 2, 8, e687.

14. Issazadeh-Navikas, S., Teimer, R. and Bockermann, R. (2011) 'Influence of dietary components of regulatory T cells.' *Molecular Medicine 18*, 1, 95–110.

15. Gomez Candela, C., Bermejo Lopez, L.M. and Loria Kohen, V. (2011) 'Importance of a balanced omega 6/omega 3 ratio for the maintenance of health: nutritional recommendations.' *Nutrición Hospitalaria 26*, 2, 323–9.

Cordain, L., Eaton, S.B., Sebastian, A., Mann, N. *et al.* (2005) 'Origins and evolution of the Western diet: health implications for the 21st century.' *American Journal of Clinical Nutrition 81*, 2, 341–54.

Simopoulos, A.P. (2008) 'The importance of the omega-6/omega-3 fatty acid ratio in cardiovascular disease and other chronic diseases.' *Experimental Biology and Medicine (Maywood) 233*, 6, 674–88.

16. Committee on the Medical Aspects of Food Policy (1991) *Dietary Reference Values for Food Energy and Nutrients for the UK. Report of the Panel on DRVs of the COMA.* London: Department of Health.

17. Horrobin, D.F. (1993) 'The effects of gamma-linolenic acid on breast pain and diabetic neuropathy: possible non-eicosanoid mechanisms.' *Prostaglandins Leukotrienes and Essential Fatty Acids 48*, 1, 101–4.

Ranieri, M., Sciuscio, M., Cortese, A.M., Santamato, A. *et al.* (2009) 'The use of alpha-lipoic acid (ALA), gamma linolenic acid (GLA) and rehabilitation in the treatment of back pain: effect on health-related quality of life.' *International Journal of Immunopathology and Pharmacology 22*, 3 Suppl, 45–50.

18. Arterburn, L.M., Hall, E.B. and Oken, H. (2006) 'Distribution, interconversion and dose response of omega 3 fatty acids in humans.' *American Journal of Clinical Nutrition 83*, 6, Suppl, 1467–76S.

Gomez Candela *et al.* 2011.

Anderson, B.M. and Ma, D.W. (2009) 'Are all omega 3 polyunsaturated fatty acids created equal?' *Lipids in Health and Disease 10*, 8, 33.

19. Jackson, A. (2004) *Scientific Advisory Committee on Nutrition. Advice on Fish Consumption: Benefits and Risks. Committee on Toxicity.* London: Stationery Office.

20. Sustain (2005) 'Like shooting fish in a barrel.' Available at www.sustainweb.org/foodfacts/like_shooting_fish_in_a_barrel, accessed on 25 September 2013.

21. Kidd, P.M. (2007) 'Omega-3 DHA and EPA for cognition, behavior, and mood: clinical findings and structural-functional synergies with cell membrane phospholipids.' *Alternative Medicine Review 12*, 3, 207–227.

22. Ratnayake, W.M.N., Behrens, W.A., Fischer, P.W.F., L'Abbé, M.R., Mongeau, P. and Beare-Rogers, J.L. (1992) 'Chemical and nutritional studies of flaxseed (variety Linott) in rats.' *Journal of Nutritional Biochemistry 3*, 232–40.

Manthey, F.A., Lee, R.E. and Hall III, C.A. (2001) 'Processing and cooking effects on lipid content and stability of alpha-linolenic acid in spaghetti containing ground flaxseed.' *Journal of Agricultural and Food Chemistry 50*, 1668–71.

23. Willett, W.C. (2006) 'Ask the doctor. I have heard that coconut is bad for the heart and that it is good for the heart. Which is right?' *Harvard Heart Letter 17*, 1, 8.

Feranil, A.B., Duazo, P.L., Kuzaka, C.W. and Adair, L.S. (2011) 'Coconut oil is associated with a beneficial lipid profile in premenopausal women in the Philippines.' *Asia Pacific Journal of Clinical Nutrition 20*, 2, 190–5.

24. Clegg, M.E. (2010) 'Medium-chain triglycerides are advantageous in promoting weight loss although not beneficial to exercise performance.' *International Journal of Food Sciences and Nutrition 61*, 7, 653–79.

St-Onge, M.P. (2005) 'Dietary fats, teas, dairy and nuts: potential functional foods for weight control?' *American Journal of Clinical Nutrition 81*, 1, 7–15.

25. Ellis, K.A., Innocent, G., Grove-White, D., Cripps, P. *et al.* (2006) 'Comparing the fatty acid composition of organic and conventional milk.' *Journal of Dairy Science 89*, 6, 1938–50.

Daley, C.A., Abbott, A., Doyle, P.S., Nader, G.A. and Larson, S. (2010) 'A review of fatty acid profiles and antioxidant content in grass-fed and grain-fed beef.' *Nutrition Journal 10*, 9–10.

26. Derbyshire, E. (2012) 'Trans fats: implications for health.' *Nursing Standard 27*, 3, 51–6.

27. Hewison, M. (2010) 'Vitamin D and the immune system: new perspectives on an old theme.' *Endocrinology and Metabolism Clinics of North America 39*, 2, 365–79.

28. Bell, D.S. (2011) 'Protean manifestations of vitamin D deficiency, part 3: association with cardiovascular disease and disorders of the central and peripheral nervous systems.' *Southern Medical Journal 104*, 5, 340–4.

29. Hewison 2010.

Zhang, R. and Naughton, D.P. (2010) 'Vitamin D in health and disease: current perspectives.' *Nutrition Journal 9*, 65.

Holick, M.F. (2008) 'The vitamin D deficiency pandemic and consequences for nonskeletal health: mechanisms of action.' *Molecular Aspects of Medicine 29*, 6, 361–8.

Kivity, S., Agmon-Levin, N., Zisapplk, M., Shapira, Y. *et al.* (2011) 'Vitamin D and autoimmune thyroid diseases.' *Cellular and Molecular Immunology 8*, 243–7.

30. Gloth F.M. 3rd and Greenough, W.B. 3rd. (2004) 'Vitamin D deficiency as a contributor to multiple forms of chronic pain.' *Mayo Clinic Proceedings 79*, 5, 696, 699; author reply, 699.

31. Gillie, O. (2006) 'A new government policy is needed for sunlight and vitamin D.' *British Journal of Dermatology 154*, 1052–61.

Gillie, O. (2011) 'Sunlight robbery: the failure of UK policy on vitamin D. In search of evidence-based public health policy.' Presentation at the Vitamin D Experts' Forum, London, April 2011.

32. Heaney, R.P. and Holick, M.F. (2011) 'Why the IOM recommendations for vitamin D are deficient.' *Journal of Bone and Mineral Research 26*, 3, 455–7.

Baggerly, C. and Garland, C. (2011) 'Vitamin D and breast cancer prevention.' Presentation at the Vitamin D Experts' Forum, London, April 2011.

33. Amsterdam, A., Tafima, K. and Sasson, R. (2002) 'Cell-specific regulation of apoptosis by glucocorticoids: implication to their anti-inflammatory action.' *Biochemical Pharmacology 64*, 5–6, 843–50.

34. Silverman, M.N. and Sternberg, E.M. (2012) 'Glucocorticoid regulation of inflammation and its functional correlates: from HPA axis to glucocorticoid receptor dysfunction.' *Annals of the New York Academy of Sciences 1261*, 55–63.

35. Nicolle, L. and Hallam, A. (2010) 'PUFA Imbalances.' In L. Nicolle and A. Woodriff Beirne (eds) (2010) *Biochemical Imbalances in Disease.* London: Singing Dragon.

36. Scotece, M., Conde, J., Gómez, R., López, V. *et al.* (2011) 'Beyond fat mass: exploring the role of adipokines in rheumatic diseases.' *Scientific World Journal 11*, 1932–47.

37. Fain, J.N. (2006) 'Release of interleukins and other inflammatory cytokines by human adipose tissue is enhanced in obesity and primarily due to the nonfat cells.' *Vitamins and Hormones 74*, 443–77.

38. Reeh, P. and Steen, K. (1996) 'Tissue Acidosis in Nociception and Pain.' In T. Kumazawa, L. Kruger and K. Mizumara (eds) *Progress in Brain Research.* Philadelphia, PA: Elsevier.

Pizzorno, J., Frassetto, L. and Katzinger, J. (2009) 'Diet-induced acidosis: is it real and clinically relevant?' *British Journal of Nutrition 103*, 8, 1185–94.

Voilley, N., de Weille, J., Mamet, J. and Lazdunski, M. (2001) 'NSAIDs inhibit both the activity and the inflammatory-induced expression of acid-sensing ion channels in nociceptors.' *Journal of Neuroscience 21*, 20, 8026–33.

39. Hale, L.P., Greer, P.K. and Sempowski, G.D. (2002) 'Bromelain treatment alters leukocyte expression of cell surface molecules involved in cellular adhesion and activation.' *Clinical Immunology 104*, 2, 183–90.

Fitzhugh, D.J., Shan, S., Dewhirst, M.W. and Hale, L.P. (2008) 'Bromelain treatment decreases neutrophil migration to sites of inflammation.' *Clinical Immunology 128*, 1, 66–74.

40. Akhtar, N.M., Naseer, R., Farooqi, A.Z., Aziz, W. and Nazir, M. (2004) 'Oral enzyme combination versus diclofenac in the treatment of osteoarthritis of the knee – a double-blind prospective randomized study.' *Clinical Rheumatology 23*, 5, 410–5.

Klein, G., Kullich, W., Schnitker, J. and Schwann, H. (2006) 'Efficacy and tolerance of an oral enzyme combination in painful osteoarthritis of the hip: a double-blind, randomized study comparing oral enzymes with NSAIDs.' *Clinical and Experimental Rheumatology 24*, 1, 25–30.

Walker, A.F., Bunday, R., Hicks, S.M. and Middleton, R.W. (2002) 'Bromelain reduces mild acute knee pain and improves well-being in a dose-dependent fashion in an open study of otherwise healthy adults.' *Phytomedicine 9*, 8, 681–6.

41.   Alternative Medicine Review (2010) 'Bromelain: Monograph.' *Alternative Medicine Review 15*, 4, 361–8.

42.   Hale, L.P., Greer, P.K., Trinh, C.T. and Gottfried, M.R. (2005) 'Treatment with oral bromelain decreases colonic inflammation in the IL-10-deficient murine model of inflammatory bower disease.' *Clinical Immunology 116*, 2, 135–42.

Onken, J.E., Greer, P.K., Calingaert, B. and Hale, L.P. (2008) 'Bromelain treatment decreases secretion of pro-inflammatory cytokines and chemokines by colon biopsies in vitro.' *Clinical Immunology 126*, 3, 345–52.

Kane, S. and Goldberg, M.J. (2000) 'Use of bromelain for mild ulcerative colitis.' *Annals of Internal Medicine 132*, 8, 680.

43.   Benhmark, S. (2006) 'Curcumin, an atoxic antioxidant and natural NFkappaB, COX2, LOX and inducible nitric oxide synthase inhibitor: a shield against acute and chronic diseases.' *Journal of Parenteral and Enteral Nutrition 30*, 1, 45–51.

Taylor, R. (2011) 'Curcumin for IBD: a review of human studies.' *Alternative Medicine Review 16*, 2, 152–6.

Aggarwal, B.B. and Harikumar, K.B. (2009) 'Potential therapeutic effects of curcumin, the anti-inflammatory agent, against neurodegenerative, cardiovascular, pulmonary, metabolic, autoimmune and neoplastic diseases.' *International Journal of Biochemistry and Cell Biology 41*, 1, 40–59.

44.   Taylor 2011.

45.   White, B. and Judkins, D.Z. (2011) 'Clinical enquiry: does turmeric relieve inflammatory conditions?' *Journal of Family Practice 60*, 3, 155–6.

Jurenka, J. (2009) 'Anti-inflammatory properties of curcumin, a major constituent of curcuma longa: a review of preclinical and clinical research.' *Alternative Medicine Review 14*, 2, 141–53.

Guimaraes, M.R., Coimbra, L.S., de Aquino, S.G., Spolidorio, L.C., Kirkwood, K.L. and Rossa, C. Jr (2011) 'Potent anti-inflammatory effects of systemically administered curcumin modulate periodontal disease in vivo.' *Journal of Periodontal Research 46*, 2, 269–79.

Aggarwal, B.B. and Harikumar, K.B. (2009) 'Potential therapeutic effects of curcumin, the anti-inflammatory agent, against neurodegenerative, cardiovascular, pulmonary, metabolic, autoimmune and neoplastic diseases.' *International Journal of Biochemistry and Cell Biology 41*, 1, 40–59.

Hsu, C.H. and Cheng, A.L. (2007) 'Clinical studies with curcumin.' *Advances in Experimental Medicine and Biology 595*, 471–80.

46.   Arthritis UK (2013) 'Osteoarthritis in General Practice'. Available at www.arthritisresearchuk. org/arthritis-information/data-and-statistics/osteoarthritis.aspx, accessed on 6 April 2014.

47.   Clauw, D.J. and Witter, J. (2009) 'Pain and rheumatology: thinking outside the joint.' *Arthritis and Rheumatism 60*, 2, 321–4.

48.   Juhl, J.H. (1998) 'Fibromyalgia and the serotonin pathway.' *Alternative Medicine Review 3*, 5, 367–75.

Caruso, I., Sarzi Puttini, P., Cazzola, M. and Azzolini, V. (1990) 'Double-blind study of 5-hydroxytryptophan versus placebo in the treatment of primary fibromyalgia syndrome.' *Journal of International Medical Research 18*, 3, 201–9.

Sarzi Puttini, P. and Caruso, I. (1992) 'Primary fibromyalgia syndrome and 5-hydroxy-L-tryptophan: a 90-day open study.' *Journal of International Medical Research 20*, 2, 182–9.

49.   Affleck, G., Urrows, S., Tennen, H., Higgins, P. and Abeles, M. (1996) 'Sequential daily relations of sleep, pain intensity and attention of pain among women with fibromyalgia.' *Pain 68*, 2–3, 363–8.

50.   Titus, F., Dávalos, A., Alom, J. and Codina, A. (1986) '5-hydroxytryptophan versus methylsergide in the prophylaxis of migraine. Randomized clinical trial.' *European Neurology 25*, 5, 327–9.

51. Wilhelmsen, M., Amirian, I., Reiter, R.J., Rosenberg, J. and Gogenur, I. (2011) 'Analgesic effects of melatonin: a review of current evidence from experimental and clinical studies.' *Journal of Pineal Research 51*, 3, 270–7.

Srinivasan, V., Pandi-Perumal, S.R., Spence, D.W., Moscovitch, A. *et al.* (2010) 'Potential use of melatonergic drugs in analgesia: mechanisms of action.' *Brain Research Bulletin 81*, 4–5, 362–71.

52. Zeidan, F., Martucci, K.T., Kraft, R.A., Gordon, N.S., McHaffie, J.G. and Coghill, R.C. (2011) 'Brain mechanisms supporting the modulation of pain by mindfulness meditation.' *Journal of Neuroscience 31*, 14, 5540–8.

53. Hassett, A.L. and Williams, D.A. (2011) 'Non-pharmacological treatment of chronic widespread musculoskeletal pain.' *Best Practice and Research Clinical Rheumatology 25*, 2, 299–309.

54. Medina-Santillan, R., Morales-Franco, G., Espinoza-Raya, J., Granados-Soto, V. and Reyes-Garcia, G. (2004) 'Treatment of diabetic neuropathic pain with gabapentin alone or combined with vitamin B complex: preliminary results.' *Proceedings of the Western Pharmacology Society 47*, 109–112.

55. Chen, J.Y., Chang, C.Y., Feng, P.H., Chu, C.C., So, E.C. and Hu, M.L. (2009) 'Plasma vitamin C is lower in postherpetic neuralgia patients and administration of vitamin C reduces spontaneous pain but not brush-evoked pain.' *Clinical Journal of Pain 25*, 7, 562–9.

Kuhad, A. and Chopra, K. (2009) 'Tocotrienol attenuates oxidative-nitrosative stress and inflammatory cascade in experimental model of diabetic neuropathy.' *Neuropharmacology 57*, 4, 456–62.

Kim, H.K., Kim, J.H., Gao, X., Zhou, J.L. *et al.* (2006) 'Analgesic effect of vitamin E is mediated by reducing central sensitization in neuropathic pain.' *Pain 122*, 1–2, 53–62.

56. England, J., Wagner, T., Kern, K.U., Roth-Daniek, A. and Sell, A. (2011) 'The capsaicin 8% patch for peripheral neuropathic pain.' *British Journal of Nursing 20*, 15, 926–31.

CHAPTER 9

1. McCormick, K. (2007) 'Osteoporosis: biomarkers and other diagnostic correlates into the management of bone fragility.' *Alternative Medicine Review 12*, 2, 113–45.

2. Ryan, J. and Ancelin, M.L. (2012) 'Polymorphisms of estrogen receptors and risk of depression: therapeutic implications.' *Drugs 72*, 13, 1725–38.

3. Hays, B. (2011) *Sex Hormones, Signalling and the Menopause Transition*. Presentation given at the Advance Functional Medicine in Clinical Practice (AFMCP) Symposium. October 2011. London: IFM

4. Bulun, S.E., Chen, D., Moy, I., Brookes, D.C. and Zhao, H. (2012) 'Aromatase, breast cancer and obesity: a complex interaction.' *Trends in Endocrinology and Metabolism 23*, 2, 83–9.

5. Vance, M.L. (2003) 'Andropause.' *Growth Hormone and IGF Research 13*, Suppl A, S90–2.

6. Bentzen, J.G., Forman, J.L., Larsen, E.C., Pinborg, A. *et al.* (2013) 'Maternal menopause as a predictor of anti-Mullerian hormone level and antral follicle in daughters during reproductive age.' *Human Reproduction 28*, 1, 247–55.

7. Cagnacci, A. Cannoletta, M., Carettok, S., Zanin, R., Xholli, A. and Volpe, A. (2009) 'Increased cortisol level: a possible link between climacteric symptoms and cardiovascular risk factors.' *Menopause 18*, 3, 273–8.

8. Nawata, H., Yanase, T., Goto, K., Okabe, T. *et al.* (2004) 'Adrenopause.' *Hormone Research 62*, Suppl 3, 110–4.

Simpson, E. and Davis, S. (2001) 'Mini-review: aromatase and the circulation of oestrogen biosynthesis – some new perspectives.' *Endocrinology 42*, 11, 4589–94.

9. Natural Medicines Comprehensive Database (NMCD) (2013) 'Menopause: Natural product effectiveness checker.' Available at http://naturaldatabase.therapeuticresearch.com/nd/Search.aspx?cs=&drg=1&s=ND&pt=&sh=3&fs=ND#7 (subscribers only).

10. Lanou, A.J. (2011) 'Soy foods: are they useful for optimal bone health?' *Therapeutic Advances in Musculoskeletal Disease 3*, 6, 293–300.

Ajdžanović, V.Z., Milošević, V.L. and Spasojević (2012) 'Glucocorticoid excess and disturbed hemodynamics in advanced age: the extent to which soy isoflavones may be beneficial.' *General Physiology and Biophysics 31*, 4, 367–74.

Rebholz, C.M., Reynolds, K., Wofford, M.R., Chen, J. et al. (2013) 'Effects of soybean protein on novel cardiovascular disease risk factors: a randomized controlled trial.' *European Journal of Clinical Nutrition* 67, 1, 58–63.

11. Gaynor, M.L. (2003) 'Isoflavones and the prevention and treatment of prostate disease: is there a role?' *Cleveland Clinic Journal of Medicine* 70, 3, 203–4, 206, 208–9.

12. Gaynor 2003.

13. NMCD 2013.

14. Akaza, H., Miyanaga, N., Takashima, N., Naito, S. et al. (2004) 'Comparisons of percent equol producers between prostate cancer patients and controls: case-controlled studies of isoflavones in Japanese, Korean and American residents.' *Japanese Journal of Clinical Oncology* 34, 2, 86–9.

15. Patisaul, H.B. and Jefferson, W. (2010) 'The pros and cons of phytoestrogens.' *Frontiers in Neuroendocrinology* 31, 4, 400–19.
    Kurzer, M.S. (2008) 'Soy consumption for reduction of menopausal symptoms.' *Inflammopharmacology* 16, 5, 227–9.

16. van Die, M.D., Burger, H.G, Teede, H.J. and Bone, K.M. (2009) 'Vitex agnus-castus in the treatment of menopause-related complaints.' *Journal of Alternative and Complementary Medicine* 15, 8, 853–62.
    NMCD 2013 from hormone slides.
    Abbaspoor, Z., Azam Hajikani, N. and Afshari, P. (2011) 'Effect of vitex agnus-castus on menopausal early symptoms in postmenopausal women: a randomized, double blind, placebo-controlled study.' *British Journal of Medicine and Medical Research* 1, 3, 132–40.

17. Abdali, K., Khajehedi, M. and Tabatabaee, H.R. (2010) 'Effect of St John's wort on severity, frequency and duration of hot flashes in premenopausal, perimenopausal and postmenopausal women: a randomized, double-blind, placebo-controlled study.' *Menopause.* 17(2): 326–31.
    Al-Akoum, M., Maunsell, E., Vereault, R., Provencher, L., Otis, H. and Dodin, S. (2009) 'Effects of hypericum perforatum (St John's wort) on hot flashes and quality of life in perimenopausal women: a randomized pilot trial.' *Menopause* 16(2): 307–14.

18. Bommer, S., Klein, P. and Suter, A. (2011) 'First time proof of sage's tolerability and efficacy in menopausal women with hot flushes.' *Advances in Therapy* 28, 6, 490–500.

19. Shams, T., Setia, M.S., Hemmings, R., McCusker, J., Sewitch, M. and Ciampi, A. (2010) 'Efficacy of black cohosh-containing preparations on menopausal symptoms: a meta-analysis.' *Alternative Therapies in Health and Medicine* 16, 1, 36–44.

20. Ofir, R., Tamir, S., Khatib, S. and Vaya, J. (2003) 'Inhibition of serotonin re-uptake by licorice constituents.' *Journal of Molecular Neuroscience* 20, 2, 135–40.

21. Kelly, J.A. and Vankrieken, L. (2000) *Sex Hormone Binding Globulin and the Assessment of Androgen Status.* Available at www.medical.siemens.com/siemens/en_GLOBAL/gg_diag_FBAs/files/news_views/spring00/techreports/zb170-b.pdf, accessed on 28 January 2014.
    Akin, F., Bastemir, M. and Alkis, E. (2007) 'Effect of insulin sensitivity on SHBG levels in premenopausal versus postmenopausal obese women.' *Advances in Therapy* 24, 6, 1210–20.

22. Lucas, M., Asselin, G., Mérette, C., Poulin, M.J. and Dodin, S. (2009) 'Effects of ethyl-eicosapentaenoic acid omega-3 fatty acid supplementation on hot flashes and quality of life among middle-aged women: a double-blind, placebo-controlled, randomized clinical trial.' *Menopause* 16, 2, 357–66.

23. Lund, T.D., Munson, D.J., Adlercreutz, H., Handa, R.J. and Lephart, E.D. (2004) 'Androgen receptor expression in the rat prostate is down-regulated by dietary phytoestrogens.' *Reproductive Biology and Endocrinology* 2, 5.

24. Bolton, J.L. and Thatcher, G.R. (2008) 'Potential mechanisms of estrogen quinone carcinogenesis.' *Chemical Research in Toxicology* 21, 1, 93–101.
    MacAlindon, T.E., Gulun, J., Chen, T., Klug, T., Lahita, R. and Nuite, M. (2001) 'Indole-3-carbinol in women with SLE: effect on oestrogen metabolism and disease activity.' *Lupus* 10, 11, 779–83.
    Kasim-Karakas, S.E., Almario, R.U., Gregory, L., Todd, H., Wong, R. and Laslev, B.L. (2002) 'Effects of prune consumption on the ratio of 2-hydroxyestrone to 16alpha-hydroxyestrone.' *American Journal of Clinical Nutrition* 76, 6, 1422–7.
    Cutolo, M., Capellino, S., Montagna, P., Villaggio, B. et al. (2003) 'New roles for estrogens in rheumatoid arthritis.' *Clinical and Experimental Rheumatology* 21, 6, 687–90.

25. Neil, K. (2010) 'Sex Hormone Imbalances.' In L. Nicolle and A. Woodriff Beirne (eds) *Biochemical Imbalances in Disease.* London: Singing Dragon.
Hays, B. (2005) 'Female Hormones: The Dance of Hormones, Part 1.' In D. Jones (ed.) *The Textbook of Functional Medicine.* Gig Harbor, WA: IFM.
Lord, R.S., Bonglovanni, B. and Bralley, J.A. (2002) 'Estrogen metabolism and the diet-cancer connection.' *Alternative Medicine Review 7*, 2, 112–29.
26. Hays 2005; Neil 2010.
27. Gasper, A., Al-Janobi, A., Smith, J.A., Bacon, J.R. *et al.* (2005) 'Glutathione-S-transferase M1 polymorphism and metabolism of sulforaphane from standard and high-glucosinolate broccoli.' *American Journal of Clinical Nutrition 82*, 6, 1283–91.
28. Felton, J.S. and Malfatti, M.A. (2006) 'What do diet-induced changes in phase I and phase II enzymes tell us about prevention from exposure to heterocyclic amines?' *Journal of Nutrition 136*, 1, Suppl, 2683–4S.
29. Shinkai, Y., Sumi, D., Fukami, I., Ishii, T. and Kumagai, Y. (2006) 'Sulforaphane, an activator of Nrf2, suppresses cellular accumulation of arsenic and its cytotoxicity in primary mouse hepatocytes.' *FEBS Letters 580*, 7, 1771–4.
30. Toyama, T., Shinkai, Y., Yasutake, A., Uchida, K., Yamamoto, M. and Kumagai, Y. (2011) 'Isothiocyanates reduce mercury accumulation via an Nrf2-dependent mechanism during exposure of mice to methylmercury.' *Environmental Health Perspectives 119*, 8, 1117–22.
31. Jeffery, E. and Araya, M. (2009) 'Physiological effects of broccoli consumption.' *Phytochemistry Reviews 8*, 1, 283-98).
32. John Innes Centre (2011) 'British research leads to UK launch of Beneforté broccoli.' Available at http://news.jic.ac.uk/2011/10/british-research-leads-to-uk-launch-of-beneforte-broccoli, accessed on 23 October 2013.
33. Women's Health Initiative (2010) Available at www.nhlbi.nih.gov/whi, accessed on 28 January 2014.
34. Harman, S.M., Brinton, E.A., Cedars, M., Lobo, R. *et al.* (2005) 'KEEPS: The Kronos Early Estrogen Prevention Study.' *Climacteric 8*, 1, 3–12.
Menon, D.V. and Vongpatanasin, W. (2005) 'Effects of transdermal estrogen replacement therapy on cardiovascular risk factors.' *Treatments in Endocrinology 5*, 1, 37–51.
L'hermite, M., Simoncini, T., Fuller, S. and Genazzani, A.R. (2008) 'Could transdermal estradiol + progesterone be a safer postmenopausal HRT? A review.' *Maturitas 60*, 3–4, 185–201.
Schierbeck, L.L., Rejnmark, L., Tofteng, C.L., Stilgren, L. *et al.* (2012) 'Effect of hormone replacement therapy on cardiovascular events in recently postmenopausal women: randomised trial.' *British Medical Journal 345*, e6409.
Lobo, R.A. (2013) 'Where are we 10 years after the Women's Health Initiative?' *Journal of Clinical Endocrinology and Metabolism 98*, 5, 1771–80.
35. Harman *et al.* 2005; Menon and Vongpatanasin 2005; L'hermite *et al.* 2008; Schierbeck *et al.* 2012.
36. American College of Obstetricians and Gynecologists Committee on Gynecologic Practice, American Society for Reproductive Medicine Practice Committee (2012) 'Compounded bioidentical menopausal hormone therapy.' *Fertility and Sterility 98*, 2, 308–12.
Pattimakeil, L. and Thacker, H.L. (2011) 'Bioidentical hormone therapy: clarifying the misconceptions.' *Cleveland Clinic Journal of Medicine 78*, 12, 829–36.
Files, J.A., Ko, M.G. and Pruthi, S. (2011) 'Bioidentical hormone therapy.' *Mayo Clinic Proceedings 86*, 7, 673–80.
37. Davidson, M.H. (1998) 'Clinical Safety and Endocrine Effects of 7-Keto™ DHEA.' Presentation at the Experimental Biology 98 Conference, 19–22 April 1998, San Francisco.
Weeks, C., Lardy, H. and Henwood, S. (1998) 'Preclinical toxicology evaluation of 3-acetyl-7-oxodehydroepiandrosterone (7-keto-DHEA).' *FASEB Journal 12*, A764,
Hampl, R., Starka, L. and Jansky, L. (2006) 'Steroids and thermogenesis.' *Physiological Research 55*, 2, 123–31.
Rose, K.A., Stapleton, G., Dott, K., Kieny, M.P. *et al.* (1997) 'Cyp7b, a novel brain cytochrome P450, catalyzes the synthesis of neurosteroids 7alpha-hydroxy dehydroepiandrosterone and 7alpha-hydroxy pregnenolone.' *Proceedings of the National Academy of Sciences of the USA 94*, 10, 4925–30.

Shi, J., Schulze, S. and Lardy, H.A. (2000) 'The effect of 7-oxo-DHEA acetate on memory in young and old C57BL/6 mice.' *Steroids* 65, 3, 124–9.

38. Hall, E. and Steiner, M. (2013) 'Serotonin and female psychopathology.' *Women's Health (London)* 9, 1, 85–97.

Albert, K. and Broadwell, C. (2011) 'Estrogen, menopause and mood regulation.' *Menopausal Medicine.* Available at http://stg.srm-ejournal.com/pdf%2FMed0%2FMenMed0811_estrogen.pdf, accessed on 28 January 2014.

39. Hall and Steiner 2013; Albert and Broadwell.

40. Chau, K., Atkinson, S.A. and Taylor, V.H. (2012) 'Are selective serotonin reuptake inhibitors a secondary cause of low bone density?' *Journal of Osteoporosis*, Epub 232061.

Wu, Q., Bencaz, A.F., Hentz, J. and Crowell, M. (2012) 'Selective serotonin reuptake inhibitor treatment and risk of fractures: a meta-analysis of cohort case-control studies.' *Osteoporosis International* 23, 1, 365–75.

41. Tan, R.S. and Pu, S.J. (2002) 'Impact of obesity on hypogonadism in the andropause.' *International Journal of Andrology* 25, 4, 195–201.

42. Vance, M.L. (2003) 'Andropause.' *Growth Hormone and IGF Research* 13, Suppl A, S90–2.

43. Frias, J., Torres, J.M., Miranda, M.T., Ruiz, E. and Ortega, E. (2002) 'Effects of acute alcohol intoxication on pituitary-gonadal axis hormones, pituitary-adrenal axis hormones, beta-endorphin and prolactin in human adults of both sexes.' *Alcohol and Alcoholism* 37, 2, 169–73.

44. Bjorntorp, P. (1997) 'Neuroendocrine factors in obesity.' *Journal of Endocrinology* 155, 2, 193–5.

45. He, F. and Feng L. (2005) 'Effects of some micronutrients on partial androgen deficiency in the aging male.' *Zhonghua Nan Ke Xue* 11, 10, 784–6.

46. Moyad, M.A. and Lowe, R.C. (2008) 'Educating patients about lifestyle modifications for prostate health.' *American Journal of Medicine* 121, 8, Suppl 2, S34–42.

47. Derby, C.A., Mohr, B.A., Goldstein, I., Feldman, H.A., Johannes, C.B. and McKinlay, J.B. (2000) 'Modifiable risk factors and erectile dysfunction: can lifestyle changes modify risk?' *Urology* 56, 2, 302–6.

48. Frattaroli, J., Weidner, G., Dnistrian, A.M., Kemp, C. *et al.* (2008) 'Clinical events in prostate cancer lifestyle trial: results from two years of follow-up.' *Urology* 72, 6, 1319–23.

Ornish, D., Magbanua, M.J., Weidner, G., Weinberg, V. *et al.* (2008) 'Changes in prostate gene expression in men undergoing an intensive nutrition and lifestyle intervention.' *Proceedings of the National Academy of Sciences of the USA* 105, 24, 8369–74.

49. Ho, E., Boileau, T.W. and Bray, T.M. (2004) 'Dietary influences on endocrine-inflammatory interactions in prostate cancer development.' *Archives of Biochemistry and Biophysics* 428, 1, 109–17.

Freeman, V.L., Meydani, M., Hur, K. and Flanigan, R.C. (2004) 'Inverse association between prostatic polyunsaturated fatty acid and risk of locally advanced prostate carcinoma.' *Cancer* 101, 12, 2744–54.

Giovannucci, E., Rimm, E.B., Liu, Y., Stampfer, M.J. and Willet, W.C. (2002) 'A prospective study of tomato products, lycopene and prostate cancer risk.' *Journal of the National Cancer Institute* 94, 5, 391–8.

Giovannucci, E. (2002) 'A review of epidemiologic studies of tomatoes, lycopene and prostate cancer.' *Experimental Biology and Medicine* Soy phytochemicals and tea bioactive components synergistically inhibit androgen-sensitive human prostate tumors in mice *(Maywood)* 227, 10, 852–9.

Zhou, J.R., Yu, L., Zhong, Y. and Blackburn, G.L. (2003) 'Soy phytochemicals and tea bioactive components synergistically inhibit androgen-sensitive human prostate tumors in mice.' *Journal of Nutrition* 133, 2, 516–21.

50. Schwarz, S., Obermüller-Jevic, U.C., Hellmis, E., Koch, W., Jacobi, G. and Biesalski, H.K. (2008) 'Lycopene inhibits disease progression in patients with benign prostate hyperplasia.' *Journal of Nutrition* 138, 1, 49–53.

51. Gaynor, M.L. (2003) 'Isoflavones and the prevention and treatment of prostate disease: is there a role?' *Cleveland Clinic Journal of Medicine* 70, 3, 203–4, 206, 208–9.

52. Wilt, T., Ishani, A. and MacDonald, R. (2002) 'Serenoa repens for benign prostatic hypertrophy.' *Cochrane Database of Systematic Reviews* 3, CD001423.

53. Chen, J., Wollman, Y., Chernichovsky, T., Iaina, A., Sofer, M. and Matzkin, H. (1999) 'Effect of oral administration of high-dose nitric oxide donor L-arginine in men with organic erectile dysfunction: results of a double-blind, randomized, placebo-controlled study.' *BJU International* 83, 3, 269–73.

54. Jang, D.J., Lee, M.S., Shin, B.C., Lee, Y.C. and Ernst, E. (2008) 'Red ginseng for treating erectile dysfunction: a systematic review.' *British Journal of Clinical Pharmacology 66*, 4, 444–50.

55. McCormick 2007.

56. Orchard, T.S., Pan, X., Cheek, F., Ing, S.W. and Jackson, R.D. (2012) 'A systematic review of omega-3 fatty acids and osteoporosis.' *British Journal of Nutrition 107*, Suppl 2, S253–60.

57. Stevenson, M., Lloyd-Jones, M. and Pappaioannu, D. (2009) 'Vitamin K to prevent fractures in older women: systematic review and economic evaluation.' *Health Technology Assessment 13*, 45.

58. Body, J.J. (2011) 'How to manage postmenopausal osteoporosis?' *Acta Clinica Belgica 66*, 6, 43–7.

59. Bolland, M.J., Barber, P.A., Doughty, R.N., Mason, B. *et al.* (2008) 'Vascular events in healthy older women receiving calcium supplementation: randomised controlled trial.' British Medical Journal 336, 7638, 262–6.

60. Aydin, H., Deyneli, O., et Yavuz, D., Gözü, H. *et al.* (2010) 'Short-term oral magnesium supplementation suppresses bone turnover in postmenopausal osteoporotic women.' *Biological Trace Element Research 133*, 2, 136–43.
    Stendig-Lindberg, G., Tepper, R. and Leichter, I. (1993) 'Trabecular bone density in a two year controlled trial of peroral magnesium in osteoporosis.' *Magnesium Research 6*, 2, 155–63.

61. Whitton, C., Nicholson, S.K., Roberts, C., Prynne, C.J. *et al.* (2011) 'National Diet and Nutrition Survey: UK food consumptions and nutrient intakes from the first year of the rolling programme and comparisons with previous surveys. Table.' *British Journal of Nutrition 106*, 12, 1899–914.

62. Bischoff-Ferrari, H.A., Willet, W.C. Wong, J.B., Stuck, A.E., Giovannucci, E., Dietrich, T. and Dawson-Hughes, B. (2005) 'Fracture prevention with vitamin D supplementation: a meta-analysis of randomized controlled trials.' *Journal of the American Medical Association 293*, 18, 2257–64.

63. Kaneki, M., Hodges, S.J., Hosoi, T., Fujiwara, S. *et al.* (2001) 'Japanese fermented soybean food as the major determinant of the large geographic difference in circulating levels of vitamin K2: possible implications for hip-fracture risk.' *Nutrition 17*, 4, 315–21.

64. Kidd, P. (2010) 'Vitamins D and K as pleiotropic nutrients: clinical importance for the skeletal and cardiovascular systems and preliminary evidence for synergy.' *Alternative Medicine Review 15*, 3, 199–222.
    Kaneki *et al.* 2001.

65. Kidd 2010.
    Katsuyama, H., Ideguchi, S., Fukunaga, M., Fukunaga, T., Saijoh, K. and Sunami, S. (2004) 'Promotion of bone formation by fermented soybean (Natto) intake in premenopausal women.' *Journal of Nutritional Science and Vitaminology (Tokyo) 50*, 2, 114–20.
    Takemura, H. (2006) 'Prevention of osteoporosis by foods and dietary supplements. 'Kinnotsubu honegenki': a fermented soybean (natto) with reinforced vitamin K2 (menaquinone-7).' *Clinical Calcium 16*, 10, 1715–22.

66. Sato, T., Schurgers, L.J. and Uenishi, K. (2012) 'Comparison of menaquinone-4 and menaquinone-7 bioavailability in healthy women.' *Nutrition Journal 11*, 93.

67. Ahmadieh, H. and Arabi, A. (2011) 'Vitamins and bone health: beyond calcium and vitamin D.' *Nutrition Reviews 69*, 10, 584–98.

68. Waynberg J. (1990) 'Aphrodisiacs: contributions to the clinical evaluation of the traditional use of ptychopetalum.' Presentation at the First International Congress on Ethnopharmacology. France, June 1990.

69. Waynberg, J. and Brewer, S. (2000) 'Effects of Herbal vX on libido and sexual activity in premenopausal and postmenopausal women.' *Advances in Therapy 17*, 5, 255–62.

70. Gonzales, G.F., Córdova, A., Vega, K., Chung, A. *et al.* (2002) 'Effect of Lepidium meyenii (MACA) on sexual desire and its absent relationship with serum testosterone levels in adult healthy men.' *Andrologia 34*, 6, 367–72.

71.　Adimoelja, A. (2000) 'Phytochemicals and the breakthrough of traditional herbs in the management of sexual dysfunctions.' *International Journal of Andrology 23*, Suppl 2, 82–4.
Gauthaman, K., Ganesan, A.P. and Prasad, R.N. (2003) 'Sexual effects of puncture vine (Tribulus terrestris) extract (protodioscin): an evaluation using a rat model.' *Journal of Alternative and Complementary Medicine 9*, 2, 257–65.

CHAPTER 10

1.　Buettner, D. (2008) *Blue Zones: Lessons for Living Longer from the People Who've Lived the Longest.* Washington, DC: National Geographic.
2.　Tregear, C., Dalle, C. and Hertoghe, T. (2006) 'Positive emotions and attitudes: precious keys to longevity.' *Journal of European Anti-Ageing Medicine 4*, 31–2.
3.　Doherty, T.J. (2003) 'Invited review: aging and sarcopenia.' *Journal of Applied Physiology 95*, 1717–27.
4.　Melov, S., Tarnopolsky, M.A., Beckman, K., Felkey, K. and Hubbard, A. (2007) 'Resistance exercise reverses aging in human skeletal muscle.' PLoS ONE 2, 5, e465.
5.　Melov *et al.* 2007.
6.　Frontera, W.R., Meredith, C.N., O'Reilly, K.P., Knuttgen, H.G. and Evans, W.J. (1992) 'Strength conditioning in older men: skeletal muscle hypertrophy and improved function.' *Journal of Applied Physiology 64*, 1038–44.
7.　Chakravarthy, M.V., Joyner, M.J. and Booth, F.W. (2002) 'An obligation for primary care physicians to prescribe physical activity to sedentary patients to reduce the risk of chronic health conditions.' *Mayo Clinic Proceedings 77*, 2, 109–13.
8.　Jonker, J.T., De Laet, C., Franco, O.H., Peeters, A., Mackenbach, J. and Nusselder, W.J. (2006) 'Physical activity and life expectancy with and without diabetes: life table analysis of the Framingham Heart Study.' *Diabetes Care 29*, 1, 38–43.
Franco, O.H., De Laet, C., Peeters, A., Jonker, J., Mackenbach, J, and Nusselder, W.J. (2005) 'Effects of physical activity on life expectancy with cardiovascular disease.' *Archives of Internal Medicine 165*, 20, 2355–60.
9.　Tuan, T., Hsu, T.G., Fong, M.C., Hsu, C.F. *et al.* (2008) 'Deleterious effects of short-term, high-intensity exercise on immune function: evidence from leucocyte mitochondrial alterations and apoptosis.' *British Journal of Sports Medicine 42*, 11–15.
10.　Boutcher, S. (2011) 'High-intensity intermittent exercise and fat loss.' *Journal of Obesity*, Epub, 868305.
11.　Stokes, K.A., Nevill, M.E., Hall, G.M. and Lakomy, H.K. (2002) 'The time course of the human growth hormone response to a 6 s and a 30 s cycle ergometer sprint.' *Journal of Sports Science 20*, 6, 487–94.
Godfrey, R., Madgwick, Z. and Gregory, P.W. (2003) 'The exercise-induced release in athletes.' *Sports Medicine 33*, 8.
12.　McEwan, B.S. (2008) 'Central effects of stress hormones in health and disease: understanding the protective and damaging effects of stress and stress mediators.' *European Journal of Pharmacology 583*, 2–3, 174–85.
Miller, M. and Cappuccio, E. (2007) 'Inflammation, sleep, obesity and cardiovascular disease.' *Current Vascular Pharmacology 5*, 93–102.
13.　Edwards, B.A., O'Driscoll, D.M., Ali, A., Jordan, A.S., Trinder, J. and Malhotra, A. (2010) 'Aging and sleep: physiology and pathophysiology.' *Seminars in Respiratory and Critical Care Medicine 31*, 5, 618–33.
14.　Miller and Cappuccio 2007.
15.　Kripke, D.F., Langer, R.D. and Kline, L.E. (2012) 'Hypnotics' association with mortality or cancer: a matched cohort study.' *BMJ Open 2*, 1, 000850.
Chien, K.L., Chen, P.C., Hsu, H.C., Su, T.C. *et al.* (2010) 'Habitual sleep duration and insomnia and the risk of cardiovascular events and all-cause death: report from a community-based cohort.' *Sleep 33*, 2, 177–84.
16.　Edwards *et al.* 2010.
17.　Roehrs, T. and Roth, T. (2008) 'Caffeine: sleep and daytime sleepiness.' *Sleep Medicine Reviews 12*, 153–62.

18. Richard, D.M., Dawes, M.A., Mathias, C.W., Acheson, A., Hill-Kapturczak, N. and Dougherty, D.M. (2009) 'L-tryptophan: basic metabolic functions, behavioral research and therapeutic indications.' *International Journal of Tryptophan Research 2*, 45–60.

19. Hartmann, E. and Cravens, J. (1974) 'Hypnotic effects of L-tryptophan.' *Archives of General Psychiatry 31*, 394–7.

    Paredes, S.D., Barriga, C.M., Reiter, R.J. and Rodríguez, A.B. (2009) 'Assessment of the potential role of tryptophan as the precursor of serotonin and melatonin for the aged sleep-wake cycle and immune function: streptopelia risioria as a model.' *International Journal of Tryptophan Research 2*, 23–36.

20. Rondanelli, M., Opizzi, A., Monteferrario, F., Antoniello, N., Manni, R. and Klersy, C. (2011) 'The effect of melatonin, magnesium and zinc on primary insomnia in long-term care facility residents in Italy: a double-blind, placebo-controlled clinical trial.' *Journal of the American Geriatric Society 9*, 82–90.

21. Saint-Hilaire, Z, Messaoudi, M., Desor, D. and Kobayashi, T. (2009) 'Effects of a bovine alpha s1-casein tryptic hydrosylate (CTH) on sleep disorder in Japanese general population.' *Open Sleep Journal 2*, 26–32.

22. Dimpfel, W., Kler, A., Kriesl, E. and Lehnfeld, R. (2007) 'Theogallin and L-theanine as active ingredients in decaffeinated green tea extract: I. electrophysiological characterization in the rat hippocampus in-vitro.' *Journal of Pharmacy and Pharmacology 59*, 8, 1131–6.

23. Fernández-San-Martín, M.I., Masa-Font, R., Palacios-Soler, L., Sancho-Gómez, P., Calbó-Caldentey, C. and Flores-Mateo, G. (2010) 'Effectiveness of valerian on insomnia: a meta-analysis of randomized control trials.' *Sleep Medicine 11*, 505–11.

24. Anderson, G.D., Elmer, G.W, Taibi, D.M., Viteiello, M.V. *et al.* (2010) 'Pharmacokinetics of valerenic acid after single and multiple doses of valerian in older women.' *Phytotherapy Research 24*, 1142–6.

    Ziegler, G., Ploch, M., Miettinen-Baumann, A. and Collet, W. (2002) 'Efficacy and tolerability of valerian extract LI 156 compared with oxazepam in the treatment of non-organic insomnia: a randomized, double-blind, comparative clinical study.' *European Journal of Medical Research 7*, 11, 480–6.

25. Bhattacharya, S.K., Bhattacharya, A., Sairam, K., Ghosal, S. (2000) 'Anxiolytic/antidepressant activity of Withania somnifera glycowithanolides: an experimental study.' *Phytomedicine 7*, 6, 463–9.

26. Lemoine, P., Wage, A.G., Katz, A., Nir, T. and Zisapel, N. (2012) 'Efficacy and safety of prolonged-release melatonin for insomnia in middle-aged and elderly patients with hypertension: a combined analysis of controlled clinical trials.' *Integrated Blood Pressure Control 5*, 9–17.

    Garfinkel, D., Zorin, M., Wainstein, J., Matas, Z., Laudon, M. and Zisapel, N. (2011) 'Efficacy and safety of prolonged-release melatonin in insomnia patients with diabetes: a randomized, double-blind, crossover study.' *Diabetes, Metabolic Syndrome and Obesity: Targets and Therapy 4*, 307–13.

27. Douillard, J. (2001) *Body, Mind and Sport*. New York, NY: Three Rivers Press.

28. Epel, E., Daubenmier, J., Moskowitz, J.T., Folkman, S. and Blackburn, E. (2009) 'Can meditation slow rate of cellular aging?' *Annals of the New York Academy of Sciences 1172*, 34–53.

29. Brook, R.D., Appel. L.J., Rubenfire, M., Ogedegbe, G. *et al.* (2013) 'Beyond medications and diet: alternative approaches to lowering blood pressure: a scientific statement from the American Heart Association.' *Hypertension 61*, 6, 1360–83.

30. Farhi, D. (1996) *The Breathing Book: Vitality and Good Health through Essential Breath Work*. New York, NY: Henry Holt and Company.

    Douillard 2001.

31. Winick, R. (1999) 'Cranial electrotherapy stimulation (CES): a safe and effective low cost means of anxiety control in dental practice.' *General Dentistry 47*, 1, 50–5.

32. McEwan 2008.

33. Lenoir, M., Serre, F., Cantin, L. and Ahmed, S.H. (2007) 'Intense sweetness surpasses cocaine reward.' *PLoS ONE 2*, 8, e698.

34. Downey, M. (2012) 'Discovering coffee's unique health benefits.' *Life Extension Magazine,*
     January. Available at www.lef.org/magazine/mag2012/jan2012_Discovering-Coffees-Unique-
     Health-Benefits_01.htm, accessed on 31 January 2014.
     Eskelinen, M.H. and Kivipelto, M. (2010) 'Caffeine as a protective factor in dementia and
     Alzheimer's disease.' *Journal of Alzheimer's Disease 20,* Suppl 1, S167–74.
35. Downey 2012; Eskelinen and Kivipelto 2010.
     Rosso, A., Mossey, J. and Lippa, C.F. (2008) 'Caffeine: neuroprotective functions in cognition
     and Alzheimer's disease.' *American Journal of Alzheimer's Disease and Other Dementias 23,* 5,
     417–22.
36. Downey 2012.
     Prediger, R.D. (2010) 'Effects of caffeine in Parkinson's disease: from neuroprotection to the
     management of motor and non-motor symptoms.' *Journal of Alzheimer's Disease 20,* Suppl 1,
     S205–20.
37. Whitton, C., Nicholson, S.K., Roberts, C., Prynne, C.J. *et al.* (2011) 'National Diet and
     Nutrition Survey: UK food consumption and nutrient intakes from the first year of the rolling
     programme and comparisons with previous surveys.' *British Journal of Nutrition 106,* 12,
     1899–914.
38. Heaney, R. (2003) 'Long-latency deficiency disease: insights from calcium and vitamin D.'
     American Journal of Clinical Nutrition 78, 912–9.
39. Cohen, S. and Cohen, S. (2008) *Drug Muggers: How to Keep Your Medicine from Stealing the Life*
     Out of You. US: Dear Pharmacist Inc.

RECIPE INDEX

SUBJECT INDEX